Medicine for Nurses

Other books by
W. Gordon Sears and R. S. Winwood

ANATOMY AND PHYSIOLOGY FOR NURSES, Fifth Edition
MATERIA MEDICA FOR NURSES, Seventh Edition

Medicine for Nurses

W. GORDON SEARS
M.D. (Lond.), M.R.C.P. (Lond.)
Honorary Consultant Physician, Mile End Hospital, London
and
R. S. WINWOOD
M.B., M.R.C.P.
Consultant Physician, Whipps Cross Hospital, London

TWELFTH EDITION

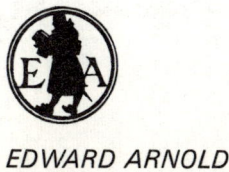

EDWARD ARNOLD

© W. Gordon Sears 1975

First published 1935
by Edward Arnold (Publishers) Ltd,
25 Hill Street, London W1X 8LL
Second Edition 1937
Third Edition 1939
Reprinted 1940, 1942 (with corrections), 1942, 1943 (twice)
Fourth Edition 1945
Reprinted 1946, 1948
Fifth Edition 1949
Reprinted 1951, 1952 (with corrections)
Sixth Edition 1954
Reprinted 1955 (with corrections)
Seventh Edition 1957
Reprinted 1959
Eighth Edition 1960
Ninth Edition 1963
Tenth Edition 1966
Reprinted 1968 (with corrections)
Eleventh Edition 1970
Reprinted 1974
Twelfth Edition 1975

Boards Edition   ISBN: 0 7131 4233 2
Paper Edition   ISBN: 0 7131 4234 0

Printed in Great Britain by
Butler & Tanner Ltd, Frome and London

Preface to the Twelfth Edition

Forty years have elapsed since this book first appeared. As the years pass Medicine tends to become more complicated and specialized although the basic principles remain more or less unchanged. However, with each edition attempts have been made to keep up with progress which, perhaps, accounts for its longevity.

Whenever possible the work has been kept within the limits of elementary anatomy, physiology and pathology but at the same time an effort has been made to include most of what the nurse is likely to see during the period of training and which may be of use afterwards both in this country and, to some extent, overseas.

In this edition, as in others, there has been little change in clinical descriptions but many established therapeutic advances have been mentioned.

We appreciate that in places technical details have been included which may be more advanced than the requirements of the average nurse. On the other hand some of these facts may be helpful to those who are faced with them.

In the first edition it was mentioned that subject matter not primarily of importance to the nurse was introduced with a view to make her contact with disease more interesting and to help her to understand what the doctor in charge of the case has in mind.

Nevertheless, the student nurse must be guided by the teacher concerning the details which she may be expected to know.

The book was originally based on a course of medical lectures to nurses and it is hoped that it still may be of use to the lecturer on the subject.

Our thanks are due to our publishers for their help and encouragement and for maintaining the standard of production at the most economical price possible.

It has been a constant source of gratification to the publishers and ourselves that the work continues to supply an increasing demand both in this country and abroad and that over 270,000 copies have been distributed. Our continued thanks are, therefore, due to the nursing profession everywhere for the loyal support they have given to this and our other works.

W. Gordon Sears
R. S. Winwood

London 1975

Contents

1 Introduction

Medicine is the Art or Science of healing disease, especially by means of internal remedies as distinct from mechanical and operative procedures which are principally in the domain of Surgery.

Health is the perfect structure of all the organs and tissues of the body, with a perfect performance of all their functions. In a broad sense, any alteration of their structure or function may be called Disease.

Definitions. It is important that certain terms, to which frequent reference will be made, should be understood and clearly defined.

Aetiology. The study of the **causes** of any disease, and the factors which influence its occurrence. Causes of disease are divided, when possible, into Exciting and Pre-disposing, e.g. Bacteria and viruses are frequently exciting causes; while age, sex, climate, unhygienic surroundings, unsuitable food, and preceding illness may be pre-disposing factors.

Pathology. The study of disease processes.

Morbid anatomy: The detailed description of the diseased structures, e.g. as seen at operation or at post-mortem.

Symptoms. What the patient complains of, e.g.
(*a*) Pain in the chest in pleurisy.
(*b*) Abdominal pain, vomiting and loss of appetite in cancer of the stomach.

Physical signs. What the physician finds on examination, e.g. in pneumonia.

Inspection: diminished movement of the affected side is seen.
Palpation: the diminished movement is felt by the hands placed on the chest.
Percussion: tapping one finger, placed firmly on the chest wall, with a finger of the opposite hand produces a dull sound in pneumonia instead of the resonant note heard over normal lung.

Auscultation: on listening with a stethoscope alteration of the normal breath sounds is heard.

The distinction between symptoms and signs is not always clear and they often overlap when the patient himself makes helpful observations.

Complications. Lesions and symptoms which are the result of the original disease and which only occur from time to time and are not necessarily part of the disease, e.g. heart block is a complication of myocardial infarction.

Sequela. A lesion or symptom persisting after the original disease or one of its complications have subsided, e.g. fibrosis of the lung is a sequela of broncho-pneumonia.

Diagnosis. The recognition of a particular ailment from the history, symptoms, physical signs and any tests which may have been performed.

Differential diagnosis. The knowledge of other diseases which resemble the disease in question and the points of difference which help to decide in a final opinion.

Prognosis. The art of foretelling the course, duration and termination of any disease.

Prophylaxis. The prevention of disease, e.g. the prevention of small-pox by vaccination.

Prophylaxis may be applied to the individual or it may affect the community at large, in which case it is in the domain of Hygiene and Public Health (Preventive Medicine).

A pathognomonic sign or symptom. A sign or symptom occurring in one disease only and not found in any other condition so that, when present, it affords a certain means of establishing a diagnosis, e.g. Koplik's spots in measles.

Syndrome. A set of symptoms and signs which occur together and constitute the manifestations of some special condition, e.g. Adams-Stokes Syndrome (p. 107).

Epidemiology. The study of disease by reference to its incidence in populations.

TYPES OF DISEASE AND GENERAL PATHOLOGY

The following table includes the commonest types of disease and is of value in answering examination questions, especially those asking the causes of any special symptoms. By running through a list of this kind, candidates are less likely to overlook diseases with which they are quite familiar, and they are able to give their answer in an orderly and well-arranged manner.

TYPES OF DISEASE

1. CONGENITAL and HEREDITARY.
2. TRAUMATIC (injury) and MECHANICAL.
3. CONDITIONS due to INFECTION and INFLAMMATION:
   (a) ACUTE (including specific fevers and virus diseases).
   (b) CHRONIC (including Tuberculosis, Syphilis and Parasites).
4. CONDITIONS due to CIRCULATORY DISORDERS and DEGENERATION.
5. NEW GROWTHS (Tumours).
   (a) Innocent.
   (b) Malignant (Cancer).
6. MISCELLANEOUS DISEASES including:
   (a) Disorders of metabolism and ductless glands.
   (b) Deficiency diseases.
   (c) Disorders due to allergy, toxins and other poisons.
   (d) Collagen and auto-immune diseases.
   (e) Iatrogenic.
   (f) Industrial disease and pollution (see chapter 15).
   (g) Psycho-somatic diseases.

1. Congenital Disease

By this it is meant that an individual is born with some defect in the structure or function of one or more organs or tissues. This may be due to some damage to the fetus especially during the first three or four months of its development and may be caused by the agency of drugs, e.g. thalidomide, virus infection, radiation or other factors which have a genetic effect, e.g. webbed fingers, faulty development of the heart (congenital heart disease), and imperforate anus.

An infection, such as syphilis, may be transmitted from the mother through the placenta to the unborn child (p. 494).

The tendency to certain diseases sometimes occurs in families and several members may be affected. These conditions often do not manifest themselves until later in life and are referred to as **familial** or **hereditary diseases.** These are due to some change in the genes in the chromosomes of one or other parent which may be handed down from generation to generation, e.g. the liability to uncontrollable bleeding (Haemophilia, p. 192). Certain diseases of the nervous system such as Friedreich's ataxia.

Diseases affecting newborn infants, but not necessarily congenital in origin, are sometimes called **'neo-natal'**.

2. Traumatic and mechanical
(Physical causes)

Trauma or injury includes damage to the tissues by:
1. Direct violence.
2. Surgical operations.
3. Excess of heat or cold, i.e. burns, scalds, frostbite.
4. Electricity, x-ray, radioactive substances and products of atomic fission.
5. Corrosive chemicals, toxic drugs and poisonous gases.

Mechanical conditions are illustrated by **obstruction** to the normal passage of the contents of hollow organs, blood vessels and ducts of the body.

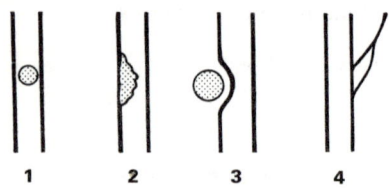

Fig. 1 Diagram illustrating obstruction. 1. Foreign body in the lumen. 2. Disease of the duct wall. 3. Pressure from outside. 4. Disorder of nerve supply.

(*a*) by the presence of some foreign body in their interior or lumen, e.g. a swallowed tooth plate in the œsophagus; a gallstone in the bile duct; a renal calculus in the ureter; a blood-clot in an artery.

(*b*) Disease of the wall of the organ itself causing narrowing of the lumen, e.g. cancer of the œsophagus in which the mechanical obstruction to swallowing produces the main symptom of the condition. The bowel may be constricted by adhesions or obstructed in a hernial orifice.

(*c*) By pressure from outside, e.g. a tumour in the glands of the thorax, cancer of the lung, etc., may press either on the œsophagus or a bronchus and narrow it. An aneurysm of the aorta may compress the trachea or a main bronchus. A tumour of the thyroid gland may press on the trachea.

(*d*) Interference with the neuro-muscular mechanism which may interrupt onward propulsion of the contents of the alimentary tract, e.g. achalasia, paralytic ileus, megacolon (Hirschsprung's disease).

Obstruction may be acute or chronic, partial or complete.

3. Infection and inflammation

Injury to the tissues may also be produced by the agency of minute living *vegetable* organisms known as bacteria, by viruses and fungi, and also by various *animal* parasites.

Bacteria, when causing disease, are present in enormous numbers, amounting to many millions at a time, but not all bacteria are harmful to the human body, so that the terms 'pathogenic' (harmful) and 'non-pathogenic' are sometimes used. When they gain entrance to the tissues or other suitable soil, such as blood-clot, unless checked, they have the power of very rapid multiplication.

Bacteria produce their effect on the body by means of special poisons known as **toxins** formed within and liberated from their bodies; each type of bacteria manufactures its own special toxin.

Some toxins produce acute or chronic inflammation, others degeneration of cells, while others have a selective action on particular tissues, e.g. diphtheria toxin attacks the heart-muscle and nerves. Tetanus toxin attacks nervous tissue.

The severity of any infection will depend on:
1. The virulence of the infecting organism and the number present.
2. The resistance of the individual to the particular infection.

A characteristic of many bacteria is their ability to acquire resistance to antibiotic drugs.

Bacteriology, microbiology and virology

I. Bacteria. The commonest infecting agents are bacteria. They can be seen under the highest magnifications of the microscope and can be grown on special media in the laboratory. They are described according to their shape.

1. A *Coccus* (plural = cocci) is a small round organism. The commonest varieties are:

Staphylococci, occurring in groups.

Streptococci, which appear in chains.

These two are responsible for most septic conditions.

Meningococci, causing cerebrospinal meningitis.

Pneumococci (*Streptococcus pneumoniae*), causing pneumonia.

Gonococci, causing gonorrhoea.

The last three occur in pairs and are sometimes called diplococci.

2.   A **Bacillus** (plural = bacilli) is a rod-shaped organism. Those commonly occurring are:

The Tubercle (Koch) bacillus.

The Diphtheria (Klebs-Loeffler) bacillus.

The Typhoid bacillus (*Salmonella typhi*).

The Whooping-cough (*Bordetella pertussis*).

The Colon bacillus (*Escherichia coli*).

The Influenza bacillus (*Haemophilus influenzae*).

The Anthrax bacillus.

The Dysentery bacillus.

The Gas Gangrene bacillus (*Clostridium welchi*).

3.   A *Spirochaete* is an organism twisted rather like a corkscrew. Syphilis, Vincent's angina and leptospiral jaundice (Weil's disease) are the only important diseases in this country caused by spirochaetes. Yaws, a tropical disease, is also due to a spirochaete. Some spirochaetes, e.g. those causing syphilis and yaws, are called treponemes.

Bacteria are recognized in the laboratory:

(i) By their reaction to certain stains, e.g.:

(a) Gram's stain. Most cocci (except gonococci and meningo-cocci) are Gram positive, that is, they take up the stain and look blue under the microscope.

Most bacilli are Gram negative and are stained red.

(b) Ziehl-Neelsen's stain used to demonstrate tubercle bacilli which retain the stain when washed with acid and are, therefore, called Acid-fast Bacilli.

(ii) By culture, that is, growing the organism on special sub-stances or media in an incubator which is kept at body tem-perature. Some organisms only grow in the presence of oxygen (aerobic); others when oxygen is excluded (anaerobic).

(iii) By agglutination reactions, e.g. the Widal test for typhoid (see p. 46).

II. Viruses. There is a group of organisms responsible for various diseases in man and animals which are too small to be seen with the ordinary microscope and which will pass through the pores of a filter so fine that it will hold up all ordinary bacteria. An organism of this nature is referred to as an ultra-microscopic or filter-passing virus.

In recent years our knowledge of the viruses has advanced. Viruses, like bacteria, vary considerably in size. There are some relatively large ones (such as that causing herpes) which are almost equal in size to small bacteria. Others, e.g. poliomyelitis, are very minute and only one twenty-fifth of the size of the larger ones. Many are spherical in shape, others are brick-shaped, and some appear to

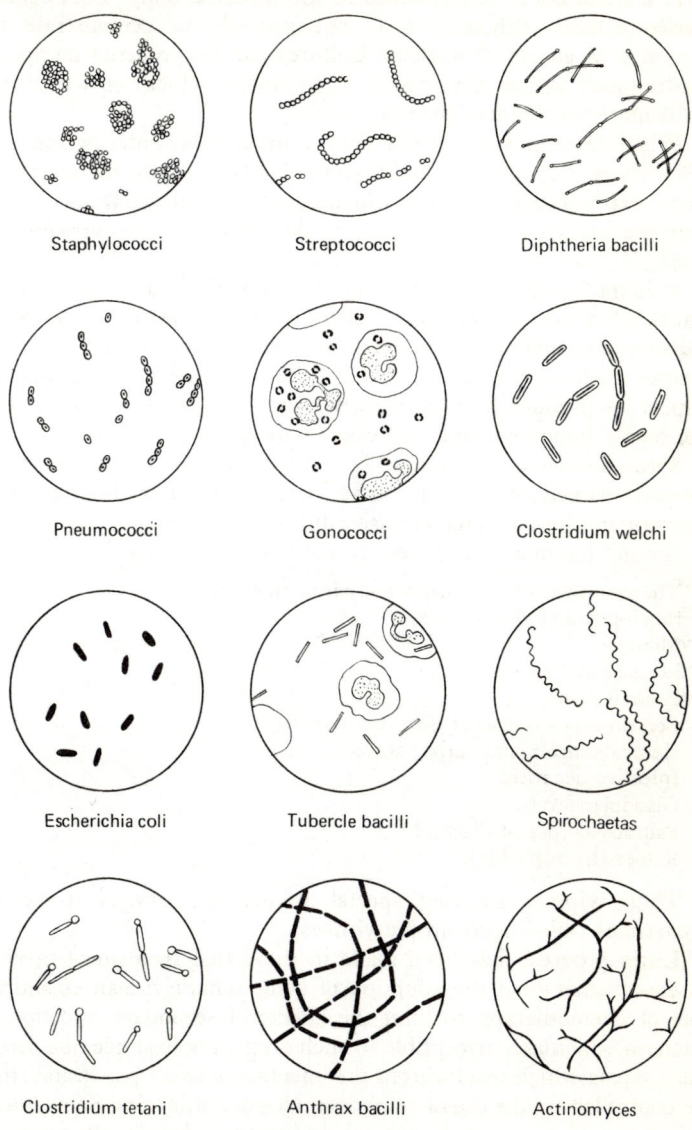

Staphylococci   Streptococci   Diphtheria bacilli

Pneumococci   Gonococci   Clostridium welchi

Escherichia coli   Tubercle bacilli   Spirochaetas

Clostridium tetani   Anthrax bacilli   Actinomyces

Fig. 2 Bacteria

have a small tail or rod attached to the spherical body. They contain nucleo-protein, although it is not possible to demonstrate the presence of an actual nucleus. Cultures can be prepared on special media (such as the egg protein of an embryo chick) on which they grow more slowly than bacteria.

When causing disease they appear to do so by entering the body cells where they multiply and injure or kill the cells. At the same time many types produce toxins which cause general symptoms. When they are known to be circulating in the blood the term **viraemia** is used.

It is interesting to note that lasting immunity may result from an attack of a virus disease. For example, second attacks of measles, chicken-pox, rubella and mumps are rare. On the other hand, other viruses such as those associated with the common cold and influenza appear to produce little permanent immunity. Many virus diseases are highly infectious and may cause widespread epidemics.

Virus disease is transmitted by similar methods to other bacterial disease, namely, by direct contact, droplet infection, fomites, food, carriers and by parasites or insect bites.

Among the diseases caused by viruses are:

The common cold, influenza and virus pneumonia.
Small-pox and chicken-pox.
Mumps.
Measles and rubella.
Poliomyelitis.
Certain types of encephalitis and meningitis.
Herpes simplex and herpes zoster.
Infective hepatitis.
Glandular fever.
Psittacosis (parrot disease).
Rabies (hydrophobia).

Those viruses showing special affinity for nervous tissue are sometimes called neuro-tropic viruses.

Little progress has been made in the actual **treatment** of virus diseases other than the adoption of symptomatic measures and the use of chemotherapy to limit the effects of secondary infection by bacteria which are susceptible to such drugs. For example, the secondary sepsis which results from the infection of small-pox lesions may be controlled by the use of sulphonamides or antibiotics. Some 'virus' infections (e.g. primary atypical pneumonia due to an organism known as *Mycoplasma pneumoniae*) are susceptible to tetracycline.

In some instances it is possible to produce a degree of immunity which may prevent the onset of a virus disease or modify its severity. Active immunity can be produced by the use of special vaccines against small-pox, poliomyelitis, measles, yellow fever, rabies and some types of influenza. Passive immunity of a temporary nature can be obtained by convalescent or adult serum, or a special preparation of serum known as immuno-globulin, in measles, mumps, polio-myelitis and infective hepatitis. Since, however, the supply of immuno-globulin is limited it cannot be used on a large scale (p. 14). It is well known that the rubella virus may cause fetal malformation if the mother is infected in early pregnancy. It is possible that other virus infections may occasionally cause similar damage. It has been suggested that influenza virus may predispose to the development of juvenile leukaemia or Hodgkin's disease under similar circumstances.

III. In addition to bacteria and viruses, other living organisms may cause disease, e.g.:

1. Protozoa, e.g. malaria, amoebic dysentery.
2. Animal parasites, e.g. scabies, intestinal worms, lice.
3. Fungi, e.g. those causing ringworm, thrush (Candida or Monilia), athlete's foot.

Acute inflammation

Inflammation is essentially a defensive process, being Nature's care-fully planned fight against the action of noxious irritants, whether they be the toxins of micro-organisms, corrosive chemicals, or forms of direct violence, but germ action is the chief cause of the commonly occurring inflammations in man.

It may be (*a*) acute, (*b*) chronic.

The aim of inflammation is to prevent further injury by counter-acting the injurious agent.

The cardinal **signs of inflammation** in any part are:

redness   pain
heat   loss of function
swelling

The main changes taking place in the tissues during the process of inflammation are:

1. Dilatation of the small blood vessels (arterioles and capillaries) producing an increase in the blood supply to the part. This accounts for the redness and increased heat.

2. Slowing of the rate of flow of the bloodstream, resulting in a local accumulation of white blood cells (leucocytes).

3. Migration of the leucocytes, that is, the white cells leave the blood vessels and enter the tissues in order that they may attack the invading bacteria.

4. Exudation of lymph from the vessels into the tissues (oedema). This produces the swelling. The stretching of the tissues by this exudate causes pain. The swelling, pain and other changes in the tissues are responsible for the loss of function.

If the bacteria are easily exterminated, the exudate and leucocytes are absorbed by the lymphatics and passed on to the nearest lymph glands where they are disposed of. This increased activity of the lymph glands accounts for those draining an inflamed area being frequently swollen and tender.

If the leucocytes and tissue cells are overcome by the bacteria, they die and the process of suppuration commences. Pus collects and an abscess is formed which, unless opened by surgical means, finds its way to the surface of the affected structure and bursts, thereby discharging its contents.

Chronic inflammation

The clinical distinction between acute and chronic inflammation is one of degree only. The onset of the latter process is usually gradual and it may follow the acute type. The bacteria responsible for acute inflammation are also capable of producing the chronic variety. Some organisms, e.g. the tubercle bacillus are particularly prone to produce chronic inflammation. If inflammation results in the loss of surface of the skin or mucous membrane leaving an open sore, the condition is referred to as an **ulcer**.

Repair of inflammation. When an open wound or ulcer heals, it does so by the formation of delicate red elevations consisting of newly-formed blood vessels and tissue cells, which gradually replace the lost tissue. This is known as **granulation tissue**. When the granulation tissue reaches the level of the skin, the latter grows over the wound and the healed area is called a scar or cicatrix.

Summary
Inflammation may be:
    (a) Acute.
    (b) Chronic (including special types, tuberculosis and syphilis).
    Results of inflammation:
    (a) Resolution, i.e. healing without permanent changes in the tissues.

(b) Suppuration, i.e. the formation of pus.

(c) Fibrosis, i.e. healing by the replacement of tissue damaged by inflammation with fibrous scar tissue.

N.B.—Whenever scar tissue is formed it shows a tendency to contract, hence many scars have a puckered appearance.

The contraction of a fibroid lung may be sufficient to pull the heart towards the affected side of the chest (see p. 308).

The contraction of a scar resulting from healing of a gastric ulcer may lead to pyloric stenosis or hour-glass stomach (p. 216).

Scarring of the valve following endocarditis due to acute rheumatism may result in mitral stenosis (p. 115).

Immunity

Immunity, or non-susceptibility, is the power of an individual to resist infection. It may be:

1. NATURAL.
2. ACQUIRED.
   (a) As a result of recovery from infection.
   (b) Artificially produced.
      (i) Active immunity (vaccine).
      (ii) Passive immunity (serum).

Immunity is dependent on two important factors: (i) the power of leucocytes (phagocytes) to destroy bacteria; (ii) the presence in the serum and tissues of antibodies which kill the bacteria, or antitoxins which neutralize their toxins.

Antibodies are present in the immuno-globulin fraction of blood protein and are formed as a response to the antigenic stimulus of an infective or other agent.

Natural immunity is inborn. Man, for example, is not liable to suffer from many bacterial diseases which affect animals, e.g. canine distemper, and some individuals are constantly exposed to infectious fevers from which they have never suffered, but do not contract them. The degree of natural immunity varies very much in different races and among individuals in the same community.

The opposite to natural immunity is a hereditary disposition to a certain disease. This liability may be transmitted from parent to child and is spoken of as a **diathesis.**

Acquired immunity

(a) As a result of recovery from infection. It is well known that second attacks of many infectious diseases, such as measles and scarlet fever, are uncommon. The majority of individuals, unless

protected by artificial immunity (vaccines), are affected by the commoner infectious fevers during childhood, and although they may be exposed frequently to the same diseases in later life, rarely contract them. They are therefore said to have acquired immunity. The mechanism of this process is important. When an individual is infected by an organism, in order to overcome the disease, the body proceeds to manufacture antibodies, which either kill the infecting agent or neutralize its toxins. When this is done the disease is cured. However, **Nature always over-produces,** and this statement may be regarded as the 'text' of the subject of Immunity. Not only are antibodies formed in sufficient numbers to counteract the disease, but also far in excess of what is required at the time. It follows, therefore, that the blood of an individual who has ceased to suffer from an infection contains a large number of antibodies to that disease, and should the same organism again attempt to attack the body, there is a sufficient reserve of antibodies ready to deal with the infecting agent at once and so prevent the development of the disease. Acquired immunity usually persists throughout life.

(b) Artificial immunity. 1. ACTIVE. If germs, which have previously been killed or specially treated in such a way that they are rendered unable to multiply in the tissues, are injected into an individual they have the power to stimulate the body to produce antibodies in the same way as living microbes. Specially made solutions of the toxins produced by bacteria have a similar effect (toxoids). Advantage is often taken of these facts to produce immunity in an individual by this artificial means and the term **vaccine** is applied to preparations of this type. A relatively small dose of killed or inactivated germs, or a very dilute solution of their toxins, is injected into the patient. The tissues immediately form antibodies to neutralize the effect of these dead germs or their toxins, but Nature over-produces, so that an excess of antibodies remains in the blood after the effect of the vaccine has passed. Another larger dose of vaccine is then given, which again stimulates the body to produce an excess of antibodies. The injection of vaccine is repeated at suitable intervals until it is considered that a sufficient excess of antibodies is present in the blood. It follows, therefore, that some weeks may elapse before full immunity is acquired. Diseases which may be prevented by the use of vaccines, i.e. in which prophylactic immunization is of value, include:

1. Small-pox	5. Diphtheria	9. Measles
2. Typhoid	6. Poliomyelitis	10. Rubella
3. Tetanus	7. Yellow-fever	
4. Whooping-cough	8. Cholera	

An example of this, is the use of typhoid vaccine (TAB) in persons who are going to districts where typhoid fever is common. Two or three injections of this vaccine produce sufficient antibodies in the blood of the individual to prevent the development of the disease, or at least to modify its severity if typhoid bacilli gain access to the body. The protection afforded by active artificial immunity usually lasts for several years but in order to maintain permanent results 'boosting' doses are usually required at stated intervals.

Generally speaking there should be an interval of some weeks between the administration of different types of vaccine. They should not be given if the individual is suffering from some acute disease, or receiving antibiotics, steroids or radio-therapy.

The bacteria or toxin which stimulates the production of anti-bodies is referred to as an **antigen.** It is possible to combine several antigens in one vaccine, thus diminishing the number of injections needed; e.g. diphtheria, pertussis and tetanus (DPT). Poliomyelitis vaccine is given by mouth.

The administration of a vaccine is sometimes followed by a feverish reaction or pain at the site of injection. It is important for the nurse to observe this, and the temperature should be charted four-hourly for at least twenty-four hours after a vaccine has been given. It may be necessary for the patient to rest during this period.

2. PASSIVE. Passive immunity is produced by introducing into an individual, **serum** containing antibodies to a disease, which is usually obtained from the horse by stimulating the animal to form antibodies by the injection of vaccine.

This type of immunity is called Passive, because the individual takes no part in the formation of the antibodies. They are actively produced by the animal and introduced ready-made into the individual and can act immediately.

It is only possible to prepare antitoxins to comparatively few bacteria. The antitoxin sera which may be used are:

    diphtheria antitoxin.

    tetanus antitoxin.

    gas gangrene antitoxin

They are usually given by intramuscular injection, but occasionally in emergency the intravenous route is used.

Passive immunity may also be produced by injecting the serum from another individual who has previously suffered from the disease under consideration and whose blood, therefore, contains antibodies to that disease which have been formed by the process of active acquired immunity already described. The more recent the recovery from the disease, the greater the amount of antibodies will the serum contain.

An example of this method is the use of convalescent serum in the prophylactic treatment of measles. The serum from an adult who has just recovered from measles contains a large amount of antibodies to the disease and, if injected into a susceptible individual who has been in contact with measles, within five days, has the power to prevent its development or of moderating its severity. The blood of any adult who has had measles in the past also has similar power but contains a smaller concentration of antibodies and, therefore, must be given in larger doses to produce the same result (p. 69).

Human immunoglobulin is obtained from human plasma and is a protein fraction in which the antibodies are concentrated. It is, therefore, especially potent and is used instead of adult serum.

It may be employed against the following conditions if the production of passive immunity is urgent:
1. Measles.
   (*a*) To help in the control of epidemics in hospitals and children's institutions.
   (*b*) Children who are ill from some other condition and in whom an attack of measles would be dangerous.
   (*c*) Children under 3 years of age (p. 69).
2. Rubella.—Women who are exposed to the disease during the first 3 to 4 months of pregnancy (p. 72).
3. Poliomyelitis.
   (*a*) Unvaccinated medical personnel who are in close contact with early cases.
   (*b*) Newborn babies who might be exposed to the infection in a maternity department.
   (*c*) Children in a hospital ward in which a case has developed, especially after recent tonsillectomy (p. 381).
4. Infective hepatitis.

Passive immunity only lasts while the artificially introduced antibodies remain in the system, usually a period of three to four weeks, and can therefore be regarded only as a temporary measure in the prevention of disease. All immunological procedures of this type do carry small risks of complications and side effects.

N.B. Both doctors and patients should keep an accurate record of all immunization procedures.

Other aspects of immunity. In addition to the immune response to infection there are other important immune responses, namely

1. Those which produce antibodies capable of acting against the patient's own tissues (**auto-immunity**, see Chapter 9).
2. Those responsible for **rejection** of transplanted tissues (homografts, organ transplants).
3. Those which are thought to destroy malignant cells arising in the bodies of normal, healthy people. According to this theory, cancer develops when the immunological 'surveillance mechanism' breaks down.

Allergy

Allergy is a term which was originally applied to the condition of over-sensitivity to foreign protein. Its meaning has now been enlarged to embrace other substances which are harmless to a normal person but which provoke abnormal reactions in sensitive people. These include carbohydrates, various chemical substances and drugs. When an individual develops this hypersensitivity, further introduction of that substance into the system is accompanied by various symptoms which are sometimes serious. A substance causing such sensitivity is called an **allergen.**

Although not invariably present, there is often a hereditary tendency to this state and allergic reactions are more common in some families than others. It is interesting to note that some emotional disturbance may occasionally predispose to the development of the allergic state (i.e. a psychosomatic phenomenon).

The chief manifestations of allergy are:

Asthma
Hay fever
Gastro-intestinal disturbances
Skin reactions, e.g. contact dermatitis, urticaria, infantile eczema
Angio-neurotic oedema
Serum sickness and anaphylaxis
Reaction to certain foods, e.g. eggs, shellfish and drugs.

Some allergic symptoms respond to treatment with anti-histamine drugs ('Benadryl,' 'Phenergan,' 'Piriton,' etc.) which may be given either by mouth or, in cases of urgency, by intravenous injections. Adrenaline and ephedrine may also be used. Cortisone and other steroids, e.g. prednisolone and corticotrophin (ACTH), are effective in some cases. Local applications of hydrocortisone ointment may be helpful for some conditions. Attempts to desensitize the individual may also be made, by giving a series of injections of very small doses of a 'vaccine' containing the offending allergen after it has been detected by special skin tests.

Hay fever which consists of seasonal attacks of sneezing and profuse running from the nose and eyes, is an allergic reaction to the pollen of certain grasses. Special vaccines (e.g. 'Alavac-P,' 'Allpyral') given early in the year and the use of antihistamine drugs during the attacks are helpful. Sodium cromoglycate ('Rynacrom') insufflated into the nostrils 4 times a day during the hay fever season may prevent or reduce attacks.

Asthma is frequently of allergic origin and is then due to oversensitivity to the protein contained in substances such as mites, house dust, animal dandruff (cats, dogs, horses), feathers, certain foods and pollens, and to the toxins of bacteria (see p. 283).

Anaphylaxis

If a patient has at any time had an injection of horse serum in any form, great care must be taken if another dose is given as the individual may have been rendered over-sensitive to the foreign proteins contained in horse serum. This over-sensitivity takes about ten days to develop and persists for a very long time. Once it has developed, a second injection of serum may cause immediate and severe collapse or even sudden death. These symptoms are known as **anaphylactic shock**. This condition is associated with the liberation in the tissues of a substance called histamine. Asthmatic patients are often sensitive to the injection of horse serum, and for these reasons all patients should be asked if they suffer from asthma or if they have previously had serum, before the injection is given. Special care is also necessary when administering anti-tetanus serum and an intradermal test dose is usually given before the main injection. Symptoms identical with those of anaphylactic shock may occasionally be produced in patients who are sensitive to penicillin and also to insect stings. All cases of anaphylaxis should be treated with intravenous hydrocortisone and subcutaneous adrenaline immediately, as first-line, life-saving treatment and an intravenous antihistamine drug, e.g. 'Piriton', should follow.

Serum sickness. Occasionally, a delayed reaction follows the injection of serum, after a period of eight to twelve days. This consists of pyrexia, swelling and pains in the joints, and the occurrence of a rash either in the form of wheals (Urticaria) or a generalized redness (Erythema). The condition is known as serum sickness. It is a form of allergy due to the protein present in the serum, and may be relieved by injection of adrenaline, 0·5 ml). Applications of calamine lotion relieve the irritation of the rash and antihistamine drugs or corticosteroids may be given.

Fever

Fever is a complex response of the body to infection and is one of the defence mechanisms, closely connected with the development of immunity. It is associated with a rise in body temperature, which is referred to as pyrexia.

Pyrexia is due to disturbance of the heat-regulating mechanism of the body by the action of toxins on the general metabolism and on the heat-regulating centre in the brain. Normally there is a balance between heat produced in the body by the chemical action (metabolism) associated with exercise, movements of muscles, activity of other organs and glands, and heat lost by conduction from the skin and the evaporation of sweat. This balance is controlled by the heat-regulating centre largely by influencing the calibre of the blood vessels in the skin. If the blood vessels are contracted, they will contain less blood. A small amount of blood in the surface of the body will result in diminished heat loss, whereas free circulation of blood in dilated vessels is associated with increased heat loss. It follows, therefore, that either increased heat production or diminished heat loss will result in a rise of body temperature.

Notes on body temperature

	Normal	
Mouth	36·7–37·0 °C	98–98·6 °F
Axilla		98–98·6 °F
Rectum	37·4 °C	99·4 °F

1. Mouth temperatures below 36·6 °C (98 °F) are referred to as subnormal, below 35·0 °C (95·0 °F) as hypothermia, above 37·2 °C (99 °F) as febrile. A very high temperature (40 °C (104 °F) and over) is called hyperpyrexia.

2. The clinical thermometer is used for taking temperatures. Remember that in order to obtain an accurate reading it is often necessary to leave the thermometer in position for a considerably longer period of time than that marked on the instrument. This is especially important in mouth temperatures of patients who are out of doors on a cold day or whose mouths have been cooled by rapid breathing (certain heart cases). **N.B.**—Special low-reading thermometers are required to record severe degrees of hypothermia.

3. Do not take a patient's temperature directly after giving either a hot or cold drink.

4. The temperature normally varies during the day, being lowest in the morning (6 a.m. 36·3–36·5 °C (97·2–97·6 °F)) and reaching its maximum in the afternoon between 3 p.m. and 5 p.m. Not infrequently there is a transient rise in temperature for a day or two before the onset of menstruation. The rectal temperature is about 0·5 °C (1 °F) higher than the mouth temperature.

The normal temperature of a newborn infant is 37·2°–37·5 °C (99–99·6 °F).

5. In addition to infection, a rise in temperature may be produced by muscular exercise, exposure to high temperature and various nervous factors.

6. Among the causes of **prolonged pyrexia** are:

Typhoid fever   Bacterial endocarditis
Malaria   Hodgkin's disease
Tuberculosis   Pyelitis
Septicaemia   Undrained pus, e.g. empyema.
Connective tissue disease.

7. Some causes of **subnormal temperature (hypothermia)** are:

(i) The direct withdrawal of heat, such as exposure to cold, immersion in water and unconsciousness from any cause, including anaesthesia, poisoning, diabetic coma and uraemia.

(ii) Great loss of fluid, e.g. diarrhoea, haemorrhage.

(iii) Surgical shock.

(iv) Heart disease.

(v) During convalescence after fevers.

(vi) Myxoedema.

(vii) Drugs, especially phenothiazines.

(viii) Artificial hypothermia necessary for some surgical operations, e.g. cardiac surgery.

Hypothermia in the elderly. This is an important winter ailment which causes some deaths every year among old people, especially those living on their own. It can develop within twenty-four hours if the heating in a bedroom or living room fails. The patient may be cold, weak, confused and the blood pressure falls.

The diagnosis is confirmed by taking the rectal temperature with a low reading thermometer, *i.e.* below 35·0 °C (95 °F). It becomes very serious at levels of 32 °C (90 °F).

Treatment. In the first instance the temperature of the room should be raised rather than applying direct heat to the patient, with a view to raising the body temperature about 1 °C per hour. Fluids should be restricted until the body temperature has returned to normal.

Efforts should be made to contact Social Services to avoid repetition of the event. A general medical check-up to detect hypothyroidism or other disease is necessary.

The course of fever. The commencement of fever is usually sudden, and is frequently accompanied by a rigor or shivering attack. In young children, temperature regulation is easily upset and the onset of pyrexia may be associated with convulsions.

The period during which pyrexia remains fully developed is referred to as the 'fastigium'. The stage of defervescence marks the termination of fever. When the fever ends rapidly it is said to resolve by **crisis**; when gradually, by **lysis** (Fig. 3).

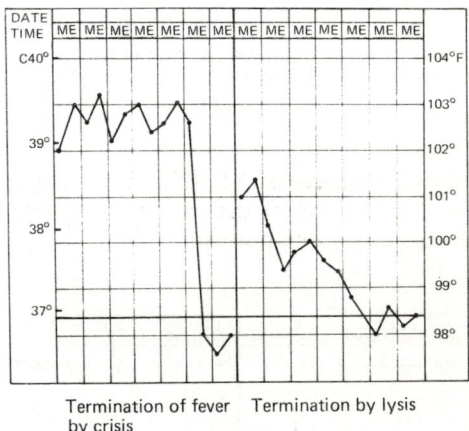

Termination of fever   Termination by lysis
by crisis

Fig. 3

There are three principal types of fever illustrated by the temperature chart (see Figs. 4 and 5).

(i) Continued, e.g. typhoid fever.
(ii) Remittent, e.g. pulmonary tuberculosis.
(iii) Intermittent, e.g. malaria.

When the temperature does not fluctuate more than 1·1 °C. (2 °F) during twenty-four hours and at no time touches normal, it is described as continuous. If it remains persistently above normal

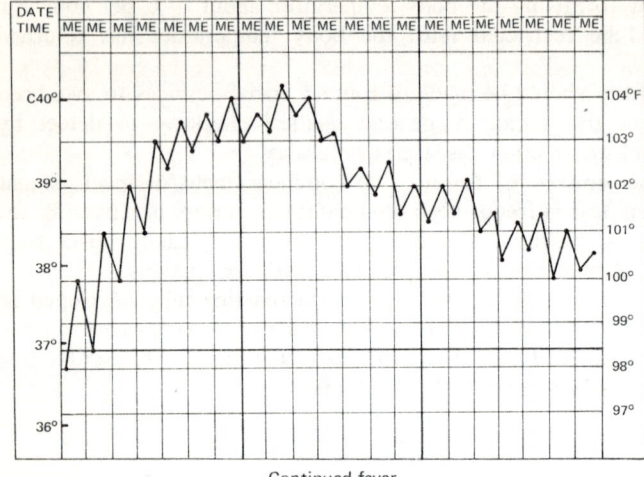

Continued fever
(Commencing in "staircase" manner characteristic)
of typhoid fever

Fig. 4

but the daily fluctuations exceed 1·1 °C (2 °F), it is known as remittent. If during some period of the day the temperature falls to or below normal, it is called intermittent.

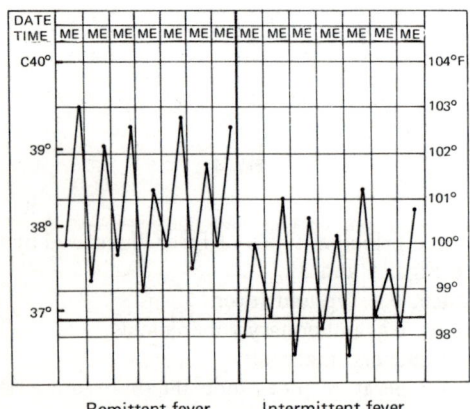

Remittent fever   Intermittent fever

Fig. 5

Effects of fever on the body. *(i) Metabolism.* The general metabolism is increased. There is increased breaking down (katabolism) especially of protein which, if the febrile condition is prolonged, leads to loss of weight.

(ii) Secretions and excretions. These are diminished in amount, particularly the saliva, the gastric and intestinal juices. This makes digestion more difficult and necessitates a light, easily digested diet in febrile cases. The amount of urine is decreased and albuminuria may occur.

(iii) Respiration. The rate is increased.

(iv) Circulation. The pulse is full and bounding and is increased in rate.

(v) Nervous system. Headache, accompanied by restlessness and delirium if the pyrexia is great.

(vi) Dehydration may result from sweating if there is an inadequate fluid intake.

The treatment of fever

   (i) Rest in bed in a warm, well-ventilated room 18·3 °C (65 °F) with isolation in the case of an infectious disease.

  (ii) Treat the exciting cause, if possible, e.g. Anti-malarial drugs; sulphonamides, penicillin or other antibiotics when indicated.

 (iii) Help the excretory organs to eliminate toxins by:

     (a) Giving plenty of fluids, to increase the quantity of urine, to flush out the kidneys, to increase the amount of toxin excreted by them and to replace fluid loss.

     (b) Giving aperients, suppositories or enema when necessary.

  (iv) Increase heat loss by cold or tepid sponging.

   (v) Maintain the general strength of the patient by administering plenty of easily digested nourishment, including milk, eggs, ice cream and glucose.

N.B.—The advantage of glucose over other sugars is that it is less sweet and therefore can be taken in considerable quantity without causing nausea.

  (vi) Care of mouth and pressure areas may be necessary.

 (vii) Treat complications as they arise.

N.B.—Slight degrees of fever do not necessarily require active treatment other than rest in bed and simple measures directed towards the patient's comfort, e.g. aspirin or similar analgesic.

Rigors

A rigor or severe shivering attack is the physiological reaction of the body to chilling of its surface, and may be described in three stages; the cold stage, the hot stage and the sweating stage.

1. THE COLD STAGE. The patient shivers violently, the teeth chatter, the skin is pale and the small papillae are raised (gooseflesh). The body surface feels cold, but the rectal temperature is elevated and the pulse is rapid. This may be associated with headache, general malaise and vomiting. If shivering is violent the temperature should not be taken in the mouth as this may result in breakage of the thermometer.

2. THE HOT STAGE. The patient becomes very hot, the skin is red and burning and the mouth temperature is raised. Thirst is marked and headache severe.

3. THE SWEATING STAGE. General profuse sweating occurs. The temperature falls rapidly to normal and the pulse becomes slower. After a severe rigor the patient may become collapsed in this stage.

Rigors commonly occur at the onset of fever, and in acute pyelonephritis, bacterial endocarditis, septicaemia and malaria.

Treatment. During the cold stage heat must be applied to the patient by means of hot or electric blankets and hot-water bottles, which are removed at the onset of the hot stage. Hot drinks are given during the cold stage and cool ones during the hot stage. Cold compresses may be applied to the forehead during the hot stage. During the sweating stage, sweat may be removed by bathing with warm water, but care must be taken to keep the patient warm and to avoid chills.

Convulsions

These are involuntary muscular movements frequently associated with transitory loss of consciousness. Epileptic fits, uraemic twitchings and the seizures of cerebral apoplexy should be regarded as convulsions of a special type, and must not be confused with infantile convulsions.

Infantile convulsions are liable to occur in children under the age of 2 years in association with pyrexia and the onset of any acute infection. They are also seen in whooping cough, rickets, in gastro-intestinal upsets, and during dentition, but do not usually show any tendency to recur after the primary cause of the condition has ceased to operate. Some cases are due to a low blood sugar (hypoglycaemia).

Although convulsions may occur in infants in similar circumstances to those in which rigors are seen in adults, the two conditions must not be regarded as identical. Rigors, though rare, may also occur in children and are due to the same reaction of the body to undue chilling of its surface. Convulsions, on the other hand, are due to excessive irritability of the nervous system. Convulsions which occur directly after birth are caused by injury to the brain during delivery.

Treatment. In the first instance a good air-way must be maintained.

Severe convulsions may be controlled by intravenous diazepam, ('Valium'), intramuscular sodium phenytoin or intramuscular injection of paraldehyde (0·2 ml per kilogram body weight).

The recurrence of convulsions may be prevented by giving phenobarbitone orally. These drugs act by depressing the sensitivity of the nervous system.

Tuberculosis and syphilis

Although these two diseases do not resemble each other in their results and their causes are entirely different they both illustrate a special type of chronic inflammation. The effects of the tubercle bacillus and the treponeme of syphilis are to produce a reaction in the diseased part which results in the formation of tissue closely resembling the granulation tissue just described and they are sometimes referred to as granulomata. (Leprosy and actinomycosis also produce similar results.)

The incidence of tuberculosis is now less in developed countries than it was half a century ago: nevertheless constant vigilance is necessary.

Tuberculosis

Two varieties of tubercle bacillus may be found in man. The **human** which is largely responsible for pulmonary tuberculosis, and the **bovine**, derived from cows, which causes most cases of bone and glandular tuberculosis. Both produce their effect on the body by the formation of the same type of specialized granulation tissue. The former is more common in towns, while the bovine form is more often found in rural districts but is now rare because of tuberculin testing of cattle and pasteurization of milk.

When the tubercle bacillus settles in any part of the body it proceeds to multiply. The defence mechanism of the body surrounds the organisms with an area of inflammation, and the tissues in the immediate vicinity are crowded with lymphocytes and other cells. The toxins liberated by the tubercle bacilli kill the infected tissue together with many of the phagocytes, and the blood supply to the area is cut off. The central part of the affected area then dies. The dead tissue has the appearance and consistency of cheese and this process is referred to as **caseation.**

The central area of caseation containing dead cells and tubercle bacilli surrounded by an inflammatory area, is referred to as a tubercle. A number of adjacent tubercles may run together and so produce a large area of tuberculous disease.

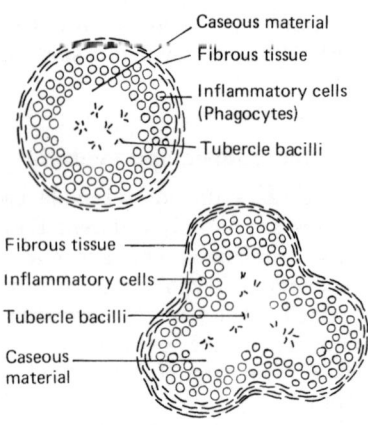

Caseous material

Fibrous tissue

Inflammatory cells (Phagocytes)

Tubercle bacilli

Fibrous tissue

Inflammatory cells

Tubercle bacilli

Caseous material

Fig. 6 Diagram illustrating: (1) A single tubercle; (2) Three tubercles running together to produce a large central area of caseation.

If the resistance of the body is sufficiently great and when aided by modern chemotherapy, the granulation tissue around the tubercles becomes converted into fibrous tissues (**fibrosis**) like a scar, completely surrounding and cutting off the affected area. Calcium salts are deposited in the caseous part (**calcification**) and healing takes place.

For many years tuberculous disease was clinically divided into two groups, viz.:

(*a*) Medical, e.g. affecting lungs, meninges, peritoneum (pp. 296, 385, 260.

(*b*) Surgical, e.g. affecting bones, joints, glands, renal tract.

Although this is still to some extent true, and surgical and orthopaedic measures may be necessary, the use of streptomycin and anti-tuberculous drugs (p. 304) is essential for all forms of the disease.

Syphilis

The treponeme of syphilis causes similar changes. The granulomatous tissue produced by this means is called a *gumma*, and occurs in the tertiary stages of the disease (see p. 493).

Leprosy

The incidence of leprosy is mainly confined to certain tropical countries but the consequences of the disease acquired there may be seen elsewhere. It is caused by the *Bacterium leprae* which causes chronic lesions of the skin and nervous systems.

Symptoms. An early symptom is the development of anaesthetic areas in the skin which may become paler in colour in dark-skinned people. The loss of sensation may lead to local tissue damage from cuts, burns, etc. with, later, mutilation and deformity particularly of feet and hands. In addition, raised nodular lesions may occur especially on the face.

Diagnosis. Apart from the clinical symptoms, the bacteria may be obtained from nasal washings or by biopsy of lesions.

Treatment. Dapsone and thiambutosine are drugs which are effective if given for several years. Segregation in leper colonies may be desirable to prevent the spread of the disease when many bacteria are found in the lesions. Corrective surgery may be helpful later when severe deformities are present.

Sarcoidosis

In this disease, the lesions are similar to tubercles but there is no caseation, the cause is unknown and the condition is not infectious. It may affect lymph nodes, lungs, parotid glands, skin, eyes, bones, liver and spleen. The subacute form of the disease usually resolves spontaneously within 2 years. Chronic sarcoidosis tends to cause permanent damage because of the fibrosis which it induces.

4. Degeneration

This means a wearing out of the cells and the gradual replacement of the normal protoplasm by fat, fibrous tissue or some other material.

It may occur as a result of the action of toxins, metabolic changes or diminution of the blood supply.

Degenerative changes are often seen in the joints, heart, arteries, liver and kidneys as a result of disease.

Circulatory disorders include

(a) Those dependent upon failure of the heart to maintain an adequate circulation to the body as a whole;

(b) local disorders due to vascular spasm or blockage of a blood vessel by thrombosis (p. 157) or embolism (p. 160).

Diminished local blood supply is sometimes called **ischaemia**, and an area of tissue which dies as a result of this, an **infarct**. Lack of oxygen is called **anoxia**.

Amyloid degeneration is the deposit of a protein-polysaccharide compound in various organs which occasionally develops in very chronic inflammatory and septic conditions (e.g. rheumatoid arthritis, tuberculosis, chronic osteomyelitis) or without obvious cause.

5. Tumours (Neoplasms)

Tumours are abnormal swellings resulting from the overgrowth of tissue cells. There are two main types:

1. Benign or innocent. 2. Malignant.

1. A **benign tumour** consists of **normal** cells resembling those of the tissue from which they arise. Its growth is usually slow; it has a capsule which limits it to the situation in which it originates, and it shows no tendency to reproduce itself in the neighbouring lymph glands, nor in distant parts of the body.

The commonest benign tumours are:

The fibrous tumour (fibroma).

The fatty tumour (lipoma).

The nerve tumour (neuroma).

The gland tumour (adenoma).

The blood vessel tumour or naevus (angioma).

The bony tumour (osteoma).

The wart (papilloma).

Their interest is mainly surgical and many of them can be removed, if necessary, by operative means.

2. *Malignant.* Malignant new growths are frequently referred to as Cancer. There are two main types of cancer.

1. Carcinoma. 2. Sarcoma (less common).

The distinguishing characteristics of malignant tumours are: (a) local invasion of normal tissue by **abnormal**, rapidly multiplying cells; (b) reproduction in distant parts of similar tumours which develop from cells detached from the parent tumour and which reach their remote destination either by means of the blood stream or the lymphatic channels.

Cancer may arise in almost any structure in the body. The tumour at the site of origin being called the primary growth. Common sites of primary cancer are the stomach, uterus, breast, lung, colon and rectum.

The tumours which are reproduced in other parts of the body are called **secondary deposits** or **metastases**. They are most common in the lymphatic glands draining the area in which the primary growth is situated. Not infrequently, however, they appear in the liver, the lungs, the brain and in bones, and give rise to various symptoms, depending upon the part in which they develop.

Malignant disease often produces a profound general effect on the body, which manifests itself by wasting, weakness and anaemia—a state sometimes referred to as **cachexia**.

The cause of the disease is still unknown. Much research is being done to endeavour to solve the mystery of this scourge. Viruses sometimes cause cancer in animals and may possibly do so in humans. A toxic agent is responsible in some cases. Cancer sometimes develops in those situations which are subject to chronic irritation. An illustration of this was the frequent association of cancer of the lip with smoking of a short-stemmed clay pipe now rarely seen.

Certain types of cancer can be produced by chemical irritants which are obtained from coal tar. There is little doubt that cancer of the lung is much more common among heavy cigarette smokers than in non-smokers, and it is now generally accepted that smoking has a causal relationship to lung cancer. A type of sarcoma affecting fowls is known to be due to a virus. The development of carcinoma of the breast and carcinoma of the prostate may be dependent on the influence of certain hormones. In some cases heredity may predispose to the condition.

The treatment of cancer is largely in the hands of surgeons, but the diagnosis of the condition frequently falls to the lot of the physician, and cases of cancer are often to be found in medical wards. The importance of early diagnosis must be stressed. It has been said that 'Delay causes as many deaths as cancer does'. People must be encouraged to report suspicious symptoms and signs to their doctors. Methods used for early and presymptomatic diagnosis include **cytology**, of which the best example is microscopic examination of the cells in a cervical smear. Obtaining the specimen for the latter examination is quick, easy, harmless and painless. Tests are now being developed in which **antigens** can be detected in the blood of patients with cancer (e.g. of the colon).

Among the methods of treatment at our disposal are complete surgical removal of the growth, if possible. In addition, deep x-ray therapy and the application of radium or other radioactive material in some form, either alone or combined with surgical measures, have been found of value. Modern developments include the use of hormones (oestrogens, such as stilboestrol) for certain types of cancer, e.g. of the prostate and breast, and the use of cytotoxic drugs which selectively kill the rapidly multiplying cells and can be given by mouth, intravenous injection or even intra-arterial injection into the region of the tumour. These are of special value in leukaemia, sometimes called 'cancer of the blood', in which abnormal white cells are present in the blood (p. 189).

A word of warning must be added. Never, under any circumstances, mention the word cancer in the hearing of a patient, for it may produce such fear and despair that the chances of the patient's recovery may be adversely influenced, especially in those cases in which operation is contemplated and especially in which the diagnosis of the condition is uncertain and the patient may not be suffering from cancer at all. It is wise, also, to avoid the words carcinoma and neoplasm, as the more educated patient may be equally familiar with these terms. The doctor may, however, decide that in certain cases the patient should be told about his disease. For psychological reasons some individuals who are perfectly healthy live in fear of cancer (cancerphobia).

Iatrogenic disease (Iatros, Gk: physician). This is disease caused by personnel who treat the patient. A physician may cause Cushing's syndrome by prescribing high doses of corticosteroids. A nurse may cause serious urinary tract infection by failing to adhere rigidly to an aseptic technique in inserting a catheter into a patient's urethra and bladder.

Medical and nursing attendants have a great responsibility in treating patients but must try to ensure that the treatment is not worse than the disease with which the patient presents.

THE MANAGEMENT OF DISEASE

Diagnosis

When a patient is suffering from an illness or injury it is first of all necessary to determine accurately the cause of the condition and to assess the alteration in both the structure and functions of the body produced by it. In order to reach a diagnosis knowledge, experience and careful observation are necessary.

History of the complaint. It is essential first of all to have accurate information about the symptoms of which the patient complains and to know how long he has had them, the order of their development and any factors which have influenced their severity. As far as possible the patient should be allowed to tell his story in his own way but careful questioning on special points is usually necessary.

Previous medical and personal history. When the detailed history of the present complaint has been given, information concerning previous illnesses, injuries, operations and admissions to hospital should be obtained. It may also be necessary to know whether the patient has had an examination for Life Insurance purposes or the Forces and whether he has travelled abroad.

Family history. This may be of more importance in some cases than others, especially when dealing with known hereditary disorders. Many diseases have a tendency to occur in families such as allergy, migraine, epilepsy and high blood pressure.

In some instances helpful information can only be obtained from a parent or relative, but as a rule this should not be sought in the hearing of the patient.

Clinical examination. Full clinical examination involves general observation of the patient and the use of hands and ears and special apparatus such as:

(a) the sphygmomanometer for measuring blood pressure.

(b) the patellar hammer to test tendon reflexes.

(c) the ophthalmoscope to examine the retina.

The mental state and intelligence of the patient is first noted and much may be gathered when taking the history. Other observations include the general physical development, state of nutrition and the appearance of the skin.

The actual physical examination of the various systems which must be carefully carried out is not a part of the nurse's duties, although some of the main points are mentioned in the chapters which follow.

Special investigations. Many special investigations may be performed according to the requirements of the individual case. They include:

X-rays

Bacteriological examinations

Chemical tests

Examinations of the blood, urine and CSF

Biopsy, i.e. taking a specimen of tissue for microscopic examination

The use of special apparatus such as the electrocardiograph and the electroencephalograph.

When the history, clinical examination and tests have been completed it is usually possible to make an accurate diagnosis and assessment of the disease and to carry out the necessary treatment. In urgent cases, however, it is not always possible to wait for confirmation of the opinion formed and treatment based on clinical experience and judgement must be commenced at once.

Treatment (therapeutics)

Treatment is the management and care of a patient whereby we endeavour to aid Nature in restoring him to health. Measures which produce this result are said to be curative. Unfortunately, it is not always possible to cure a disease, but in these cases it is often possible to do something to relieve pain and obviate distressing symptoms; treatment of this kind is referred to as palliative or symptomatic.

There are a number of methods at our disposal for attaining these ends.

1. Rest. The chief natural curative agent we have is rest. Hilton (1863), in his work on *Rest and Pain*, says: 'Under injury pain suggests the necessity of, and indeed, compels man to seek for rest. Every deviation from this necessary state of rest brings with it, through pain, the admonition that he is straying from the condition essential to his restoration.'

Rest may be local or general. Local rest refers to resting the damaged part or organ by means of splints, plaster or strapping or the adoption of a posture affording the greatest mechanical advantage. General rest includes sleep with muscular and mental relaxation. If this cannot be obtained by natural means, 'sedation' is obtained by giving drugs, either of the barbiturate or 'tranquillizing' type.

On the other hand, it must be remembered that unnecessary confinement to bed may be a bad thing, especially in old people. The muscles become weak, the joints stiff, the circulation defective and the bowels sluggish. Bedsores may develop and the patient may become dull and apathetic. Thrombosis of the calf veins may occur (see p. 157).

In fact, the modern tendency is towards early ambulation both in medical and surgical cases whenever possible. 'Arm-chair' rest may often be a good substitute for 'bed rest'.

2. Diet. Food is required by the body for purposes of growth, for the renewal of tissues and to produce energy for the work performed by the individual. The essential constituents of food are proteins, fats, carbohydrates, vitamins, mineral salts and water which, in health, should be taken in balanced proportions according to bodily requirements. The diet must be of a sufficient calorific value to supply the necessary amount of energy and there should be present an adequate supply of unabsorbable residue or 'roughage' to stimulate the action of the large bowel and ensure a daily evacuation of its contents.

In disease it is often necessary to vary the proportions of the main constituents of a diet. For example, in diabetes the amount of carbohydrate is reduced or strictly controlled. In some cases of kidney disease the amount of protein may be diminished. A low salt diet is given when oedema is present and special diets are used in the treatment of peptic ulcer, nephritis and ulcerative colitis.

Fluid and electrolyte balance are matters of great importance in many medical and surgical conditions (p. 426).

3. Drugs. There are an enormous number of substances at our disposal for the treatment of disease. Some of these are of vegetable origin and are obtained from plants (e.g. digitalis from the Foxglove), others are prepared from animals (e.g. extract of thyroid gland) and an ever-increasing number are made by chemical processes in the laboratory, e.g. tranquilizers, barbiturates and sulphonamides.

Drugs may be administered in several ways:

1. By the mouth (orally) or the rectum.
2. By injection:
    (*a*) Hypodermic or subcutaneous.
    (*b*) Intramuscular.
    (*c*) Intravenous.
    (*d*) Intrathecal (into the spinal canal).
    (*e*) Intra-articular, e.g. hydrocortisone.
3. By inhalation, e.g. anaesthetics, oxygen, aerosols, friar's balsam.

4. By local application, e.g. lotions, ointments and plasters.

A **placebo** is a medicine given for the sole purpose of pleasing or satisfying the patient. It usually consists of a simple mixture free from powerful drugs, e.g. a tonic, or gentian mixture.

4. Anti-Microbial agents. These include chemical substances such as the sulphonamides and co-trimoxazole ('Septrin'), the use of which may be described as 'chemotherapy,' and the antibiotics.

An **antibiotic** may be defined as a substance made and excreted by an organism (usually a mould) which kills or prevents the growth of other organisms. Those in common use are penicillin, streptomycin, the tetracyclines ('Aureomycin,' 'Terramycin'), cephaloridine and chloramphenicol ('Chloromycetin').

5. The Corticosteroids. These are hormones which may be given internally, by injection or applied locally. Corticotrophin (ACTH) is an extract of the anterior pituitary of animals which stimulates the suprarenals to secrete hydrocortisone. Tetracosactrin ('Synecthen') is a synthetic compound which has the same action. Most of the steroids (cortisone, prednisolone and hydrocortisone) can be prepared synthetically. They may be used in such conditions as rheumatoid arthritis, asthma, skin conditions and connective tissue diseases. (As there are many preparations available, for brevity, they will be referred to as '*steroids*'.)

6. Vaccines (p. 12). These are usually given by subcutaneous or intramuscular injection. They are made from live attenuated (weakened) organisms, killed organisms or toxoids, and they promote active immunity against the corresponding live virulent organisms.

Vaccines are used in the prevention of certain diseases rather than in the actual treatment of the condition.

7. (*a*) **Sera** (antitoxins). These are given by injection; either subcutaneous, intramuscular, intravenous or, rarely, intrathecal. Their use is limited.

(*b*) **Human immunoglobulins**

Like animal sera, these confer passive immunity. *Human Normal Immunoglobulin Injection, B.P.* is made from pooled plasma and contains globulins which confer immunity to a number of infections. *Human Specific Immunoglobulins* are obtained from patients convalescent from specific infections.

8. Various Physical Agencies including:

(*a*) Heat—radiant heat, infra-red rays, hot-air baths, short-wave diathermy.

(*b*) Light—Artificial sunlight (ultra-violet rays).

(*c*) Hydrotherapy—Special baths, cold or tepid, sponging, etc.

(*d*) Electricity—Galvanism, faradism and ionization.

(*e*) X-rays— } particularly in cancer.
(*f*) Radium—

(*g*) Radioactive substances (isotopes), e.g. Iodine (^{131}I), Phosphorus (^{32}P).

9. Rehabilitation. This is a subject of great importance and one of the aims of Modern Medicine is to return the patient to the maximum degree of mental and physical fitness which his condition will permit in as short a time as possible. This is called 'rehabilitation'. In some cases return to full normal work is possible, in others only partial restoration can be obtained, but even in such instances patients may be able to lead a happy, useful life and become economically self-supporting. To attain this end three major methods of treatment are employed, viz.

Physiotherapy,

Occupational therapy,

Psychotherapy,

which may be combined or appropriately modified to meet the needs of individual cases.

A great deal can be done, not only in hospital but also in the patient's home. It may be desirable to send certain cases to special rehabilitation centres where the necessary facilities and special apparatus are available and where the spirit of team-work and competition are added incentives to recovery.

Occupational therapy may be of three kinds:

(*a*) *Diversional*, that is something which the patient is given to do which will keep his mind occupied and interested and prevent him from becoming bored and obsessed by his illness while he is in hospital.

(*b*) *Remedial.* By this is meant some form of occupation specially designed to re-educate damaged muscles or disordered joint movements such as may occur after fractures or dislocations and poliomyelitis. It is closely linked with physiotherapy and routine exercises which the patient supplements by his own efforts.

(*c*) *Training.* When a patient's illness or disability is such that he will be prevented from returning to his original occupation, teaching him some other craft or trade will enable him to earn his own living. For this purpose it may be necessary to send him to a special occupational therapy and rehabilitation unit where this can be carried out by skilled instructors. Physically handicapped individuals may require special apparatus and adaptations in their homes.

The physiotherapist and the occupational therapist give instruction in their respective departments but the nurse can help enormously by encouraging the patients to carry on their good work.

10. Psychotherapy. Although the sciences of psychology and psychiatry and the special methods of treatment, such as the use of psychotropic drugs, electroconvulsive therapy (ECT), insulin coma, abreaction, aversion therapy, psychoanalysis and hypnosis, practised by the psychiatrist are not always applicable in general medical work, it is very important to remember the psychological aspects of each case. The mental outlook of every patient is to some extent influenced by bodily disease, and it is essential to bear this in mind. A sick person may be 'faddy' or irritable and generally difficult to manage. Firmness tempered by sympathy, kindness and understanding must be the watchword of all case management. Recovery is often determined by the will to get well and it is the duty of all those who attend the sick to be optimistic and to encourage them in every way, in addition to performing conscientiously the routine duties of nursing and treatment.

Much of the interest of the Science of Medicine is found in studying the cause of illness, the methods and effects of disease processes and the results of treatment, but the essential aim of the Art of Medicine is to procure the happiness and comfort of the patient, whether it be by curing his disease, or by relieving his symptoms, and if neither of these are possible, by helping him to live in bright and cheerful surroundings and to forget, as far as he is able, his sufferings.

2 Infectious Diseases

Introduction. There is a large group of diseases due to infection in which the whole economy of the body is disturbed. Important features of most of these maladies are that they are accompanied by fever, are contagious or transmissible from one person to another, and that one attack usually protects the individual against subsequent attacks. Some of these conditions are caused by ordinary bacteria; others are virus infections.

It is generally convenient to consider a number of these together under the heading of acute infectious diseases, especially those which are liable to occur in epidemic form; while other diseases, although of bacterial or virus origin, such as pneumonia, influenza, poliomyelitis, meningitis and pulmonary tuberculosis, are dealt with in connection with the particular system of the body on which the brunt of the attack falls.

[In giving the classical description of these diseases it must be remembered that the course and general management of many of them may be greatly modified by the use of antibiotics or previous vaccination. Also, because some are more common in other countries some detailed descriptions are included.]

Modes of entrance

Bacteria and viruses may gain entrance to the body in the following ways:

1. Directly through the skin, especially if there is a local abrasion of surface (**inoculation**), e.g. erysipelas, syphilis.
2. Via the alimentary tract (**ingestion**), e.g. typhoid fever.
3. Via the respiratory tract, including the nasal mucous membrane and the tonsils (**inhalation**), e.g. tuberculosis, and diseases due to droplet infection.

Modes of spread

Infection is commonly conveyed by the following agencies:
1. Water, milk and food.
2. Direct contact with the patient or articles infected by the patient (fomites), dust, etc.
3. Droplet infection.
4. Insects or other animals.
5. Carriers.

1. Water, milk and food. These are important vehicles of infection. Water, ice or shellfish obtained from a source which is contaminated by sewage are particularly liable to be dangerous. Typhoid fever, cholera and dysentery may be spread in this manner. Milk and food may carry infection if they are obtained from a diseased animal—e.g. milk from a tuberculous cow may contain large numbers of tubercle bacilli. Food may also be contaminated by flies or by human beings, who are carrying disease germs, and who handle it during the course of its preparation. Typhoid fever is sometimes conveyed in this way. Some cases of poliomyelitis and infective hepatitis are also due to water-borne infection.

2. Direct contact. A susceptible individual who comes into direct contact with a patient suffering from an infectious disease, or with a third person who has been in contact with the patient, or with articles used by the infected person, is very liable to contract the disease. Germs also accumulate in dust which may be spread through the air. Fortunately, however, many germs in dust or air are rapidly killed by the action of sunlight.

Fomites may be defined as any objects or substances which harbour and transmit infectious particles.

3. Droplet infection. Every time an individual breathes air out of the lungs, that air contains a large number of minute droplets of moisture, which remain in the atmosphere immediately surrounding the individual for some time and then gradually evaporate. When that person speaks the droplets are projected a greater distance from the body—possibly as much as a yard. If coughing or sneezing should occur they are conveyed a distance of several yards.

It is clear, therefore, that if a patient harbours disease germs in the mouth, nose, throat or other air passages, they will be present in the droplets of moisture expelled by that person, and any susceptible individual within the range of the expelled droplets is liable to acquire the infection. Hence the importance of wearing masks in the operating theatre and when attending to maternity cases and young children. Also when the droplets fall to the floor and evaporate their contained organisms may accumulate in dust.

The diseases commonly transmitted in this way include:

the common cold	mumps
scarlet fever	influenza
measles	meningococcal meningitis
rubella	poliomyelitis.
whooping-cough	

4. Insects and other animals. The part which flies may play in the spread of disease by infecting food has already been pointed out. Some organisms are actually carried by insects in their bodies and conveyed from one individual to another, by means of their bite. Malaria is carried by the mosquito, plague by rat fleas and typhus by lice. Pets and other animals may occasionally convey disease, e.g. ornithosis (birds) and toxocariasis (dogs and cats).

5. Carriers. Certain individuals harbour in their bodies virulent pathogenic organisms which are capable of producing disease in other persons. These individuals are called disease carriers. They do not suffer from the disease themselves, either because they have natural immunity to the particular organisms concerned, or because they have acquired immunity as a result of previous infection. Typhoid fever, diphtheria and meningococcal meningitis are frequently conveyed in this way.

Harmful staphylococci may be harboured in the nose and on the skin of the perineum.

It is very important that known germ carriers should take no part in the preparation of food to be eaten by other individuals. They should avoid contact with children, and every effort should be made to eradicate the germs from their bodies.

Definitions

Epidemic (from the Greek, upon the people)

A disease occurring in outbreaks and attacking many people simultaneously in a community.

Endemic (Gk., in the people)

A term used to describe a disease which is always present in a community.

Pandemic (Gk., all the people)

A disease which breaks out simultaneously in many countries.

Sporadic (Gk., scattered)

A term used to describe the distribution of a disease in which cases occur singly instead of in groups.

Prevention of infection
(for details, see books on communal health, etc.)

1. Notification of infectious diseases. The medical practitioner is required by law to notify cases of certain infectious diseases to the local District Community Physician (Medical Officer of Health). The Public Health Authorities then take necessary steps to ascertain the source of infection and to ensure proper isolation of the patient and disinfection of infected articles.

2. Isolation. It is essential that cases of infectious disease should be isolated, either in a separate room or in a special hospital, until all risk of infection has passed. In order to prevent the spread of disease, it is sometimes necessary, also, to isolate those who have been in contact with an infectious case.

Disease	Usual incubation Period	Day of eruption	Quarantine Period	Isolation Period
	Days		Days	
Scarlet Fever	2–4	1st or 2nd	Nil	With penicillin, 5 days: otherwise 4 weeks, provided there is no sore throat and no discharge from the nose, ear or any open wound.
Diphtheria	2–4	No rash	Nil	4 to 5 weeks, provided all discharges have ceased and no bacilli can be found in the nose and throat.
Influenza	2–4	No rash	Nil	Until acute symptoms have subsided (3 to 4 days).
Whooping-cough	10–14	No rash	Nil	4 to 5 weeks.
Typhoid Fever	10–14	6th–12th	*	When examination shows the bacilli are absent from the stools and urine—usually about 6 weeks.
Measles	10–14	4th	Nil	7 days from the appearance of the rash.
Small-pox (Variola)	10–14	3rd	18	Until all scabs have separated and all scars healed.
Chicken-pox (Varicella)	14–21	1st	Nil	Ditto.
Rubella	14–21	1st	Nil	5 days.
Mumps	21	No rash	Nil	9 days from onset of swelling.

* Quarantine unnecessary but surveillance of contacts is required for three weeks.

NB. It will be seen from the table that a quarantine period is no longer considered necessary for most infectious diseases.

The length of time sometimes necessary to isolate contacts is called the **period of quarantine** and is slightly greater than the incubation period of the disease.

Disinfection. It may be necessary to disinfect or burn clothes, letters, books, toys, etc. at the end of isolation.

In some diseases (e.g. typhoid and poliomyelitis) the excreta must be chemically disinfected. Lysol, 5%, phenol or a proprietary disinfectant may be used.

4. Immunization of contacts. The use of typhoid vaccine, vaccination against small-pox and the administration of immunoglobulin in preventing measles and rubella, have already been mentioned.

Incubation period. The period of incubation in acute infectious diseases is the time intervening between the entrance of the infecting organism into the body and the first manifestation of the disease in the individual (not necessarily the appearance of a rash). This varies in different maladies, and is related to the rate of multiplication of the germ in the tissues.

For practical purposes it is easy to remember that, of the common fevers, four have a **short incubation period** of 2 to 4 days, viz. scarlet fever, diphtheria, influenza and poliomyelitis; three have a **long incubation period** of up to 21 days, viz. mumps, chicken-pox and rubella, whilst the remainder (measles, whooping-cough, small-pox and typhoid) take 10 to 14 days to develop. In exceptional cases, the figures may be greater or less than those given.

Rashes. A number of the acute infectious diseases are characterized by an eruption on the surface of the body, which is called a rash. These diseases are sometimes referred to as acute **exanthemata** (from a Greek word meaning 'I blossom out'). Rashes are not necessarily the first symptoms of illness.

The following table gives the usual time of appearance of the rash.

Rubella	1st	day of disease
Chicken-pox	1st	,, ,, ,,
Scarlet fever	1st or 2nd	,, ,, ,,
Small-pox	3rd	,, ,, ,,
Measles	4th	,, ,, ,,
Typhus fever	5th	,, ,, ,,
Typhoid fever	6th–12th	,, ,, ,,

The characteristics of each rash will be described with the various diseases (see also p. 467).

Toxaemia. This is the result of toxins, elaborated by bacteria in some local site in the body, gaining access to the circulation and to the tissues.

The symptoms produced depend upon the nature of the toxins. The general effects are fever, vomiting, headache, pains in the limbs and back and sweating. In severe cases the so-called 'typhoid state' may develop (see p. 43). Some toxins have a special affinity for nervous tissues (e.g. diphtheria toxin produces paralysis, tetanus produces spasms). Diphtheria toxin may also damage the heart muscle.

Septicaemia. In this condition the invading organisms spread from the local site of infection and enter the bloodstream where they multiply. The organisms chiefly responsible for septicaemia are streptococci and staphylococci. In cases of typhoid fever, bacteria may be present in the blood from which they may be obtained by blood culture. In the case of virus infections when the organism is present in the blood the term **viraemia** is used.

The local infections which may give rise to septicaemia include tonsillitis, puerperal sepsis, septic abortion, wounds of the subcutaneous tissues of the hands and feet and osteomyelitis.

The symptoms include high remittent temperature associated with rigors, progressive anaemia and enlargement of the spleen. The condition is a very serious one and may prove fatal.

The treatment is the same as that for fever (p. 21). Attention is given to any local condition and one of the antibiotic drugs is administered according to the sensitivity of the organism.

Pyaemia. When septicamia is complicated by the formation of multiple abscesses in various parts of the body, the term pyaemia is used. It is also very serious and the treatment is similar to that of septicaemia. Abscesses are opened as they appear.

Blood culture. If organisms are present in the bloodstream they may be demonstrated in the following way:

Fifteen ml of blood are withdrawn from a vein, with careful aseptic precautions, by means of a dry sterilized syringe. The blood is then injected into 3 bottles containing a suitable sterile culture medium such as broth. These are placed in an incubator and kept at body temperature. One bottle is incubated with oxygen (aerobically), one without oxygen (anaerobically) and one with oxygen plus 5–10% of carbon dioxide. In 2 or 3 days any organisms present multiply and form a growth in the medium, from which they can be obtained and identified.

Blood culture is carried out to confirm the diagnosis:
(*a*) During the first week of typhoid fever.
(*b*) In cases of septicaemia.
(*c*) In cases of bacterial (infective) endocarditis (p. 134).

Typhoid fever

Definition. An acute infectious fever marked clinically by intestinal upset, usually diarrhoea, and rose-coloured spots; running a course of 3 to 5 weeks and ending by lysis. It is accompanied by ulceration of the small intestine and enlargement of the spleen. Typhoid and paratyphoid are known as the **enteric** fevers.

Cause. The disease is due to the typhoid bacillus (*Salmonella typhi*). It is frequent in tropical countries and although it cannot now be regarded as a very common disease in Britain, epidemics do occur from time to time. Any age may be affected, but second attacks are rare.

Mode of infection. The germ may be conveyed by contaminated water or ice, infected food and milk, shellfish from beds which have been contaminated by sewage, and the agency of flies: by direct contact with the excreta, bed linen and other articles coming from an infected patient, and by means of carriers.

Some cases arising in Great Britain occur in holiday-makers returning from abroad. Other outbreaks have resulted from the consumption of tinned foods, such as corned beef, which have been prepared abroad.

The portal of entry into the body is the alimentary tract.

Morbid anatomy and pathology. *First week.* During the first week of the illness there is swelling and inflammation of the Peyer's patches and lymphoid tissue of the small intestine.

Second week. During the second week, sloughs form in the inflamed Peyer's patches.

Third week. In the third week the sloughs separate, leaving ulcers in the bowel wall. The floor of the ulcer is formed, either by the muscular coat of the intestine or, in the deepest ulcers, by the peritoneum—hence their liability to perforate the bowel and allow the intestinal contents to reach the peritoneal cavity, thereby causing peritonitis.

If the ulcer happens to involve a blood vessel in the bowel, severe haemorrhage may occur when the sloughs separate.

Perforation and haemorrhage are the most important and serious complications of typhoid fever.

At the end of the third week the ulcers commence to heal by the formulation of granulation tissue (p. 10), and the process is usually complete by the end of the fifth week.

The toxins formed by the typhoid bacilli produce a profound effect on all the tissues of the body. Prostration is very marked and the heart is weakened.

It is important to remember that the germs are not confined to the intestine. During the early stages of the disease typhoid bacilli are present in the bloodstream (septicaemia) and may settle in almost any organ in the body and cause inflammation. This accounts for the fact that many complications may occur. It also explains why not only the faeces are infectious but also the sputum and urine, for the typhoid bacilli on reaching the lung cause bronchitis or pneumonia and are present in the sputum. Organisms carried to the kidneys by the blood are excreted in the urine.

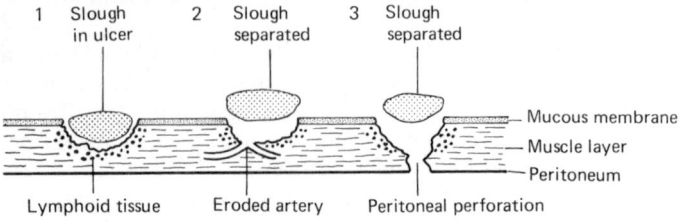

Fig. 7 1. Typhoid ulcer in Peyer's Patch. 2. Erosion of blood vessel, with separation of slough, causing haemorrhage. 3. Perforation of ulcer through peritoneum.

Bacilli may persist in various situations in the body, such as the gallbladder, for many years after the illness, without causing any symptoms. Individuals thus affected are liable to be typhoid carriers.

Symptoms. The incubation period is approximately 14 days (limits 5 days to 4 weeks).

It is convenient to describe the course of the disease in weekly periods, but it must be understood that the stages merge gradually into each other.

First week. The onset of the disease is gradual, the symptoms increasing in intensity until the patient is compelled to take to his bed at the end of 3 to 4 days. The common symptoms are:

1. Headache—persistent and severe.
2. Increasing weakness and languor.
3. Epistaxis (bleeding from the nose).
4. Loss of appetite.
5. Diarrhoea or constipation.

6. Rise of temperature by steps (the so-called staircase type), rising approximately 1·1 °C (2 °F) in the evening and falling 0·5 °C (1 °F) in the morning, and reaching 39·4 °C (103 °F) about the fourth day (Fig. 4).

7. The pulse rate is slightly accelerated, but is slow in proportion to the degree of fever.

8. Increasing deafness.

Second week. There is a further increase in the intensity of the symptoms. The malaise becomes more marked and the exhaustion increases. The temperature remains constantly high and the pulse, although still relatively slow, becomes more rapid towards the end of the week.

SPECIAL POINTS. 1. The abdominal symptoms become more obvious. If diarrhoea is present the stools rapidly assume their characteristic 'pea-soup' appearance and are yellow and offensive. The abdomen is distended and sometimes tender in the right iliac fossa. The tongue is furred and sordes accumulate on the lips and gums. The spleen is enlarged.

2. The **rash** appears between the seventh and twelfth days. The spots occure most frequently on the abdomen and chest, less often on the back and thighs and consist of slightly raised pink or rose-coloured papules, 2 to 4 millimetres in diameter, which fade when pressure is applied to them. They are usually scanty in number and appear in successive crops. Each spot persists for about three days and then fades, leaving a slight brown stain. It is often possible to demonstrate the occurrence of the rash in crops by surrounding all the spots visible at one time by an ink mark, and observing the appearance of fresh spots on succeeding days. In some instances no spots are visible.

Third week. (The period of the dangerous complications—haemorrhage and perforation.)

The patient remains very ill and weak. The temperature becomes remittent, and in favourable cases commences to decline. The pulse is weak and rapid because the heart muscle is weakened by the toxins of the disease, and is unable to contract as forcibly as usual.

SPECIAL POINTS. 1. The abdomen is distended (tympanites).

2. There is congestion of the lungs and bronchitis.

3. The **typhoid state**, which in severe cases may have started to develop in the second week, is present.

The main features of this condition are:

(*a*) Rapid, soft pulse.

(*b*) Dry, brown, tremulous tongue.

(c) The collection of sordes (dried mucus and bacteria) on the lips and gums.

(d) Great muscular prostration, with tremors of the limbs and picking of the bedclothes (carphologia).

(e) A tendency to slip down to the end of the bed and lie curled up.

(f) Profound lethargy or semi-coma, sometimes accompanied by quiet delirium in which the patient mutters incoherently.

(g) Incontinence of faeces and urine. (Occasionally retention of urine occurs.)

This so-called typhoid state, although characteristic of typhoid fever, may occur in other severe forms of fever, such as small-pox or pneumonia, and is evidence of very marked toxaemia.

Fourth week and onwards. Convalescence now commences. The temperature falls to normal by lysis, and may even become subnormal. The general condition and nutrition of the patient improves gradually.

During the period of convalescence (fourth to sixth weeks) **relapses** may occur even after treatment with chloramphenicol. In these there is a repetition of the whole illness, with a rise in temperature and a liability to the occurrence of complications, such as haemorrhage and perforation which may prove fatal.

Complications. It has been pointed out that typhoid fever is associated with septicaemia and that bacilli circulating in the blood may settle in almost any tissue or organ of the body, producing inflammation or abscesses. It is not necessary to discuss all these complications in detail. The most important are:

1. Haemorrhage.
2. Perforation.

1. Haemorrhage from the bowel, due to erosion of a blood vessel by a typhoid ulcer, is present in 7% of cases. It is most likely to occur at the end of the second or during the third week, when the sloughs separate leaving a deep ulcer. The onset is sudden. The patient complains of faintness, which is followed by pallor and symptoms of collapse. There is often a sharp fall in temperature and an increase in pulse rate. These symptoms indicate internal haemorrhage. The stools contain bright blood or may be tarry in character, but their passage is frequently delayed for some hours after haemorrhage has occurred. It is important, therefore, to recognize the initial symptoms.

2. Perforation. Rupture of the ulcer through all coats of the bowel, at the time of the separation of the slough, is the most serious complication of typhoid fever. The contents of the intestine are able to enter the general peritoneal cavity, and, being infected, cause peritonitis. In about one out of every three fatal cases, death is due to perforation of the intestine. The perforation is usually situated in the last two feet of ileum, where the ulceration is always most severe. The condition is seen most frequently in those cases in which diarrhoea and abdominal distension have been excessive, and occurs during the third or fourth weeks of the disease.

The main signs and symptoms of perforation are:

(a) Sudden, severe abdominal pain, usually in the right iliac fossa, with local tenderness and rigidity of the abdominal wall on examination.

(b) Sudden, temporary fall in temperature with an increase in the pulse and respiration rates. (Collapse.)

(c) Rapidly increasing distension of the abdomen.

(d) Frequency of micturition due to irritation of the bladder.

In view of the fact that the chief hope of recovery in these cases is early recognition of the condition and immediate operation in order to close the perforation, it is of very great importance that the nurse should recognize these signs when they occur and report them at once to the doctor.

If the initial signs and symptoms of perforation are overlooked, the pain becomes less severe for a few hours. This latent period is followed by the development of general peritonitis, during which the temperature rises again, the pulse becomes very rapid, the pain increases, vomiting may occur and the patient becomes very ill.

3. Other well-known complications include pneumonia, laryngitis, toxic myocarditis, meningitis, parotitis, abscesses and boils.

Thrombosis of the femoral vein may occur in the convalescent stage of the disease. The vein becomes tender and the leg is swollen and painful. The condition is associated with a rise in temperature.

Diagnosis. A correct diagnosis of typhoid fever is not always possible when the patient is first seen. The condition may be mistaken for pneumonia, septicaemia, bacterial endocarditis, or tuberculosis in various forms including peritonitis and meningitis.

Its recognition is dependent upon the following facts:

1. Symptoms and signs including the character of the temperature, the appearance of spots and enlargement of the spleen, etc.

2. Bacteriological examination. (a) During the first week it is often possible to grow the typhoid bacillus from blood taken from the patient (Blood culture, page 40). This method affords the earliest proof of the disease.

(*b*) Later in the disease the organisms may be obtained from the stools, rectal swab, the urine, and sometimes the sputum. A white cell count shows leucopoenia.

3. Serological examination. Widal test. By this is meant examination of the blood serum of the patient for the presence of antibodies to the typhoid germs. When the typhoid bacilli enter the body they stimulate the tissues to form antibodies in the same manner as other germs, and, after about ten days, the blood of a patient suffering from typhoid fever contains sufficient antibodies to cause typhoid bacilli, when mixed with the patient's serum on a glass slide, to run together in clumps. This is called agglutination.

Agglutination tests are carried out in other diseases, e.g. undulant fever, typhus and glandular fever.

The test becomes positive after the first week of the disease, reaches its maximum about the fourteenth day and remains positive for months or even years after the attack. It also becomes positive in persons who have been inoculated against typhoid fever with TAB.

Prognosis. Typhoid fever is a severe illness and, although it varies in intensity in different epidemics, the mortality may be as high as 15 per cent. Haemorrhage and particularly perforation are responsible for a number of deaths.

Sudden death may occur from heart failure. The outlook in cases with very severe nervous symptoms is bad.

Treatment of typhoid fever

1. PREVENTION
     (*a*) Control of epidemics.
     (*b*) Prophylactic inoculation.
     (*c*) Prevention of direct infection from patients.
2. TREATMENT PROPER
     (*a*) General management.
     (*b*) Diet.
     (*c*) Medicinal treatment.
3. TREATMENT OF COMPLICATIONS
     (*a*) Haemorrhage.
     (*b*) Perforation.
     (*c*) Venous thrombosis, etc.

1. Prevention

(a) Control of epidemics. This is largely a matter for the Public Health Authorities, who endeavour to trace the origin of the infection and to prevent further dissemination of the disease from that source.

(b) Prophylactic inoculation. The use of a vaccine consisting of the following heat-killed bacilli (in 1·0 ml):

Typhoid	1000 million
Paratyphoid A	500 ,,
Paratyphoid B	500 ,,

produces a high degree of immunity lasting for up to 2 years. This immunity may be sufficiently great to prevent the development of the disease or, at any rate, to diminish greatly its severity and death rate.

It is specially important for those nursing typhoid fever in an epidemic and for persons who are going abroad including holidays in certain areas. The first dose of 0·5 ml is followed by 1·0 ml 4 to 6 weeks later but never less than 10 days. A third injection of 1·0 ml should be given between 6 and 12 months after the second. A reaction is liable to occur after each injection but tends to be less severe if the vaccine (specially labelled) is given intracutaneously, in which case the dose is only 0·1 ml.

(The abbreviation TAB Vac. is sometimes used to describe this vaccine.)

(c) Prevention of direct infection from patients. This is essentially a matter of nursing. It is important to remember that the stools, urine, sputum, and pus from abscesses, together with any object which may be contaminated by them, are all highly infectious. Disposable protective gloves should be worn by the nurse.

1. The stools, urine and sputum must be covered with 1 in 20 phenol (carbolic) or lysol for at least 2 hours. Avoid spilling urine. Bedpans must be scalded after use.

2. Linen must be soaked in 1 in 20 phenol (carbolic) for 2 hours and then boiled.

3. All feeding utensils must be marked and kept separate. The patient must have a separate thermometer.

4. The sleeves should always be rolled up when attending to the patient. The nails must be kept short. The hands and arms must be carefully scrubbed with soap and water every time the nurse leaves the patient. Merely dipping the hands in antiseptic lotions is quite useless.

2. Treatment

(a) General management. The patient is kept at absolute rest in bed with one pillow in a warm, well-ventilated room at an even temperature of 15 °C (60 °F). Great care must be taken to keep the sheets smooth on account of the liability to bed-sores. A spongy

rubber mattress should be used. The patient should be turned from one side to the other every 4 hours in order to diminish the liability to congestion of the lungs and bed-sores. (Except after haemorrhage, when the patient must not be moved.) The usual treatment, with spirit and powder, is applied for the care of the skin, and pressure points are watched carefully. For constipation, give enemata on alternate days. On no account must an aperient be given, lest a violent action of the bowels should precipitate the occurrence of perforation or haemorrhage. It may be necessary to catheterize the bladder for retention of urine. A 4-hourly temperature chart should be kept and the intake of fluid and output of urine recorded, together with the number of stools passed.

(b) Diet. 1. It must be remembered that in any severe febrile illness the intestinal juices are diminished in quantity, and the power of the alimentary tract to digest and assimilate food is impaired.

2. Typhoid fever is frequently a long and debilitating disease and sufficient nourishment to maintain the strength of the individual must be administered.

3. Any matter which is solid and undigested by the time it reaches the lower end of the ileum may increase peristalsis, or actually cause an abrasion of the ulcerated areas, thereby predisposing to haemorrhage or perforation.

The diet now allowed in typhoid fever is more liberal than formerly. The essential points are that the food shall be easily digested and in a liquid state by the time it reaches the lower end of the ileum and that it shall not produce an excessive amount of gas resulting in distension of the bowel.

DURING THE FEBRILE PERIOD. Milk is the basis of the diet. For an adult, 3 pints daily are necessary, given diluted in 150 ml (5 oz) feeds every 2 hours. (4-hourly during the night is sufficient if the patient be asleep.) A little tea or coffee may be added to the milk as a flavouring. When curds appear in the stools the milk must be peptonized.

The following additional articles are allowed: Arrowroot, Benger's Food, custard, junket, jellies, eggs, plain or milk chocolate, plain toffee, ice-cream. Sugar or glucose is of great value as it is of high calorific value and is easily digested and absorbed. It may be administered with any of the above or given in lemonade. Fluids, such as plain water, barley water, soda water and lemonade, must be given plentifully, but in small quantities at a time.

In mild cases, mashed potatoes and crustless bread and butter may be given throughout the disease, if the patient desires them. Meat extracts and minced meats are sometimes allowed, and alcohol may be ordered by the doctor.

Diarrhoea calls for stricter dieting than constipation.

At the end of the fourth week, the diet is gradually increased by the addition of pounded fish and, later, minced chicken. A normal diet is generally resumed during the sixth week.

The mouth must be cleaned after each feed with Glycothymolene or weak phenol lotion, etc.

(c) Medical treatment. The treatment at present generally used is to give full doses of chloramphenicol (e.g. 0·5 gram by mouth every 6 hours for 14 days. Co-trimoxazole ('Septrin'), 2 tablets 12-hourly for 10 days, may also be highly effective. Purgatives must be avoided. Individual symptoms sometimes demand treatment. Severe headache may be relieved by cold compresses to the forehead and the administration of aspirin in mixture form. Abdominal distension (tympanites), which is due to the presence of gas in the bowel, is usually caused by excessive fermentation of carbohydrate and milk. It necessitates dilution or peptonization of milk, and diminution in the sugar intake. If this is unsuccessful, albumen water and whey are substituted for milk, and sugar is omitted from the diet. Turpentine enemata relieve distension. Sedatives may be required for delirium and sleeplessness.

Tepid sponging is of some value when the temperature is high and if nervous symptoms are marked. It is contra-indicated in the presence of cardiac weakness, abdominal pain, haemorrhage, peritonitis and venous thrombosis.

3. Treatment of complications

(a) Haemorrhage. The aim of treatment is to allow the blood to clot in the exposed blood vessel. The patient must, therefore, be kept at absolute rest. The bedpan is dispensed with for the time being and the motions passed on to large pads of wool or tow.

Morphine (15 mg, gr $\frac{1}{4}$) is usually injected. An ice-bag may be applied to the lower part of the abdomen and ice is given to suck.

If collapse is very severe the foot of the bed is raised in order to increase the blood supply to the vital centres in the brain.

Blood transfusion is necessary in severe cases.

(b) Perforation. Formerly the treatment was almost invariably surgical, the abdomen being opened and the perforation closed by sutures. However, in view of the high surgical mortality, medical treatment with gastric suction, intravenous fluids (including blood) and antibiotics to combat peritonitis is now preferentially employed.

(c) Venous thrombosis. The patient is kept at rest in bed, and cotton-wool is wrapped round the limb which is kept elevated on pillows or some other suitable inclined plane. Anticoagulants such as heparin or 'Dindevan' might be used, but are dangerous except in the late convalescent stage owing to the risk of haemorrhage from the bowel, which would be difficult to stop if these drugs had been given.

4. Carriers

Carriers may often be cleared of infection by a long course (e.g. 12 weeks) of ampicillin (given with probenicid) or co-trimoxazole.

In some cases cholecystectomy may be advised, since gallstones may form a reservoir of infection which cannot be penetrated by chemotherapeutic agents.

Paratyphoid fever

There are two germs, resembling the typhoid bacillus, but which can be distinguished from it and each other by bacteriological methods.

They are responsible for the conditions known as paratyphoid A and paratyphoid B. These diseases resemble typhoid fever in every way and a separate description of them is unnecessary. Generally speaking, they run a milder and shorter course and the incidence of complications is lower. They may be recognized by the Widal test.

In all enteric infections the patient is isolated until bacteriological examination of the stools and urine shows that bacilli are no longer present.

Other enteric infections

Typhoid and paratyphoid bacilli belong to a group of organisms known as the Salmonella. Others of this group, including the *Salmonella typhimurium,* are not infrequently responsible for outbreaks of **food poisoning**, especially those due to duck eggs, cream, etc. Calves and chickens are reservoirs of infection and now account for most cases of human food poisoning. The animals themselves may show no signs of illness. Pigs harbour a particularly dangerous salmonella bacillus which may find its way into pet meat and be a source of human infection if, for example, the pet's dish is washed in the same washing-up bowl as other dishes. The onset is not so acute as that caused by staphylococcal toxins but the main symptoms are headache, nausea and vomiting followed by diarrhoea which is often very severe. The diagnosis is established by stool culture or rectal swab. Apart from the routine treatment of dehydration and the other symptoms, Colistin is useful. The organisms are often insensitive to sulphonamides but may be sensitive to co-trimoxazole (see p. 516).

Scarlet fever (scarlatina)

Definition. An acute infectious fever characterized by a sore throat and a rash which is scarlet in colour.

Cause. The disease is due to the haemolytic streptococcus. It occurs in epidemics especially during the autumn. The commonest age incidence is 2 to 10 years. Infants under a year are rarely affected.

Mode of spread. Direct contact with the patient, droplet infection or by fomites.

Symptoms. The incubation period is 2 to 4 days. The disease is conveniently divided into stages:

1. The stage of onset. The onset is sudden with headache, vomiting, sore throat and pains in the back. The temperature rises and rigors or convulsions may occur. The tongue is coated and the bowels are constipated.

2. The stage of eruption. The **rash** appears within 24 to 36 hours after the onset of the fever. It is seen first on the neck and chest and then spreads over the body. It consists of a general redness of the skin (erythema) associated with minute red elevations (puncta) which can be seen with a magnifying-glass and which impart a sensation of roughness when the hand is passed over the skin. The rash of scarlet fever is therefore described as a **punctate erythema**. It lasts for several days and has usually faded by the end of a week.

The area around the mouth is seen to be exceptionally pale when contrasted with the rest of the face, an appearance referred to as circum-oral pallor.

The throat is inflamed, the tonsils are red and swollen and frequently covered with an exudate.

The tongue is at first coated with a white fur through which the red papillae protrude. This is sometimes described as the 'white strawberry' tongue. In the course of 2 or 3 days the fur peels off, leaving the swollen papillae easily visible. By contrast, this is referred to as the 'red strawberry' or peeled tongue.

The temperature depends on the severity of the disease and is usually between 38·3 and 39·4 °C (101 and 103 °F) during the first 3 days. Except in the severe cases it is normal at the end of a week. The pulse tends to be rapid and is commonly 120–130 per minute.

3. The stage of desquamation. This corresponds with the period of convalescence. After the rash has faded the superficial layers of skin begin to peel off. The process commences on the cheeks as a fine powdering; later it spreads to the trunk and limbs where the dead skin may come off in large strips. It occurs last on the palms of the hands and soles of the feet, which are often not affected for 2 to 3 weeks. The whole process of peeling or desquamation may take from 2 to 6 weeks.

Varieties of the disease. The term **surgical** scarlet fever is sometimes used to indicate those cases in which the germ enters the system during or after a surgical operation such as tonsillectomy, or as a result of injuries or burns. This variety is essentially the same as ordinary scarlet fever.

Complications. Four important complications may occur in scarlet fever. These are inflammation of the middle ear, nephritis, rheumatism and inflammation of glands. They are now less frequent than formerly.

(a) Inflammation of the middle ear (otitis media). It will be remembered that the middle ear communicates with the pharynx by means of the Eustachian tube. In scarlet fever and other conditions in which the throat and naso-pharynx are inflamed infection may spread up this tube to reach the middle ear and there cause suppuration. This may result in:
1. Perforation of the drum, with the discharge of pus into the external auditory meatus (otorrhoea).
2. Spread of the inflammation to the bone of the mastoid process behind the ear. This is known as mastoiditis and is accompanied by pyrexia, pain, tenderness and swelling over the mastoid process.
3. Some degree of permanent deafness.

In some instances the otorrhoea continues for many weeks, and it must be remembered that the pus from the ear contains the germs of scarlet fever and may be infectious for up to 3 months after its onset.

(b) Nephritis. Inflammation of the kidneys ranks with otitis media as the most serious complication of scarlet fever. It is as liable to occur after a mild attack as a severe one. Some albumin may be found in the urine during the stage of eruption, but this must not be confused with nephritis which occurs during the third week of the disease (22nd to 23rd day) when the temperature is normal. With the onset of nephritis the temperature may rise abruptly. Albumin and blood are found in the urine. The eyelids are 'puffy' and there is nausea or vomiting. As a rule, complete recovery takes place in 3 to 6 weeks, but occasionally permanent damage is done to the kidney.

The nephritis of scarlet fever resembles acute nephritis described on p. 331.

(c) Rheumatism. The rheumatism following scarlet fever is similar to that associated with tonsillitis or other streptococcal infection (p. 163). It tends to be milder in character but may be followed by cardiac complications.

The condition consists of pain in one or more joints which often become tender, swollen and inflamed. It usually occurs after the 13th day of the disease.

(d) Inflammation of glands. The glands of the neck are swollen and painful (cervical adenitis) in the early stages of the disease. These glands are involved because they drain the inflamed area of the throat. Cervical adenitis may also occur during the third week, when the glands occasionally suppurate and form an abscess.

Diagnosis. The diagnosis of the disease is made on the symptoms, combined with the appearances seen in the throat and the character of the rash.

Prognosis. The severity of scarlet fever varies in different epidemics, but in recent years the disease has been of a very mild type. The foregoing account describes a moderately severe case untreated with antibiotics.

Treatment

The use of penicillin or one of the other antibiotics has considerably modified the traditional treatment of scarlet fever, for it has been found that by giving appropriate doses for 5 or 6 days not only do haemolytic streptococci disappear from the throat but also that the incidence of complications is reduced to a minimum. It is, therefore, possible to treat many cases at home when isolation conditions are suitable. Uncomplicated cases treated in this way in hospital may be sent home after about a week.

General management. In cases not treated with antibiotics it was customary to keep the patient in bed for 3 weeks with a view to avoiding the onset of nephritis. The urine is tested on alternate days, especially for the presence of albumin. Patients treated with antibiotics should remain in bed only whilst febrile and feeling ill.

Diet. During the febrile stage a fluid diet, including milk, eggs and custard, is usually required and the patient is encouraged to drink fluids. The diet can be increased rapidly as the temperature falls and most patients can take a full diet within a few days. Special dietetic measures are necessary if nephritis occurs.

Other measures. If the nose is sore it should be cleaned carefully, and ointment applied to the nares. For mild cases gargles of glycerin of thymol may be used. In severe cases antiseptic paints and lozenges (e.g. 'Dequadin') may help.

Nephritis. Fluids in limited amounts are given at first. A farinaceous diet is allowed later, but the intake of protein is restricted if the blood urea is elevated. The bowels are kept comfortably open by means of Epsom salts or other suitable aperient. For details of treatment, see p. 333.

Otorrhoea requires constant attention. Pus must not be allowed to collect in the ear and frequent cleansing of the meatus with wool swabs followed by the instillation of glycerin and phenol or other antiseptic drops is necessary. The occurrence of earache should be reported as it is some-times considered advisable to puncture the drum (tympanic membrane) and evacuate the pus before the abscess bursts. This procedure relieves pain and is referred to as paracentesis of the middle ear, or myringotomy. Anti-biotics are useful in this complication of scarlet fever.

Mastoiditis. An operation to drain or remove the inflamed bone is necessary. This operation is called mastoidectomy.

In scarlatinal **rheumatism** the joints may be wrapped in cotton-wool and kept at rest. Methyl salicylate liniment may be applied. Sodium salicylate or aspirin usually controls the pain.

Cervical adenitis is treated by the application of kaolin poultices. If an abscess forms, incision is delayed as long as possible because premature opening is followed by slow healing in this condition.

It is very important to remember that all discharges from the nose, ear, throat or open wounds in scarlet fever are highly infectious, and any material soiled by them, including handkerchiefs, swabs and dressings, must be burnt.

In cases not treated with penicillin the period of isolation is about 4 weeks. The scales of desquamation unless contaminated by dis-charges are not considered to be infectious. In cases of persistent otorrhoea isolation must be carried out for longer periods. **Return cases** of scarlet fever or diphtheria are those which develop the disease after coming into contact with a patient who has recently been discharged from hospital.

Erysipelas see p. 473

This is a contagious skin infection caused by streptococci.

Diphtheria

Definition. An acute infectious disease characterized by local exudate on the mucous membrane of the nose, throat, or larynx. (Greek, diphtheria = membrane.)

Cause. The disease is caused by a bacillus known as the diphtheria or Klebs-Loeffler bacillus (*Corynebacterium diphtheriae*).

Any age may be attacked, but the greatest incidence and highest mortality occurs between 1 and 5 years. Owing to improved hygiene and the widespread use of immunization it has now become an uncommon disease in this country but cases do occur from time to time and it is still seen in many parts of the world hence a full description of the disease is given.

Mode of infection
1. Direct contact and droplet infection.
2. By means of infected objects.
3. By the agency of carriers.

Pathology and morbid anatomy
(a) Local lesion. The bacilli cause the formation of an exudate or membrane consisting of dead cells and fibrin, in the locality in which they are situated.

(b) Toxaemia. The bacilli themselves remain in this situation, but they produce a toxin which is absorbed into the blood. This toxin has a special liability to poison the heart muscle and the nerves, which accounts for occurrence of important complications.

Types of the disease. There are three main clinical varieties of diphtheria, depending on the part affected.
1. Faucial
2. Laryngeal
3. Nasal.

These will be described separately.

1. Faucial diphtheria. After an incubation period of 2 to 4 days the disease commences with general malaise, slight fever, occasional vomiting, swelling of the glands in the neck and sore throat. The temperature rarely rises above 38·4 °C (101 °F) and the sore throat is not severe. Young children may not complain of the throat at all— hence the importance of examining the throats of all sick children. Yellowish-white patches appear on one or both tonsils. This diphtheritic membrane covers either part or the whole of the tonsil, and has a 'wash-leather' appearance. If removed with a swab a bleeding surface remains.

In severe or untreated cases the membrane spreads from the tonsils and may cover the uvula and soft palate. It assumes a dirty grey colour and, in such instances, the illness is very severe. There is evidence of great toxaemia; the colour is poor, the pulse rapid and weak, albuminuria develops and haemorrhages may appear under the skin. The cervical glands may become very swollen, causing a 'bull-neck' appearance.

In ordinary cases, with adequate treatment, the membrane disappears in the course of 2 or 3 days.

The breath has a peculiar foetid odour which some people can recognize very readily.

2. Larygeal diphtheria. This may occur independently or it may be associated with the faucial type. Diphtheritic membrane forms in the larynx and over the vocal cords. The first symptoms, due to involvement of the vocal cords, are hoarseness, combined with a characteristic harsh and noisy cough, described as a 'croupy cough'. Later, inspiration becomes noisy (stridor) since the presence of membrance in the larynx causes obstruction to the entry of air into the lungs. Respiration becomes laboured and all the respiratory muscles come into action. These violent inspiratory efforts cause sucking in of the spaces between the ribs which is called recession.

The symptoms at first occur in attacks or paroxysms and are associated with blueness of the lips and cheeks (cyanosis) and a good deal of restlessness. Later, the dyspnoea becomes continuous and, in severe cases, unless the laryngeal obstruction is relieved, death occurs from suffocation.

3. Nasal diphtheria. In this variety of the disease the exudate is situated on the mucous membrane of the nose. The symptoms are nasal obstruction, blood-stained or mucopurulent nasal discharge from one or both nostrils, and soreness of the nares and upper lip.

Very little diphtheria toxin is absorbed into the blood when the membrane is confined to the nose, consequently constitutional disturbances are not marked and serious complications do not occur but the patient is a dangerous source of infection to others.

4. Other situations. Occasionally the vulva, the conjunctiva or wounds may be infected with diphtheria bacilli.

Haemorrhagic diphtheria. This is fortunately a rare form of the disease, for it is nearly always fatal. The throat is extensively involved and the membrane spreads to the nose, causing much bloodstained nasal discharge. The toxins in this type are especially powerful and injure the capillaries. Blood leaks out into the tissues and produces a haemorrhagic rash under the skin. (Purpura.)

Complications. The important complications of diphtheria follow the faucial type of the disease, and are dependent on the action of diphtheria toxin. In severe cases, they may occur at the end of the first week but, as a rule, they develop between the second and fourth weeks.

(a) Cardiac complications. Diphtheria toxin poisons the heart muscle, but leaves the valves unaffected. (This poisoning of the

heart muscle is a form of acute myocarditis, see p. 111.) In severe cases, therefore, the action of the heart becomes weak, blood pressure falls and heart-block and irregularities of the pulse may occur. Actual heart failure, which may prove fatal, supervenes in some instances, and is associated with vomiting and enlargement of the liver.

(b) Nervous complications. The toxin may also produce degeneration of the nerves of the body in that part of their course which lies outside the brain and spinal cord (peripheral neuritis). The damage to the nerves results in paralysis of the muscles which they supply. The commonest parts affected are the palate, pharynx, eyes and limbs.

If the soft palate is paralysed, it is impossible to shut off the nasal portion from the rest of the pharynx. This produces an alteration in the voice which becomes nasal in character. It can be detected by making the patient say such phrases as 'plum pudding', 'Billy Buttons', and 'kiss the cook', and is similar to that of patients who have a cleft palate. Some difficulty in swallowing usually occurs from associated paralysis of the pharyngeal muscles, and liquid food is regurgitated through the nose.

Paralysis of the eye muscles results in difficulty in reading and the occurrence of squints. Paralysis of the limbs may be of varying degree. Paralysis of the diaphragm causes difficulty in breathing. If the patient recovers from the disease, the paralysis eventually clears up completely.

Diagnosis. The diagnosis of the condition is made on the appearance of the throat and nose, or the characteristic symptoms of laryngeal diphtheria. It may be confirmed by taking a swab of the affected part and growing the organism in the laboratory.

Faucial diphtheria must be distinguished from simple tonsillitis and the tonsillitis due to scarlet fever. Apart from the appearances seen, the other varieties of tonsillitis are usually accompanied by high fever, whereas in diphtheria the temperature is, as a rule, only slightly raised.

Laryngeal diphtheria must be distinguished from simple laryngitis, the laryngitis associated with measles before the rash appears, and laryngeal obstruction from any other cause.

Prognosis. The chances of recovery from diphtheria are almost entirely dependent upon early recognition of the condition. Those cases which are treated with adequate doses of diphtheria antitoxin on the first day of the disease have practically no mortality. In the faucial type, if antitoxin has not been administered by the fourth day, the mortality rises to 10%. Death may occur within the first few days from the severity of the toxaemia or later, in the second or third week, as a result of heart failure the onset of which may be sudden and unexpected. In laryngeal diphtheria the outlook in those cases treated early is also much better.

Treatment

General management. The usual measures concerned with isolation are adopted. The most important point in the nursing of faucial diphtheria is rest, the mildest case being kept in bed, for at least 3 weeks. In all other cases, rest in bed must be absolute for considerably longer. The more severe the attack, or if complications arise, the longer the period of rest which must be enforced. Six weeks to 3 months in bed is often necessary.

The patient must not be allowed to do anything for himself. He is fed and must not lift his head from the pillow in order to drink. The nurse may raise the head a little with her hand, or fluids may be sucked out of a feeder by means of a short piece of glass or rubber tubing. When the bed is made he must be rolled from side to side, and he must be lifted on to a bedpan. It is the nurse's duty to carry out these details and to see that the instructions are obeyed.

The importance of this can be realized if it is understood that the amount of damage done to the heart by toxins in any case of diphtheria cannot be estimated. The patient may look well and feel quite strong, and yet the degree of myocarditis be so severe that any slight strain will cause heart failure or even sudden death.

When it is considered that the danger of cardiac complications has passed, the patient is permitted to feed himself. He must not, however, raise himself from the pillows until permission is given. After sitting up, walking and additional exercise are gradually allowed. During all this time the regularity, rate and strength of the pulse are most carefully observed. Any abnormality may demand further rest and must be reported.

In the acute stages, the mouth needs careful attention. Cleansing is performed by wiping with pieces of soft rag or damp wool swabs which are burnt after use. Nasal discharge is removed in the same way.

Local treatment, such as syringing the throat, generally causes the patient some distress, and gargles, which cannot be given to young children, necessitate more muscular movement than is desirable in a diphtheria patient. Both these measures, therefore, should be avoided unless specially ordered.

On no account must aperients be given unless ordered by the

doctor. Except in mild cases, enemata are given on alternate days or when required during the first few weeks.

The toxin of diphtheria also causes a disturbance of carbohydrate metabolism, and improvement occurs after the administration of glucose, especially in severe cases. This may be given intravenously or by mouth for about 10 days.

Diet. In mild cases, solid food may be allowed from the beginning; in all other cases, a fluid diet, with milk as a basis, is used; this is increased by the addition of eggs, custard and semi-solids until a full diet is reached in the course of 2 to 4 weeks.

The diet and feeding of patients with palatal and pharyngeal paralysis requires special consideration. In order to minimize nasal regurgitation, the milk feeds are thickened with gruel or cornflour. If this is unsuccessful, feeding with a nasal tube must be employed.

Antitoxin. The essential method of treating the disease is by the administration of antitoxin. After its use became general in 1894, the mortality from diphtheria fell steadily from 30% to less than 5% and is now much lower. The antitoxin is obtained from horses which have been immunized by injections of diphtheria toxin (see p. 13).

The serum is concentrated so that it contains a standard amount of antitoxin which is measured in units. It is usually administered subcutaneously into the abdominal wall or intramuscularly into the buttock or the outer side of the thigh. Intravenous injection is sometimes employed in severe cases:

Dosage
10,000 to 100,000 units according to the severity of the disease.

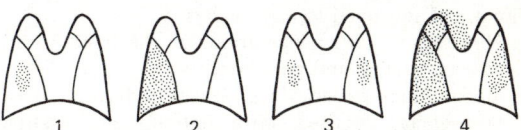

Fig 8. Diagram of the fauces and tonsils illustrating the approximate initial dosage of antitoxin as estimated by the extent of the diphtheritic membrane.

1. Dosage 10,000 units (approx.).   3. Dosage 20,000 units (approx.).
2. Dosage 20,000 units (approx.).   4. Dosage 40,000 to 100,000 units (approx.).

The dose may be repeated in 12 to 24 hours if necessary.

Diphtheria bacilli are sensitive to penicillin which, however, has no effect on the toxaemia. Its use is advisable in severe cases, in addition to antitoxin.

Treatment of complications

Salt restriction and diuretic therapy is required for heart failure.

In palatal paralysis, in addition to special care in feeding, the foot of the bed must be raised in order that saliva and mucus which the patient is unable to cough up or swallow, may drain into the mouth and be removed by swabbing or suction. Diaphragmatic paralysis may require artificial ventilation by means of a mechanical ventilator (p. 537).

Treatment of laryngeal diphtheria. Early administration of antitoxin is frequently sufficient to relieve this condition and may be combined with inhalations of steam. Penicillin is given. This may sometimes prevent the necessity of tracheostomy and even if this should become necessary will help to avoid the development of a secondary pneumonia. If laryngeal obstruction persists or increases, it must be treated in one of the following ways to allow sufficient air to reach the lungs and prevent suffocation.

1. Tracheostomy. 2. Removal of the membrane from the larynx by a suction apparatus.

Tracheostomy. The operation of tracheostomy consists of opening the trachea by an incision in the mid-line of the neck, below the cricoid cartilage, and inserting a tube made either of silver or, preferably, plastic material. The term 'tracheotomy' is also used for this procedure.

The following is a list of the more common conditions requiring tracheostomy:

1. Laryngeal diphtheria.
2. Oedema of the glottis due to inflammation or scalds of the mouth and throat.
3. Tumours or syphilis of the larynx.
4. Cut throat and impacted foreign bodies.
5. As a preliminary to certain operations on the throat.
6. Some cases of tetanus and poliomyelitis.
7. Deeply unconscious patients, e.g. severe barbiturate poisoning, head injury, especially if used with intermittent positive pressure respiration apparatus (p. 535).
8. Some cases of tracheo-bronchitis in infants.
9. In any serious condition in which there is inability to cough up mucous secretion.
10. Severe crush injuries of the chest.

The aim of tracheostomy is to permit an adequate supply of air to reach the lungs, and it is clear, therefore, that the opening must be made below the level of the obstruction. Sometimes the operation can be performed deliberately in the operating theatre; at other times, it has to be done as an emergency in the ward. The latter method will be described. The nurse may have the following important duties to perform in connection with the operation:

1. Preparation of the instruments.
2. Preparation of the patient.
3. Holding the patient's head.
4. Assisting at the operation.
5. After-treatment.

1. INSTRUMENTS REQUIRED. Two scalpels (one narrow-bladed for opening the trachea, the other for incising the skin), two pairs of dissecting forceps, several pairs of artery forceps, small single hook retractors, tracheal dilator, tracheostomy tube and tapes, swabs. A local anaesthetic may be used.

TRACHEOSTOMY TUBES. Each tube consists of four main parts—the outer tube; the inner tube; the pilot or introducer; and the collar, to which tapes are attached, so that they can be tied round the neck of the patient to keep the tube in place.

Tubes are made in various sizes, the number being marked on the collar, and it is important that a complete set should be at hand, in which the inner tubes and pilots all fit their respective outer tubes. The size of the tube used depends on the age of the patient.

Infants sizes 1 to 3 (18–22 French gauge)
Children sizes 4 to 6 (24–28 French gauge)
Adults 7 to 10 (30–40 French gauge)

A special tracheostomy tube with an inflatable rubber cuff is used in connection with a positive pressure artificial ventilator in some conditions including poliomyelitis.

2. PREPARATION OF THE PATIENT. In emergency tracheostomy, the operation is sometimes performed without the use of any form of anaesthesia. It is important to control struggling and the patient is therefore wrapped tightly in a blanket which binds the arms firmly to the sides.

The top of the blanket reaches just below the shoulders and may be secured with a large pin.

The patient is laid on a table with a sand-bag, small pillow, or stuffed stocking if the others are not available, placed under the shoulders. This is done in order to stretch the neck as much as possible.

The head must be held steady and kept absolutely straight, for it is important that the incision should be made directly in the middle line, and any rotation of the head will deflect the trachea slightly to one side.

The assistant at the operation, together with the operator, should wear masks covering the mouth and nose, because infected material may be coughed out violently when the trachea is opened. The assistant must be ready to hand instruments and swabs to the operator immediately he requires them, and must also swab away blood from the field of operation.

A third person, if available, stands at the lower end of the table and holds the patient's limbs.

AFTER-TREATMENT. Immediately after tracheostomy the patient is placed flat in bed and allowed to rest for some minutes in order to recover from the strain of the operation. In the case of a child, spints are placed on the arms in order to prevent his touching the tube.

The nurse must remain in constant attendance and never, under any circumstances, must she let the patient be out of her sight or hearing. She should be provided with a bell in order to summon immediate assistance if necessary.

The secret of nursing a case of tracheostomy is to interfere with the patient as little as possible.

The important duties are:

(a) To wipe away mucus as fast as it appears at the outlet of the tube.

(b) To keep the inner tube clean, by removing and cleansing it as often as is necessary.

(c) To summon assistance at once if an efficient airway is not being maintained.

(d) Only in cases of great emergency, when the airway is blocked and assistance is not forthcoming, to remove the outer tube and insert the tracheal dilator.

(e) Rubber gloves should be worn when attending to a tracheostomy dressing as there is a possible risk of herpetic infection of the fingers.

Mucus is removed from the opening of the tube by swabbing it away with squares of moist gauze.

The inner tube is removed every 3 hours or whenever breathing becomes noisy and the patient is encouraged to cough up as much mucus as possible. When removing the inner tube, the collar of the outer tube is steadied with the thumb and forefinger of the left hand. Great care must be taken that the outer tube is not dislodged from the trachea. The inner tube must be washed well in a solution of sodium bicarbonate 4 g in 0·5 litre (one drachm in a pint) and cleansed inside and out. Any mucus in the outer tube may be removed by wisps of moist wool. The opening of the tube is kept covered by a layer of gauze moistened in boric acid or sodium bicarbonate lotion.

The collar of the outer tube is separated from the wound by placing under it a square 'bib' of sterile lint or gauze which has been cut down the centre in order to encircle the tube.

Failure to maintain an efficient airway is accompanied by urgent dyspnoea and may be due to:

1. Blocking of the inner tube by diphtheritic membrane.

2. Slipping of the tube out of the trachea.

3. Blocking of the trachea below the opening of the tube.

1. Blocking of the inner tube by membrane is easily remedied by removing and cleaning the inner tube.

2. There are 3 common causes for the tube slipping out of the trachea:

(a) The tube is too short.

(b) The tapes have been tied loosely.

(c) The child has pulled on the tapes, or tube. (This should not occur if the arms are properly splinted and the child watched continuously.)

It can be detected by the fact that the tube is obviously displaced and that no air is passing through it. The patient's voice returns to some extent.

Medical aid must be summoned at once and, if not forthcoming, the nurse is justified in cutting the tapes, removing the tube and inserting the dilating forceps into the trachea.

If the condition of the patient is so serious that breathing ceases, artificial respiration must be commenced even though the child appears dead.

3. If the trachea is blocked by membrane below the opening of the tube, it is usually possible to remove the membrane by means of specially curved membrane forceps or by a suction apparatus to which a sterile soft rubber catheter is attached if excess of mucus is causing obstruction.

ADDITIONAL POINTS. Tracheal dilator. If it is found necessary to insert the dilator, it must be held by the blades close to the joint and not by the handles. If the handles are compressed, the dilating portion of the blade opens prematurely and cannot be inserted into the trachea. The tracheal dilator, a spare tube and pilot and a pair of scissors must always remain by the bedside.

A steam kettle may be used in order to loosen the mucus and to humidify the air. Care must be taken that the spout of the kettle is in such a position that it cannot be knocked over by the patient.

Tracheostomy does not, as a rule, interfere with swallowing, but patients should be given fluids for a few days and then semi-solids. Occasionally nasogastric feeding is necessary. Broncho-pneumonia may be a complication.

The tube is removed as soon as possible but this is rarely attempted until 48 hours have elapsed.

In cases in which the cricoid cartilage has been injured at the operation, it may be impossible for the patient to dispense with the tube until special treatment has been instituted. These cases are spoken of as having a retained tube.

N.B.—A temporary emergency opening into the trachea is called a tracheotomy. For a more permanent opening the correct term is tracheostomy (see above). *Complications of tracheostomy* include ulceration of the trachea which may progress to uncontrollable *haemorrhage*, by perforating a large blood vessel, or to *stricture* formation.

Removal of membrane by suction. A special laryngoscope is passed into the larynx, and by means of a semi-soft or metal catheter attached to a suction apparatus, the membrane is removed from the larynx. This is preferable to tracheostomy if the necessary instruments are available.

Immunization (prophylaxis)

Active immunization should be afforded to all children. From a practical point of view, in order to minimize the number of injections, this should be part of a general scheme in which whooping cough and tetanus are included. (See p. 90.)

In spite of the fact that diphtheria is now quite an uncommon disease it is still our duty to emphasize to parents the importance of having all children immunized.

The Schick Test. If a minute dose of diluted diphtheria toxin is injected intradermally into the skin of the forearm and no local reaction occurs, it indicates that the individual has sufficient antibodies in the blood to render them immune to diphtheria. However, this test is not now carried out as a routine before active immunization.

Whooping-cough (Pertussis)

Definition. An acute infectious disease characterized by respiratory catarrh and paroxysms of coughing terminating in a 'whoop'.

Cause. The disease is due to the whooping-cough bacillus, sometimes called after its discoverers, the Bordet-Gengou bacillus (*Bordetella pertussis*). It is most prevalent in winter and spring and frequently occurs in epidemics. Children under the age of 6 are mostly affected but adults occasionally contract the disease, which is spread almost entirely by droplet infection.

Symptoms. The incubation period is approximately 7 to 14 days. The disease may be described in stages.

1. The catarrhal stage. The malady commences as an ordinary attack of upper respiratory catarrh which may be associated with some bronchitis, dry cough and slight fever. This continues for a week to 10 days and is the most infectious period. It is followed by:

2. The paroxysmal stage. Bronchitis persists, the cough becomes more frequent, especially at night, and tends to occur in spasms or paroxysms. In a few days the characteristic whoop develops. If a paroxysm of coughing is carefully observed it will be seen to consist of the following stages:

(i) A long inspiration.

(ii) A series of 10 to 20 short expiratory coughs, occurring rapidly one after the other without an intervening inspiration, until the lungs are almost emptied of air and the child's face is congested and cyanosed. Incontinence may occur.

(iii) A long noisy inspiration. This noisy inspiration or whoop is produced by air being drawn in through the partially closed vocal cords.

Two or three paroxysms may occur in rapid succession and as many as 20 may be observed in 24 hours. They are frequently followed by retching and vomiting of food or mucus which may be bloodstained. They are very disturbing both to the child and its parents. Strong paroxysms, though distressing, do help to expel mucus and diminish the liability to pulmonary collapse and pneumonia.

3. The stage of convalescence. The general condition of the child improves, the temperature remains normal and bronchitis subsides. The paroxysms of coughing become less frequent and less severe. The period of infection lasts for 4 weeks after the onset of the whoop, but the whoop often continues for 6 to 8 weeks or even longer.

Complications. (a) The most serious complication is **broncho-pneumonia**, due to secondary invasion of the lungs by other organisms and developing at the height of the paroxysmal stage. It is associated with an increase in pyrexia and a rapid pulse and respiration rate. The characteristic whoop often disappears with the onset of broncho-pneumonia.

Collapse of part of the lung (atelectasis) may occur and can be detected by x-rays. If allowed to persist this may lead to permanent lung damage, i.e. fibrosis and bronchiectasis.

(b) Nervous complications, including convulsions and various types of paralysis and other forms of brain damage sometimes occur and must always be regarded as serious.

(c) Haemorrhage from the nose, under the conjunctiva, or into the skin is not uncommon.

(d) Sublingual ulcer, which consists in the formation of an ulcer on the under surface of the tongue and is caused by abrasion of the tongue on the lower incisor teeth during paroxysms, is frequent.

(e) The mechanical strain of coughing may produce inguinal or umbilical hernia or prolapse of the rectum.

Sequelae. Chronic chest troubles, such as bronchitis, fibrosis of the lungs and bronchiectasis may follow whooping-cough and very rarely tuberculosis occurs.

Diagnosis. This is difficult during the catarrhal stage but is usually clear when the paroxysms have commenced. A white cell count is of considerable diagnostic value. The white cells generally rise to 20,000 per cubic millimetre, of which about 60% are lympho-cytes. The sedimentation rate is not raised in uncomplicated cases. The organism may sometimes be obtained by means of a post-nasal swab or the 'cough plate' method. The development of a paroxysmal cough followed by vomiting is always a suspicious symptom.

Prognosis. Whooping-cough is a much more serious malady among the children of the poor and in those suffering from malnutrition than among those in comfortable circumstances. Apart from this, age is the most important factor. The mortality is relatively high in infants under 1 year, considerable under the age of 3, and low after 5 years. The disease is highly dangerous among newborn and very young infants so that every effort should be made to keep them away from infection if this happens to occur in other members of the family. Broncho-pneumonia is responsible for most deaths. Repeated convulsions are also serious. The development of gastro-enteritis in a whooping-cough ward is also very dangerous. Immediate segregation of such cases is essential. With antibiotics to control respiratory complications, the death rate has diminished considerably in recent years.

Treatment. The child should be kept away from other children for 4 weeks. While the temperature is raised or the paroxysms are severe, he must be kept in bed in a warm room with free ventilation and abundant fresh air. After the temperature has become normal and the bronchitis has subsided, he is allowed in the open air provided isolation can be maintained.

During paroxysms the child will usually sit up. The head should be inclined forwards and held firmly by the nurse. It is wise to have a receiver at hand in case the paroxysm terminates in vomiting or the expectoration of mucus. It should, however, be kept out of sight until required, as its presence acts as an encouragement for the child to vomit.

Diet. A light, nourishing and easily digested diet must be given. Food should be given frequently and in small quantities, as a large meal will overload the stomach and aggravate the cough. A feed should be given about 10 minutes after a paroxysm which has terminated in vomiting in order that the stomach may digest the food before the next attack occurs. Dry and crumbling food, such as biscuits, which may irritate the pharynx and provoke coughing, should be avoided, but ice-cream is useful.

Drugs. A number of drugs have been used in the treatment of whooping-cough, the commonest being belladonna and phenobarbitone. 'Eumydrin' (atropine methonitrate) may help to diminish the severity and frequency of paroxysms. Linctuses are best avoided as it is undesirable to suppress the cough, but simple expectorant mixtures may be given. Inhalations of oxygen with carbon dioxide sometimes shorten a paroxysm. Tetracycline or chloramphenicol may be used in the treatment of the disease, but cases of agranulocytosis have followed the use of chloramphenicol which is, therefore, generally contra-indicated. As a rule antibiotics are reserved for very young children and cases which develop pneumonia. Severe cases may need an oxygen tent.

Breathing exercises and postural drainage are required if pulmonary collapse occurs.

Immunisation. Vaccines provide a considerable degree of immunity and have reduced the incidence and severity of the disease. They are most conveniently given in the combined diphtheria-tetanus pertussis form (DTP) (p. 64).

Rarely neurological complications appear to result from vaccines, but their incidence is probably not greater than those which have always, but rarely, occurred in the unvaccinated.

Measles (morbilli)

Definition. An acute infectious disease characterized by a rash and catarrh of the air passages.

Cause. The disease is due to a virus known to be present in the secretions of the nose and throat, and, therefore, disseminated by droplet infection. The disease is particularly infectious during the catarrhal stage, before the appearance of the rash. Epidemics are frequent and tend to occur every 2 years usually in late winter and early spring. Although no age is entirely immune, few individuals escape an attack in childhood. The commonest incidence is under 5 years and second attacks are rare.

Symptoms. The incubation period is 10 to 14 days (limits 7 to 21 days).

The disease may be described in stages.

1. The catarrhal stage or *stage of onset.* The onset is abrupt and resembles a severe cold in the head. Pyrexia is moderate (39 °C, 102 °F), cough, sneezing with a watery nasal discharge, redness of the eyes (conjunctivitis) and objection to bright light (photophobia) are present. On the 2nd or 3rd day there is usually some bronchitis, the nasal catarrh and conjunctivitis increase in severity and the child appears very miserable. Hoarseness of the voice, due to laryngitis, is sometimes present. Convulsions may occur in severe attacks.

KOPLIK'S SPOTS are seen during the catarrhal stage. They consist of minute bluish-white spots resembling grains of salt surrounded by an area of redness, which appear on the mucous membrane of the mouth and inner surface of the lips. Their number is variable, but they are most frequent on the mucous membrane opposite the lower molar teeth and can only be seen properly in good daylight. They persist for several days but vanish shortly after the rash appears. They are not found in any other condition and are, therefore, characteristic of measles.

2. Stage of eruption. On the 4th day of the disease there is an increase in the severity of the symptoms. Bronchitis is marked and the eyelids appear puffy and swollen.

RASH. The rash commences on the forehead, temples and behind the ears; it spreads rapidly over the face, trunk and limbs. It consists of slightly raised dusky red spots, called macules, which are at first separate from each other. Later a number of macules may run together, producing a diffuse, blotchy rash on the skin. A rash of this type is called a macular or morbilliform rash. The eruption lasts 3 or 4 days and is followed by staining of the skin and sometimes by fine, powdery desquamation.

The temperature, after rising steadily during the catarrhal stage, reaches its maximum with the appearance of the rash, remains high for a day or two and then, in the absence of complications, subsides to normal by the end of a week.

3. Stage of convalescence. If no complications are present, convalescence is rapid and the child is free from infection 10 days after the appearance of the rash.

Complications. The disease tends to increase susceptibly to infections due to streptococci, pneumococci and *H. influenzae* hence:

(a) Bronchitis and broncho-pneumonia. A certain amount of bronchitis is always present in measles and must be regarded as a symptom rather than a complication. If, however, the bronchitis is very severe the inflammation may spread further into the lungs and develop into broncho-pneumonia (p. 289), a serious complication which may lead to bronchiectasis. The temperature remains high and the respiration rate is greatly increased.

(b) Laryngitis sometimes occurs at the onset of the disease and may be so severe as to necessitate tracheostomy.

(c) Otitis media, following otorrhoea, is not uncommon, and mastoiditis occasionally develops.

(d) Inflammation of the mouth (*stomatitis*) is common.

(e) Encephalomyelitis (rare).

In very debilitated children sloughing of the lips and cheeks may follow *(cancrum oris)*, but this is now very rare.

(f) Severe conjunctivitis and corneal ulcers sometimes occur. The latter may lead to blindness.

(g) Inflammation of the brain (**encephalitis**) is rare but dangerous.

Diagnosis. In the catarrhal stage this is often difficult unless Koplik's spots can be recognized. After the rash has appeared the condition must be distinguished from scarlet fever, rubella and various eruptions caused by drugs.

Prognosis. Measles causes some deaths among young children every year and must be regarded as a serious disease in infants and debilitated children. Broncho-pneumonia is responsible for most of the fatalities but the death rate has diminished greatly during the past 30 years.

Treatment. The patient may be nursed in bed in a well-ventilated room during the first few days, the usual precautions to prevent the spread of infection being taken. The room should be kept warm and a temperature of 18 °C (65 °F) must be maintained. In view of the photophobia, bright light should be excluded, but this must not interfere with adequate ventilation. Bedclothes should be warm but light, and draughts are to be avoided.

A bronchitis kettle is sometimes used and is particularly valuable if laryngitis be severe. Various cough medicines may be ordered. The mouth must be kept clean and nasal discharge removed with a swab. Frequent bathing of the eyes with sodium chloride eye lotion may be followed by the application of an eye ointment to the lids if these are sore. Sulphacetamide or antibiotic drops every 2 hours may be necessary if conjunctivitis is severe.

The patient should remain in bed until the bronchitis has subsided and the temperature has been normal for a few days. A light diet is given at first and gradually increased.

Antibiotics may be used in the prevention and treatment of complications but have no effect on the course of the main disease.

Prophylaxis. A measles vaccine is available and should be given after the age of 8 months. Mild reactions may occur. If vaccination were universally employed major epidemics might well disappear. Serum collected from adult patients who are convalescent from the disease (convalescent serum) or who have suffered from measles in childhood (adult serum) contains antibodies to the germ (see p. 14). If this serum is administered to an individual who has been in contact with measles and who is incubating the disease, it has the power to prevent the development of the malady, or at least to modify its severity. Human Normal Immunoglobulin is generally used

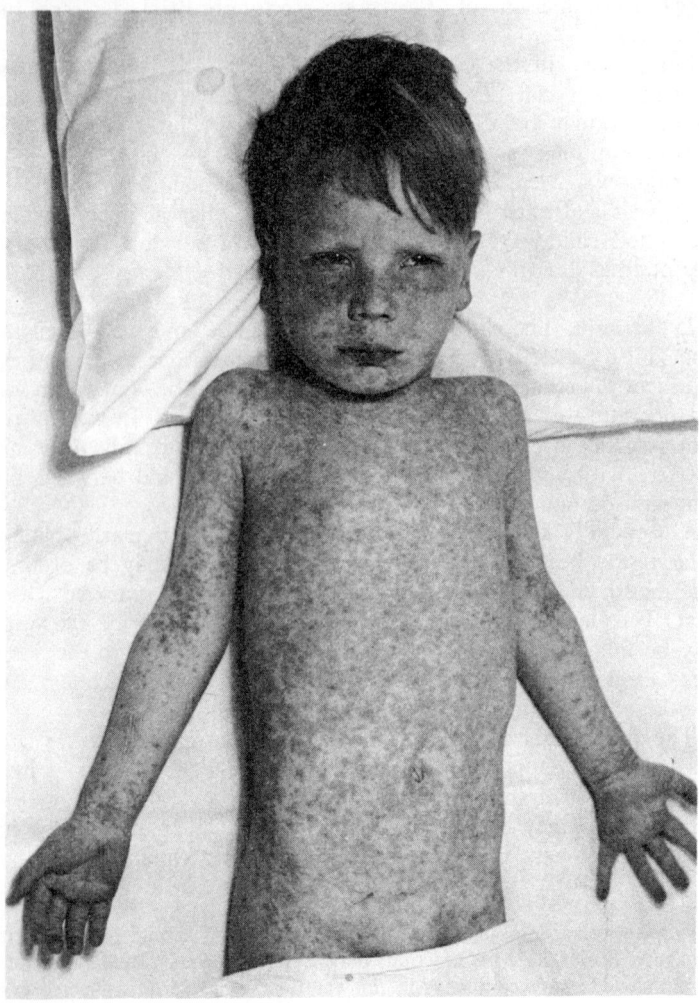

Fig. 9 The rash in measles

instead of adult serum. The dose, given intramuscularly, varies with the age of the patient.

If the immunoglobulin is given early in the incubation period, the disease is prevented (sero-prevention). If given after 5 days of the incubation period have elapsed, the disease is modified, and a mild attack occurs (sero-modification). The immunity conferred by sero-prevention only lasts for a few days and when it has passed off the individual is again liable to contract measles, if re-exposed to the infection. That following sero-modification of the disease is permanent.

In view of the prevalence of measles it is therefore preferable that a patient should acquire permanent immunity by suffering from a modified attack which is unlikely to prove serious, unless some other condition makes postponement essential.

German measles (rubella)

Definition. An acute infectious disease, characterized by a rash and enlargement of the lymphatic glands, usually mild in children and even in adults but dangerous to the fetus during the first 3 or 4 months of pregnancy.

Cause. The causal organism is a virus which is present in the blood (viraemia). The disease tends to occur in epidemics. Any age may be affected although it is uncommon in very young children and second attacks are rare but it should be remembered that a previous history of rubella is not always reliable. It is spread by direct contact and by droplet infection.

Symptoms. The incubation period is 14 to 21 days. There is often mild fever, headache, malaise and slight sore throat at the onset of the condition. The **rash** appears on the first or second day, commencing on the face and then spreading to the trunk and limbs. It consists of numerous rose-pink macules, which are smaller, less raised and lighter in colour than the spots of measles. It lasts one to 3 days and leaves very little staining.

A characteristic feature of the malady is swelling of the **lymphatic glands.** Those most frequently involved are situated in the neck, over the mastoid process and in the occipital region. The enlargement is slight and the glands feel firm and 'shotty'. They are rarely painful and never suppurate. Adults may complain of joint pains. The only important complication, which occurs very rarely, is encephalitis and the malady is generally regarded as a very mild one. If, however, it occurs early in pregnancy, i.e. before the end of the 4th month, there is a very considerable risk that the child will be born with some congenital defect such as cataract, deafness (usually bilateral), mental deficiency, or a cardiac defect. A clinical diagnosis of congenital rubella is confirmed by finding rubella antibody in the child's serum between the age of 6 months and the 4th birthday. Before the age of 6 months, maternal rubella antibody may persist in the child's blood. After the 4th birthday, the presence of rubella antibody may be due to postnatal rubella infection. The antibody is called HI antibody because in the test it inhibits agglutination of blood (haemagglutination-inhibition). The young fetus is also susceptible to other viruses and some chemical agents.

Diagnosis. The rash must be distinguished from that of measles and scarlet fever. The absence of catarrh and Koplik's spots excludes measles. The changes in the throat and tongue characteristic of scarlet fever are absent. The diagnosis may be confirmed by isolation of the virus or by testing the patient's serum, at the onset and again a week later, for HI antibody against rubella virus.

Treatment. It may be necessary to confine the patient to bed for a day or two, if the temperature is raised, but no special nursing is required. Isolation is maintained for a week but in the case of young girls no special steps should be taken to prevent them acquiring the disease, since one attack will usually produce immunity, and will avoid the fetal risks mentioned above.

Immuno-globulin (1·5 g) may be given to pregnant women who have not previously had rubella and who become contacts during the first 4 months of pregnancy but its efficacy cannot be guaranteed. A vaccine is available which, given before, but never during, pregnancy, produces a high degree of immunity. It is ideally administered to girls between their 11th and 14th birthdays.

Should rubella occur during the first 4 months of pregnancy, termination should be considered after the facts have been presented to the patient. Midwives should undergo rubella vaccination so that they do not become hazardous to their patients.

Mumps (epidemic parotitis)

Definition. An acute infectious disease, characterized by swelling of the parotid glands.

Cause. Mumps is due to a virus which can be identified in the laboratory but which has little vitality outside the body, so that infection is rarely carried by fomites. The mode of spread is by droplet infection and by direct contact with the patients. Epidemics occur every few years, and boys between the ages of 5 and 15 are most often affected. Second attacks are very rare.

Symptoms. The average incubation period is between 14 and 21 days. The disease commences with pyrexia (e.g. 38·5 °C, 101 °F), malaise, and pain below and behind the angle of the jaw, causing some stiffness of the neck. Later the parotid gland becomes swollen and tender and swallowing is painful. The swelling may be confined to one side (unilateral), but in many cases the parotid gland of the opposite side is similarly affected at the same time or during the course of the next 5 days. (The condition is then said to be bilateral.) The enlargement of the parotid glands, which have a peculiar elastic,

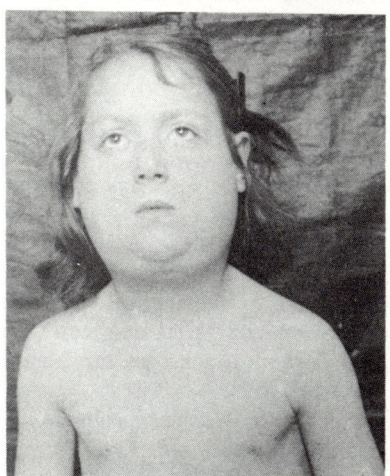

Fig. 10 Mumps, showing swelling
of both parotid glands.

doughy feeling, increases for 2 or 3 days, and then subsides gradually, until the normal appearance is reached by the end of a week or 10 days. Very occasionally the other salivary glands, viz. either the sublingual or submaxillary, are involved. Suppuration is very rare indeed.

Complications. *Orchitis,* or inflammation of one or both testicles, is liable to occur about the 8th day but is rare before puberty. The testicle is swollen and very painful and may remain permanently damaged and atrophied after the disease has subsided. Inflammation of the ovaries, pancreas or breasts sometimes occurs. Meningism and encephalitis are rare.

Diagnosis. This is, as a rule, simple, and the prognosis is almost invariably favourable.

Treatment. Adults may be confined to bed while there are marked constitutional symptoms. A light diet consisting of semi-solids is taken more easily than fluids. Frequent mouth washes are employed. If pain in the glands is severe it may be relieved by applications of glycerin of belladonna; kaolin poultices are comforting. When orchitis occurs, the testicle is wrapped in cotton-wool and supported on a pillow or sand-bag. Cold applications, e.g. lead and opium lotion, may be used and analgesic drugs, such as pethidine, nepenthe or morphine may be needed. Corticosteroids usually hasten the subsidence of testicular pain and tenderness but antibiotics are not indicated.

The patient is isolated for 3 weeks, including one clear week from the subsidence of all swelling.

Small-pox (variola)

Definition. An acute infectious disease characterized by a typical eruption which passes through successive stages.

Cause. The organism causing the disease is a virus which survives for a considerable time outside the body. Small-pox is prevalant in various parts of the world (e.g. India, Africa and the East) and occurs in epidemics which vary greatly in severity. Any age may be affected, but second attacks are rare. The modes of spread are:

(*a*) By direct contact with a patient, probably by droplet infection from the respiratory tract.

(*b*) By means of infected articles.

(*c*) By the agency of a third person who has been in contact with the disease.

Symptoms. The incubation period is 12 to 15 days, therefore, air travel may start epidemics.

1. Stage of onset. The onset is sudden, with 'influenza-like' symptoms, e.g. pyrexia, headache, vomiting and pains in the back which may be severe and persistent. Rigors or convulsions are frequent.

PRODROMAL RASHES: During the first 2 days various atypical rashes may occasionally appear and are particularly likely to affect what used to be called the 'bathing drawers' area. These prodromal or 'warning' rashes may be scarlatiniform or purpuric.

2. Stage of eruption. TEMPERATURE. In a moderately severe attack the temperature rises to 39·5 °C (103 °F) during the stage of invasion but, on the 3rd day, falls to normal with the appearance of the rash. When the rash becomes pustular, about the 8th day, the temperature again rises and remains elevated for 'a week. This is called the 'secondary fever'.

RASH. The typical eruption appears on the 3rd day. It is seen first on the face and then on the chest and back; later the abdomen, arms and legs are involved and finally the hands and feet.

The distribution of the rash is important. When fully developed it is thickest on the face, the forearms and hands, and on the distal portions of the legs; and least marked on the trunk and adjacent parts of the limbs (proximal parts).

The eruption always tends to be particularly abundant in those areas of skin which are subject to pressure or irritation (e.g. by a garter, wrist-watch or the upper part of the boot). Protected areas such as the axilla are avoided. Lesions may also occur on the mucous membrane of the mouth. The rash passes through successive stages but, at any one time, all the lesions have reached the same stage (cf. chicken-pox).

1. *Papules*. (3rd day of disease.) The eruption commences with the appearance of flat pimples, which feel like small lead shot under the skin.

2. *Vesicles*. (6th day of disease.) Clear fluid develops in the papules which, when thus distended, are called vesicles. A small depression is present in the centre of each vesicle which is referred to as umbilication (like the umbilicus).

3. *Pustules*. (8th day of disease.) The fluid in the vesicles becomes turbid and consists of pus.

Such lesions are called pustules, and are surrounded by an area of redness and oedema.

4. *Scabs*. (10th day of disease.) The pustules rupture and pus is discharged. The process of drying up or desiccation, with the formation of crusts or scabs, then commences and continues for about 2 weeks. By this time the scabs fall off, leaving scars which are referred to as pock-marks.

Varieties of the disease. Various types of the disease are seen, and are described in the order of their severity.

1. Modified small-pox. When small-pox happens to occur in a previously vaccinated individual it follows a very mild course and may be difficult to diagnose. The eruption is scanty and ill-developed. Subsequent pitting is unusual. A person, unprotected by vaccination, coming in contact with such a case may, however, develop one of the severe forms of the disease.

2. Discrete small-pox. This is the ordinary type of the disease, which has been described. It is called discrete because all the pocks remain separate. A very mild type (alastrim, variola minor) sometimes occurs.

3. Confluent small-pox. This is a severe variety. Numbers of pocks run together producing extensive lesions. The constitutional symptoms are very marked.

4. Haemorrhagic small-pox. This is the most severe form of all, and is usually fatal. Haemorrhages occur under the skin and into the rash or even before the typical rash appears. Bleeding from the mouth and nose may occur.

Complications. Delirium, with the development of the typhoid state and coma, may occur. Laryngitis, bronchitis and bronchopneumonia are not uncommon. Other complications are boils, inflammation of the eyes and corneal ulcers leading to blindness, and otitis media which may cause permanent deafness. Inflammation of the brain (encephalitis) is occasionally seen.

Diagnosis. The diagnosis in the prodromal stage is often difficult but during an epidemic cases of illness with severe headache and backache, in the absence of an obvious cause, should be regarded with suspicion and, if possible, isolated for 4 days. The presence of a prodromal rash strongly supports the suspicion. When the eruption has appeared, the condition must be distinguished from chicken-pox. This is often very difficult in mild cases and in cases modified by vaccination. (The main distinctions will be pointed out under chickenpox, p. 81.)

Laboratory tests may help and be essential to establish the diagnosis. The virus can be cultivated on special media (in chick embryo and in tissue cultures) from material taken from the lesions and viral antigen can be demonstrated in the fluid from vesicles. An electron microscope also shows the differences between the viruses of small-pox and chicken-pox.

Prognosis. The severity of the disease varies in each epidemic. The mortality is always greatest in young unvaccinated children, while in adults who have been vaccinated the disease runs a milder course and has a lower mortality. The more recent the vaccination, the less severe will be the attack.

Treatment. The treatment of small-pox is almost invariably carried out in special isolation hospitals, situated outside a town in an unpopulated district. Important public health measures are taken on the discovery of a case. Careful search is made for all contacts, who are urged strongly to be vaccinated. In epidemics of a severe type contacts should be isolated for the quarantine period of 14 days.

The general principles employed in the management of a case are to keep the patient in bed, to maintain the room at an even temperature and to ensure abundant ventilation. Bright light should be excluded and all superfluous furniture must be removed. The bedclothes should be light; tepid sponging or warm baths night and morning, regulation of the bowels and administration of a fluid diet are necessary. In severe cases the patient should be nursed on an air or water bed, and, if lung complications are present, should at intervals be turned from side to side. The mouth must be cleansed frequently with weak phenol lotion. The eyes need constant attention in severe cases and should be bathed with sodium chloride eye lotion. Antibiotic eyedrops may be instilled into the conjunctiva and ointment applied to the lids. Care of the eyes will help to avoid serious complications. Antibiotics may be used for septic complications but have no effect on the main disease.

Delirious patients must not be left unattended. A sheet passed loosely over the patient and fastened to each side of the bed is helpful in controlling violence. Sedative drugs such as paraldehyde, barbiturates or morphine may be ordered for this condition.

Local treatment. A very offensive odour accompanies severe cases of the disease. Frequent hot baths or sponging the skin with water to which a little eau de Cologne has been added reduces the odour and helps to relieve itching. Alternatively, the skin lesions may be painted with a solution of potassium permanganate. It is on account of the odour that adequate ventilation is so essential.

The hair should be cut short. The face in the early stages is covered by a lint mask moistened with water or 2% phenol lotion and the hands are encased in lint gloves in order to minimize the effect of scratching. Moist wool, which is subsequently burnt, should be used for wiping away discharges. Irritation in the healing stage may be relieved by application of lead lotion.

The patients are regarded as infectious until all scabs have separated and the sores are completely healed.

Vaccination (small-pox)

Vaccinia is an acute infectious disease affecting cows and characterized by a pustular eruption which is confined to the udder and teats. It is believed that the condition is due to the infection by the virus of small-pox, the virulence of which is so modified by its passage through the body of the cow that only a localized lesion results.

It was found that human beings who contracted cow-pox as the result of milking infected cows remained immune to small-pox. Edward Jenner, in 1780, made use of this fact and commenced the practice of deliberate vaccination with vaccinia as a prevention against small-pox.

Vaccination. The material used for purposes of vaccination is prepared in the following way. A healthy calf or sheep is inoculated with the virus of vaccinia. Vesicles of cow-pox develop on the udder of the animal. The lymph from these vesicles is then collected and mixed with glycerin, which acts as a preservative and kills any other germs which may be present. The final product, after tests have been employed to ensure its sterility, is placed in small plastic tubes and is known as **glycerinated (calf) lymph.**

The usual technique of vaccination is as follows:

1. The site chosen for inoculation is cleaned with soap and water. Antiseptics are not used as they may cause the lymph to become inactive. Vaccination is usually performed on the upper and outer part of the left arm. The thigh is sometimes selected for cosmetic reasons.

2. The lymph is squeezed out of its container on to the skin in one or more places. Originally separate inoculations were made, but now one is generally considered to be sufficient.

3. Multiple pressure technique. Using a triangular pointed (cutting) needle or the flat surface of the point of a scalpel which is held almost parallel with the skin, 15 to 30 applications of firm pressure are made through the drop of lymph. This is just sufficient to roughen the skin without drawing blood. The lymph is allowed to dry for about 5 minutes. The area is then covered with a square of gauze, kept in position by tapes or strapping. Some operators do not use any dressing but dust with an antiseptic powder when the pock develops.

4. An older method is to make a scratch through the lymph about 1·25 cm ($\frac{1}{2}$ in) long.

The following sequence of events takes place at the site of a first or primary inoculation. On the 3rd day a red papule appears, by the 6th day it has become a vesicle which reaches its maximum development on the 8th day and has a central (umbilicated) depression. By the 10th day a pustule is formed, with some surrounding redness and tenderness of the skin. The axillary glands may be painful. Slight fever and general malaise are often present. In the course of 2 or 3 days the pustule dries up leaving a scab which separates at the end of 3 weeks. Re-vaccination usually produces less definite results and such cases should be inspected on the 3rd day.

After-treatment. It is essential to keep the vaccinated area dry, and for this reason it should not be immersed while bathing. Frequent changing of the dressing is undesirable and, provided it remains in place, need not be touched for the first 10 days.

If the arm is painful it may be necessary to obtain rest and support by means of a sling. Care should be taken that the lesion is not accidentally injured.

Maximum distribution of rash

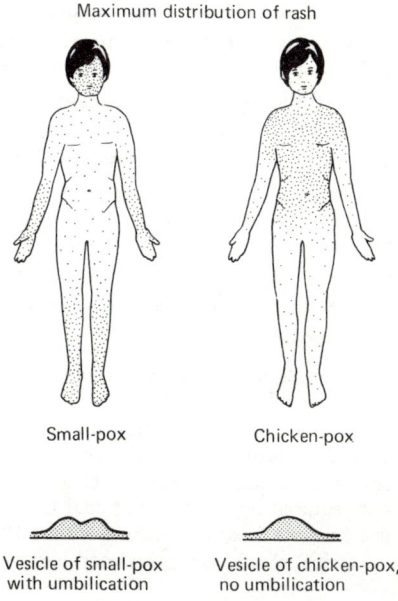

Small-pox   Chicken-pox

Vesicle of small-pox   Vesicle of chicken-pox,
with umbilication   no umbilication

Fig. 11

Complications. (*a*) **Local sepsis**, which should not occur if the subject is in a good state of health and proper cleanliness is observed.

(*b*) Inflammation of the brain, or **post-vaccinal encephalitis** very occasionally develops in children who are vaccinated for the first time between the ages of 3 and 13. This is a fatal condition (mortality 30–40%). It may be possible to treat this with human vaccinia immuno-globulin.

(*c*) *Generalized vaccinia* in which lesions spread extensively over the body. This is very rare but can prove fatal.

The law no longer demands that vaccination shall be performed on infants before the age of 6 months nor is it recommended as a routine measure. In view of the possibility of post-vaccinal encephal-itis in older children it is, however, advisable for vaccination to be carried out between the ages of 1 and 2 years.

The immunity conferred by vaccination lasts about 3 years but revaccination should be performed at intervals of 1 year in individuals who are likely to come in contact with the disease. A lesser degree of immunity may persist for about 7 years. Recent successful vaccina-tion produces complete immunity to small-pox, which develops in 9 days from the time of inoculation. The incubation period of small-pox is approximately 14 days. It follows, therefore, that an individual vaccinated within 3 or 4 days of exposure to small-pox will obtain some degree of protection provided the vaccination 'takes.' In view of possible genetic and other effects, routine vaccination should be avoided during the first 3 months of pregnancy and, unless essential, in any stage of pregnancy. It should not be done in cases of infantile eczema, during steroid administration or in any intercurrent illness.

A new drug, 'Marboran' (methisazone), has given promising results in preventing small-pox when given to contacts during an epidemic but it is liable to have some toxic effects. It has no part in the treat-ment of established disease.

In view of certain international travel requirements the following should be noted:

1. Small-pox vaccination within 3 years may be required. Primary vaccination is best performed during the 2nd year of life. Re-vaccina-tion should then be carried out during school life and subsequently every 3 years if required by the International Certificate.
2. For certain areas yellow fever inoculation within 10 years.
3. Yellow fever vaccine should be given not less than 5 days before small-pox vaccine.
4. If primary small-pox vaccination has been done, 3 weeks must elapse before yellow fever vaccine is given.

Chicken-pox (varicella)

Definition. An acute infectious disease characterized by a vesicular eruption appearing in successive crops.

Cause. The disease is due to a virus and is highly infectious. A connection exists between chicken-pox and a condition which is more liable to affect adults, known as shingles or herpes zoster (page 480). Both are due to the same virus.

Any age may be affected, but the disease is most frequent in children under the age of 10. Second attacks are rare. The mode of spread is by direct contact or by contact with infected articles.

Symptoms. The incubation period is about 15 days and the appearance of the eruption is the first sign of the disease. The constitutional disturbances are very slight and include mild pyrexia and headache.

Rash. The eruption consists of typical 'tear drop' vesicles containing clear fluid which appear first on the trunk and later are seen on the scalp, face and limbs but may also appear on mucous membranes. Within 48 hours the vesicles have become pustules which rupture and dry up to form scabs. In some cases small ulcers develop under the scabs, but as a rule separation and healing takes place in a few days.

The spots may be scanty or very numerous. Their distribution on the body is of importance. In chicken-pox the maximum number of spots is on the trunk (proximal parts), whereas in small-pox they are thickest on the distal parts.

In addition, the rash appears in successive crops on different days which leads to the presence at the same time on a given area of

Differential diagnosis between small-pox and chicken-pox

	Small-pox	Chicken-pox
General symptoms	May be severe, with pyrexia, bachache, etc., for 3 days before appearance of eruption.	Mild. Appear at same time as rash
Eruption	3rd day of illness.	1st day.
Type	Papules before vesicles. Deep, often 'shotty'.	Vesicles from start. Superficial.
	Umbilication of vesicles.	No umbilication.
Shape	Circular.	May be oval.
Appearance	All spots at same stage of development	Successive crops, therefore all stages present at the same time.
	Pustules appear on the 8th day.	Pustules on second day.
Distribution	Maximum on distal parts, not in axillae or groins.	Maximum on trunk, present in axillae.

skin, of lesions, in all stages of development (e.g. vesicles, pustules and scabs). Small vesicles are sometimes seen in the mouth. Umbilication of the vesicles does not occur. Complications are rare.

Diagnosis. The chief difficulty arises in connection with small-pox. The main points of difference are given in the table above.

Prognosis. As a rule the disease is a very mild one, and serious complications rarely occur although occasionally the lesions become infected or gangrenous. Rarely, adults develop pneumonia.

Treatment. Isolation must be maintained until all scabs have separated and the skin healed, usually a period of three weeks. Infants must be prevented from scratching the lesions, if necessary by splinting the arms. Itching may be allayed by bathing with calamine lotion or dusting with a powder of starch and zinc oxide. A mild sedative and anti-histamine drugs may be desirable. A light diet is required during the eruptive period.

Influenza

Definition. An acute infectious disease affecting mainly the respiratory system, which tends to occur in epidemics, usually during the winter months, which may spread widely from country to country.

Cause. The organism causing the disease is a virus of which there are several different strains. (Basic types are A, B and C. A types cause the most serious epidemics.) Secondary organisms, such as the influenza bacillus (*Haemophilus influenzae*), streptococci or staphylococci may also play a part in producing complications. It is common practice for any severe cold associated with constitutional symptoms to be called influenza but this is not strictly correct. True influenza occurs in epidemics which may be very extensive. In some epidemics the disease is mild in character while in others it is very severe, depending on the strain of virus present. No age is immune, and one attack affords no protection against subsequent infection. The mode of spread is probably by means of droplet infection.

Symptoms. The incubation period is 2 to 4 days, and the onset is striking in its abruptness. The symptoms are very variable and on this account it is usual to describe 3 types of the disease. As a rule, one type predominates in an epidemic.

The febrile type. In this variety the main features are severe headache, pains in the back and limbs, marked prostration and pyrexia lasting about 4 days. There may also be a cold in the head and slight soreness of the throat.

The respiratory type. After 2 or 3 days of the symptoms just described, the catarrhal process becomes more developed with definite involvement of the larynx, trachea and bronchi.

The bronchitis may be marked and is associated with severe cough and expectoration. Pleurisy or pneumonia sometimes develop and it is the latter condition which is responsible for the majority of deaths in a serious epidemic.

The gastro-intestinal type. Less commonly, abdominal symptoms with diarrhoea and vomiting develop.

Complications. The most serious complication is the development of pneumonia. In all varieties of the disease nervous symptoms, including restlessness and delirium or even meningitis, may be present. Acute myocarditis sometimes occurs and may lead to heart failure.

As a rule, the temperature subsides in the course of a week, but in some instances it may be prolonged. There is a marked tendency for prolonged nervous depression to follow the condition which, in some instances, is sufficiently intense to render the patient suicidal.

Treatment. Apart from the possible use of amantadine in A_2 influenza, this is symptomatic. The patient should remain in bed and isolation maintained until the temperature has been normal for several days and the lungs are clear. Adequate ventilation is essential. Copious fluids are given in the febrile stages and a light nourishing diet during convalescence.

The bowels should be kept open and drugs such as aspirin and paracetamol ('Panadol') are useful.

Any marked symptoms, such as headache, insomnia and cough, or complications such as broncho-pneumonia, will require special treatment as they arise.

The effects of sulphonamides, co-trimoxazole ('Septrin'), penicillin and other antibiotics are variable, but they are used in the treatment of pneumonia due to secondary infection.

The importance of retiring to bed at the onset of symptoms, especially when an epidemic is prevalent, and remaining there until the temperature has been normal for at least 48 hours, cannot be over-emphasized.

A suitable vaccine given in the autumn may afford some degree of protection and is specially desirable for the elderly and in patients already suffering from chronic respiratory or cardiac disease, but should be avoided in allergic subjects, especially those sensitive to eggs.

Malaria

Malaria is a disease caused by a parasite which is transmitted to man by the bite of a mosquito. It is common in tropical countries and in most of the cases seen in England the disease has been acquired abroad.

The malarial parasite (*Plasmodium*) is a protozoal organism, larger than bacteria, which is present in the salivary glands of certain mosquitoes (*Anopheles*). When an infected mosquito bites an individual in order to suck blood, saliva, containing parasites, is injected at the same time. Each parasite gains entrance to a red blood corpuscle where it multiplies (erythrocyte cycle, schizogony) and, when a new generation is fully formed, the young parasites are discharged into the bloodstream, and in turn attack more red cells. This process is repeated indefinitely. The degenerated red cells are finally destroyed by the spleen. It follows, therefore, that anaemia develops and the spleen becomes enlarged. Except in malignant tertian malaria, the parasites also undergo development in the liver (exo-erythrocytic cycle). This reservoir of infection renews the erythrocyte cycle when that dies out either naturally or as the result of treatment. Acute attacks of malaria are due to the erythrocyte cycle and relapses are due to the exo-erythrocytic cycle. Each cycle is vulnerable to different drugs and both cycles must be attacked in order to eradicate the infection.

The characteristic and important symptom of the disease is the occurrence of rigors at regular intervals of 48 or 72 hours, depending on the variety of parasite present. The rigors of malaria are identical with those occurring in any other condition, and their description and treatment is the same (see p. 22).

Quinine will quickly control an acute attack of malaria but the drug of choice is chloroquine. In malignant tertian malaria, in which there is no exo-erythrocytic cycle, chloroquine alone is adequate. In benign tertian malaria, and in other varieties of malaria infection, a second drug is required to eradicate the parasites in the liver. Primaquine is usually preferred for this purpose.

Drugs used for prophylaxis include proguanil ('Paludrine'), chloroquine ('Nivaquine') and pyrimethamine ('Daraprim'). In some areas the parasites are resistant to one or more of these drugs; local knowledge is therefore necessary before the best drug for prophylaxis can be chosen.

Dysentery

This is a disease conveyed by infected food and water, by carriers who pass the organism in their stools, by flies, and also by those who are attending to patients suffering from the condition. It is common in the tropics but may be seen in various forms in this country. The main symptom is frequency of the stools which contain blood and mucus. This is due to ulceration of the intestine. There are two distinct types—one caused by the dysentery bacillus (bacillary dysentery); the other due to an amoeba (amoebic dysentery).

Bacillary dysentery

The various forms of bacillary dysentery are classified according to the organism found on bacteriological examination, viz. the Flexner, Shiga or Sonne bacilli.

The symptoms vary in severity with the virulence of the organism, but are usually most marked in the Shiga type. They are diarrhoea with the passage of blood and mucus in the stools, which are sometimes as frequent as 20 in 24 hours. The temperature is usually raised and vomiting may be present. Sometimes there is abdominal pain and often severe straining at stool (tenesmus). If the attack is a severe one the tongue will become dry and furred and the loss of fluid from the body will cause marked dehydration with sunken eyes, depressed fontanelle in the case of infants, and diminished urinary output.

Outbreaks of **Sonne dysentery**, in particular, are not infrequent. Both adults and children may be affected. In infants the condition may resemble gastro-enteritis, but the presence of blood and mucus in the stools is suspicious. The diagnosis is confirmed by bacteriological examination of the stool or a rectal swab.

The treatment to some extent depends on the severity of the case. Strict isolation with disinfection of bed linen and stools is important. A gown should be worn when attending to the patient and handwashing most carefully carried out.

In the acute stages a fluid diet is given which includes water, albumin-water, barley-water, meat-juice and clear soups. Milk is often best avoided at first. Later a low-residue diet is gradually introduced.

Intravenous glucose and saline or subcutaneous saline with hyalase are employed for dehydration.

Stool cultures must be tested to determine the sensitivity of the organism to various drugs. Most strains of the Sonne bacillus found in Britain are resistant to sulphonamides. Against sensitive organisms, either 'non-absorbable' sulphonamides (e.g. sulphaguanidine 10–20 g daily) or sulphadimidine 1 g 6-hourly may be given for 5 days. Effective alternatives are ampicillin, streptomycin, neomycin and nalidixic acid ('Negram'). Resistance to tetracycline is common.

Antidysentery serum can be given in severe cases of Shiga infection. Warmth, starch and opium enemata and morphine suppositories may be required for tenesmus and abdominal pain.

Chronic or relapsing cases sometimes occur. In addition to chemotherapy, a high-calorie, high-vitamin, low-residue diet is then required.

Amoebic dysentery is due to a single-celled organism or protozoon known as the *Entamoeba histolytica*, which has the power of forming itself into small cysts. In addition to causing ulceration of the intestine, the organisms sometimes pass to other structures, such as the liver, where they form abscesses. It is spread by the ingestion of contaminated water or vegetables. The main drugs used in treatment are **emetine**, metronidazole ('Flagyl') and diloxanide ('Furamide'). In addition, symptomatic treatment is required. Abscesses are aspirated. Chloroquine may be used when amoebic hepatitis is present.

Food poisoning. See p. 233.

Tetanus (lockjaw)

This is an acute infection characterized by muscular spasms. It is due to the toxin of a bacillus (*Clostridium tetani*) which itself remains at the site of an entrance wound. The bacillus and its spores, both of which grow in the absence of oxygen, is found in soil and in animal faeces. The toxin probably enters the central nervous system by travelling up the peripheral nerves and having reached the central nervous system becomes fixed in the nerve cells.

The incubation period varies from a few days to 2 weeks or more. The earlier the symptoms occur the more serious does the condition become. Under 10 days most cases may be described as severe and often fatal. Over 14 days many cases are relatively mild.

The initial symptom is usually stiffness of the jaw (trismus) and is followed by spasm of the facial muscles and general stiffness of abdominal, neck and back muscles. Later, painful convulsions, often producing opisthotonos (p. 372) may develop and may be initiated by noise or shaking of the bed etc. Difficulty in swallowing may occur and the spasms may involve the larynx and glottis causing cyanosis and asphyxia which may prove fatal.

Prevention. Active immunization with tetanus toxoid affords protection for some years and should be universally adopted with booster doses at intervals of 5 to 10 years.

Treatment. The earlier treatment is commenced the better even in those cases which appear to be relatively mild. It is usual to commence tetanus antitoxin with a trial dose of 0·1 ml subcutaneously and, if there is no untoward reaction within half an hour, to give 50,000 to 100,000 Units intramuscularly. Serum sickness and serious anaphylactic shock may occur in sensitive individuals so that adrenaline should be available when the injection is given. Human tetanus immuno-globulin is preferable if it is available.

Penicillin, 1 mega-unit, is given by intramuscular (IM) injection twice daily for 5 days to destroy organisms which could produce more toxin. Surgical excision or opening of the wound may be necessary. Dead tissue and foreign bodies must be removed.

Muscle spasms and convulsions may be treated by IM injection of chlorpromazine ('Largactil'), 50 to 100 mg every 4 to 6 hours. If this proves inadequate, muscle relaxants (curarine or gallamine) are used together with tracheostomy and mechanical ventilation via a cuffed tube. The patient is fed with a naso-gastric tube. Hyperpyrexia is treated by exposing the patient, wearing only a loin cloth, to electric fans.

Erysipelas. p. 473
Glandular fever. p. 195
Meningitis. p. 381.

Rabies (Hydrophobia)

Rabies is a virus disease of the central nervous system carried by the saliva in the bite of an infected animal, usually a dog. Occasionally a cat, fox, bat, or very rarely some other carnivorous animal may be responsible.

The incubation period can vary from about 1 month to as long as 6 months (usually 1 to 2 months).

The virus attacks the neurones of the central nervous system and spreads to the spinal cord and brain (an encephalo-myelitis).

The main symptoms are severe muscular spasms, particularly of the throat involving swallowing, hence the name hydrophobia or fear of drinking water. Attempting to drink or swallow food induces the spasms. Death finally ensues from exhaustion and dehydration while consciousness is maintained until paralysis and coma terminate the agony.

Strict quarantine of imported animals has eliminated the acquisition of the disease in Britain.

Dogs can be immunized by a vaccine which is employed on the continent and in quarantine kennels. Humans can also be protected by vaccine if travelling to an area at risk.

If bitten by a suspected animal, the human wound should be carefully cleaned but not cauterized, and a course of vaccine commenced followed by anti-rabies horse serum.

Typhus fever

This is a contagious disease lasting about 14 days, characterized by marked nervous symptoms (delirium) and a rash, now very rare in this country but still endemic abroad. It is conveyed from man to man by the body louse, and must not be confused with typhoid fever. The disease is due to minute organisms (Rickettsia bodies) found in infected lice. Other varieties of typhus are conveyed by ticks and fleas.

After an incubation period of about 12 days, the temperature begins to rise and remains high until it falls by crisis about the 14th day. There is marked prostration, headache is severe, while drowsiness and delirium followed by coma are common during the 2nd week. The rash consists of general mottling of the skin together with purplish spots about the size of a pin's head which become petechial and will not disappear on pressure after 3 days. It appears on the 4th or 5th day, first on the backs of the hands, folds of axillae and front of chest and abdomen.

The diagnosis may be confirmed at the end of the 1st week by the Weil-Felix serum agglutination test. The mortality is high (20%). Bronchopneumonia is a serious complication. Prophylactic vaccines are used. Tetracycline or chloramphenicol may be given.

Plague

A rare infectious disease of high mortality, conveyed by rat fleas and characterized by swellings in the groins and axillae (bubonic plague), or which may affect the lungs (pneumonic plague). It is due to a bacillus, the *Pasteurella pestis*. In addition to the spread by rat fleas, the pneumonic form may be conveyed from man to man by the sputum and by droplet infection. After a century of decline, plague is increasing again in Asia, Africa and Latin America.

The incubation period is 2 to 5 days. Prostration is marked and may be associated with severe giddiness (vertigo), producing a state resembling alcoholic intoxication in the early stages. The spleen and liver may be enlarged. Swelling of the glands appears on the 2nd or 3rd day, those of the inguinal region being most commonly affected and, if the patient survives, progresses to suppuration about the 10th day. Bacilli can be obtained from the glands and sometimes in blood culture. The pneumonic form is very often fatal, usually about the 3rd to 5th day. The treatment consists of careful nursing, local treatment of the buboes with fomentations or kaolin poultices until they are ready for incision, and the injection of serum. Vaccines are used for prophylaxis. Sulphadiazine is of value but the best drugs are streptomycin and tetracycline. Insecticides are used to destroy fleas.

Cholera

This disease is due to a bacillus or vibrio (comma bacillus) and is characterized by violent vomiting, purging, cramps and suppression of urine. The stools are described as being like rice-water. It is conveyed by drinking water, flies, contaminated food and milk and by carriers.

After an incubation period of 3 to 6 days, the disease commences with severe diarrhoea and vomiting which is later followed by the stage of collapse. If the patient survives, a stage of reaction ensues during which the pulse improves, the colour is less cyanotic and corpse-like, and the surface temperature of the body rises.

The complications included pneumonia, nephritis, ulceration of the eyes and gangrene of the toes.

The treatment consists of the immediate intravenous infusion of isotonic saline or Hartmann's solutions, as much as 2 litres being necessary to raise the blood pressure to normal. Isotonic sodium lactate can also be used. Oral fluids follow. When urinary excretion is normal potassium may be added. Antibiotics help to destroy the bacillus and steroids help to overcome shock. Vaccines are used in prophylaxis and produce an immunity lasting up to six months.

Undulant fever (brucellosis)

This is a bacterial disease, common in the Mediterranean countries but occasionally seen in Great Britain. It is due to the *brucella abortus* or *melitensis,* an organism which may be found in cow's and goat's milk and which may also be conveyed by handling animal carcases or hides. The incubation period is about 3 weeks. The symptoms consist of headache, general malaise, drenching sweats, profound weakness, anorexia, gastrointestinal disturbances, muscle and joint pains and a characteristic temperature chart. This shows periods of high fever lasting about 14 days, with a few days' interval of normal temperature. The pulse tends to be slow for the degree of fever. The illness may be a long one, with severe debilitation and weakness.

The diagnosis is confirmed by a rising titre of antibodies detected by serum agglutination tests and blood culture. General symptomatic treatment is required. At least 3 weeks of treatment is given with tetracycline 500 mg 6-hourly and streptomycin 2 g intramuscularly each day or co-trimoxazole may be used.

Preventive measures are the vaccination of calves and the pasteurization or boiling of milk. Besides brucellosis, raw milk may convey the organisms of tuberculosis, Q-fever and salmonella infection.

Hydatid disease

This condition is common in Australia and New Zealand. It is due to a parasite which enters the alimentary tract of man by means of food or water contaminated by faeces containing the eggs (ova) of the *taenia echinococcus,* a tape worm which infests the dog. The egg develops into a small embryo which is carried from the alimentary tract via the portal vein to the liver, where it forms cysts of varying sizes surrounded by a fibrous capsule. These hydatid cysts contain colourless fluid and often form secondary or daughter cysts. Cysts are sometimes found in other organs. The treatment is surgical. The Casoni test (intradermal injection of hydatid fluid) may confirm the diagnosis.

Immunization schedule

There are a number of diseases which can be prevented by immunization. Not only can the individual be protected but also some conditions can be practically eliminated from a community if the practice is sufficiently widespread.

In most instances, the procedures should commence in infancy with subsequent 'booster' stimuli at suitable intervals.

As a rule the first antibody stimulus consists of 3 injections of a vaccine containing diphtheria, tetanus and pertussis antigens (DTP or Triple antigen). Doses of oral poliomyelitis vaccine are usually given at the same time. This course is normally commenced at the age of 6 months. The 2nd dose is given 6 to 8 weeks after the first. The 3rd dose is given 4 to 6 months after the 2nd.

A boosting dose is given at the age of school entry (e.g. 5 years). In the latter instance the pertussis antigen is omitted but poliomyelitis vaccine is included.

Booster doses of tetanus vaccine (not DTP), poliomyelitis, and small-pox vaccine are recommended at school-leaving age (15 to 19).

Primary small-pox vaccination may be desirable between the ages of 1 and 2 years. In countries where the disease is endemic infant vaccination is necessary.

Severe reactions to immunization procedures are rare. They should not be carried out if the child is not in good health or is subject to allergic conditions such as asthma or eczema.

In addition to the vaccines mentioned it may be necessary to administer tuberculosis vaccine (BCG) to infants who are in contact with the disease. This is usually done as soon after birth as possible, and does not necessarily interfere with the routine schedule of immunization. The usual age for BCG vaccination in Mantoux-negative children in UK is between 13 and 14 years.

Other vaccines available which are not necessary in Britain but may be required in travellers and residents abroad, are those against typhoid, small-pox, cholera and yellow fever.

The following is a suggested vaccination schedule:—

Age	Immunization
4–6 months (1st dose)	DTP + Pol/Vac (Oral)
6–8 months (2nd dose)	DTP + Pol/Vac (Oral)
12–16 months (3rd dose)	DTP + Pol/Vac (Oral)
16–24 months	Measles, Small-pox 4–8 weeks later
5 years (school entry)	Tetanus + Diphtheria + Pol/Vac (Oral) Small-pox—if necessary
10–13 years	BCG if necessary. Rubella vaccine (girls)
11–13 years	Tetanus + Pol/Vac (Oral)
15–19 years	Small-pox revaccination if necessary

N.B.—DTP = Diphtheria, Tetanus and Pertussis vaccine.
Pol/Vac (Oral) = Oral Poliomyelitis vaccine.

3 Diseases of the Circulatory System

Introduction. The life of every tissue in the body is dependent upon its receiving an adequate supply of food and oxygen. One of the most important functions of the blood is to convey these necessities and, at the same time, to remove carbon dioxide and waste products formed in the tissues during the process of metabolism. The heart and blood vessels furnish the mechanism by which constant circulation of the blood throughout the body is maintained. The heart acts as a pump, driving blood through the arteries and capillaries, which returns to the heart by way of the veins.

The cardiac output or the volume of blood expelled from each ventricle is approximately 5 litres per minute or 70–80 ml per beat when the heart rate is 72 per minute.

General anatomy. The heart is a hollow muscular organ situated in the thorax behind the sternum and extending outwards to the left for 9 cm ($3\frac{1}{2}$ in). It is divided by a partition (septum) into right and left halves, which do not communicate directly with each other. Each half consists of two chambers, an upper thin-walled atrium and a lower thick-walled ventricle. Venous blood enters the right atrium from the superior and inferior venae cavae, passes through the tricuspid valve to reach the right ventricle, whence it is pumped, via the pulmonary arteries, to the lungs. In passing through the lungs it absorbs oxygen and is collected, as arterial blood, in the pulmonary veins. These veins pass to the left atrium which is separated from the left ventricle by the mitral valve. Contraction of the left ventricle forces blood, past the aortic valve, into the aorta.

From a structural point of view the heart consists of three parts:

The pericardium
The myocardium or heart muscle.
The endocardium.

The **pericardium** is a sac consisting of two layers, the parietal or outer and the visceral or inner, which glide smoothly over each other when the heart contracts.

The **myocardium** or heart muscle is the portion which contracts and acts as the pump. Its integrity is therefore most important if an efficient circulation is to be kept up. A healthy myocardium has enormous reserve power and, when called upon can cope with very considerable athletic demands.

The **endocardium** lines the chambers of the heart and also forms the valves.

The heart muscle receives its blood supply from the coronary arteries which are the first branches to leave the aorta.

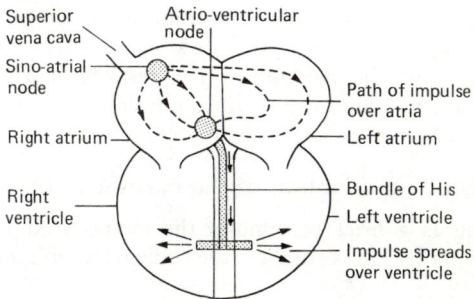

Fig. 12 Diagram illustrating the spread of the impulse for contraction from the sino-atrial node over the atria to reach the atrio-ventricular node, whence it passes down the bundle of His, and is distributed to the ventricles.

General physiology. The function of the heart muscle is to contract rhythmically (about 72 beats per minute at rest), and it is necessary for the chambers to pass on their contained blood in regular sequence. The atria contract first and empty their blood into the ventricles which then contract in their turn. The period of contraction is called systole, the period of rest and relaxation, diastole. This regularity is maintained by electrical impulses which pass along special conducting paths in the heart muscle. It is important that this conducting mechanism be understood if the disorders of cardiac rhythm are to be appreciated.

The impulse starts in a specialized collection of tissue, lying close to the entrance of the superior vena cava into the right atrium, known as the **pace-maker,** or **sino-atrial node.** It then passes, in a wave-like manner, over the atria and is, as it were, collected up at the **atrio-ventricular node.** It then passes down the **atrio-ventricular bundle** of His, which divides into right and left branches in order to convey the impulse to the ventricles. This bundle is situated in the inter-ventricular septum and is the only means by which the impulse can spread from the atria to the ventricles.

Directly after an impulse has been transmitted along the bundle of His, a period of rest is required before another impulse can pass. This period of rest is called the **refractory period**. Any impulse which happens to arrive during the refractory period fails to pass along the bundle of His and, therefore, will not produce a contraction of the ventricles.

The sino-atrial node receives two sets of nerve fibres derived from the autonomic nervous system, impulses from which influence the rate of cardiac action. Those conveyed by the vagus nerve slow the heart rate, while the accelerator impulses from the sympathetic increase the rate of contraction. These nerve fibres arise from the cardiac centres in the medulla. Their respective actions can be altered by drugs in addition to various physiological and pathological conditions.

Methods of examination of the cardiovascular system

The following is a brief account of the methods employed by the physician in order to estimate the efficiency of the heart and circulation.

I. Physical examination of the heart

(a) Inspection and palpation. Notice is taken of any bulging in that part of the thoracic wall overlying the heart which is known as the precordium. The position of the apex beat is ascertained. Normally this is situated in the 5th intercostal space 9 cm ($3\frac{1}{2}$ in) from the middle line.

In certain instances when the valves are narrowed a definite vibration can be felt in addition to the ordinary beat of the heart. This vibration is called a thrill (e.g. in aortic stenosis).

(b) Percussion. The heart is dull to percussion. The area of cardiac dullness indicates the heart's size and position.

(c) Auscultation. When the various valves of the heart close during the process of the heart beat, sounds are produced which can be heard with a stethoscope. The sound produced by the mitral valve is heard best over the apex beat; that produced by the tricuspid valve over the lower end of the sternum. Closure of the aortic valve is heard best in the second right intercostal space, and that of the pulmonary valve in the second left intercostal space. It is for this reason that the stethoscope is placed over these four areas in turn.

Normally two sounds are heard in each area, which resemble the words 'lubb dup'. Damage to the valves will produce alteration of the sounds which, instead of being sharp and clear, are replaced by musical or blowing noises called **murmurs**. If a murmur occurs during contraction of the heart it is referred to as systolic; if during relaxation, as diastolic.

e.g. Systolic murmur = 'lubbsssh dup'.

Diastolic murmur = 'lubb dup ssh'.

When the pericardium is inflamed the two surfaces become roughened and can be heard rubbing against each other. The sound thus produced is called a pericardial rub or pericardial friction sound.

II. Examination of the radial pulse

Contraction of the left ventricle forces blood into the aorta, which, being elastic, expands in order to accommodate the additional amount of blood. This wave of expansion is transmitted all over the arterial system and constitutes the pulse.

It may be felt, and sometimes seen, in the radial artery at the wrist, in the temporal artery in front of and above the ear, in the facial artery over the lower jaw, in the carotid artery in the neck and in the dorsalis pedis artery on the dorsum of the foot. In infants it is most easily felt over the anterior fontanelle. It is customary to examine the radial pulse in all cases.

Accurate examination of the pulse is of great importance both to the doctor and the nurse, for not only may valuable diagnostic information be obtained but also evidence as to the progress of the case.

Examination of the pulse is made so frequently by the nurse that she should be thoroughly familiar with both the theoretical and practical aspects of the subject.

Method of taking the pulse. Two or 3 fingers of the right hand are placed on the radial artery just above the wrist. In examining the pulse of a patient for the first time both radial arteries should be felt simultaneously, and the pulses on each side compared. Differences between the two sides are sometimes caused by aneurysm or tumours in the thorax.

Observations to be made
1. The rate
2. The rhythm
3. The quality

   (*a*) volume; (*b*) tension; (*c*) state of the artery.

1. THE RATE

Normal rates.	Adults at rest	60– 80 beats per minute		
	Infants „ „	100–120	„	„	„
	Children (6–10)	80–100	„	„	„

Increased frequency is called **tachycardia** (p. 106). Exercise may double the frequency of the heart beat, but with cessation of effort the pulse returns to its normal rate in 2 or 3 minutes. Also, as a results of nervous or emotional states, the rate may be increased. Other causes of increased frequency are fever, thyrotoxicosis, tobacco poisoning and some forms of heart disease. Atropine, adrenaline and isoprenaline are drugs which increase the heart rate.

Undue slowness (30–50 per minute) is called **Bradycardia** (p. 106). As age advances the pulse rate normally tends to become slower.

The apex rate. It will be noticed that some extra-systoles may be so small that they fail to produce a beat which can be felt in the radial pulse. Likewise, some of the ventricular contractions in atrial fibrillation fail to produce a pulse beat. In such cases it is clear that the actual rate of the heart beat will be more rapid than the rate of the pulse counted at the wrist. In order to assess this difference in rate or **'pulse deficit'** it is necessary to count and record the respective rates at the apex and the wrist. The apex rate is determined by listening to and counting the heart beats with a stethoscope or by palpation. (Most nurses will have the opportunity of observing the effect of digitalis in decreasing the pulse deficit during the treatment of atrial fibrillation.)

2. RHYTHM.   The normal pulse is regular in rhythm. Any irregularities in the beat of the heart produce corresponding changes in the pulse. The common causes of irregularity of the pulse rhythm are (p. 102):

1. Sinus arrhythmia.
2. Extra-systoles (ectopic beats).
3. Atrial fibrillation.

It will be seen that extra-systoles (premature or ectopic beats) sometimes produce the phenomenon of 'dropped beats'. Atrial fibrillation results in a pulse which is completely irregular in rate, rhythm, and volume, while in sinus arrhythmia there is an increase of frequency during inspiration and a slowing during expiration.

There are three other alterations in the pulse which, though rare, may be mentioned for completeness. (See Fig. 13.)

1. Pulsus bigeminus consists of two beats followed by a pause and is

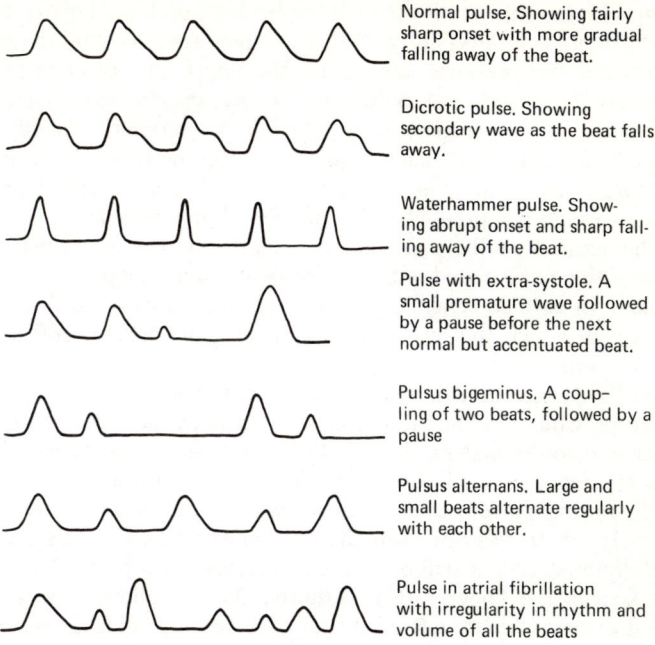

Normal pulse. Showing fairly sharp onset with more gradual falling away of the beat.

Dicrotic pulse. Showing secondary wave as the beat falls away.

Waterhammer pulse. Showing abrupt onset and sharp falling away of the beat.

Pulse with extra-systole. A small premature wave followed by a pause before the next normal but accentuated beat.

Pulsus bigeminus. A coupling of two beats, followed by a pause

Pulsus alternans. Large and small beats alternate regularly with each other.

Pulse in atrial fibrillation with irregularity in rhythm and volume of all the beats

Fig. 13 Diagram illustrating the common types of pulse.

due to a regular series of extra-systoles, each following a normal beat. It occurs, for example, in digitalis poisoning.

2. Pulsus alternans is a serious sign of left ventricular failure in which large and small beats alternate regularly with each other. This can rarely be detected by the finger, but can be demonstrated by the sphygmomanometer.

3. Pulsus paradoxus, in which the pulse disappears during inspiration, is sometimes found in pericardial effusion.

3. THE QUALITY OF THE PULSE. (a) The **volume** must first be considered. When the degree of expansion of the artery is greater than normal the pulse is said to be full. A full pulse is commonly met with in febrile conditions. On the other hand, the expansion may be poor and the pulse difficult to feel. Such a pulse is called a weak or small pulse and is most frequently encountered in conditions of dehydration and blood loss and when the action of the heart is enfeebled by disease, e.g. after severe myocardial infarction.

(b) The **tension** of the pulse may be high or low. This is determined by its compressibility. If three fingers are placed on the radial artery and the pressure applied by the upper and lower fingers is gradually increased, the pulse, as felt by the middle finger, will disappear. With practice, it is possible to estimate roughly the amount of pressure normally required to stop the pulse. If increased pressure is required, it is said to be hard and of high tension; if the pulse is easily compressed, it is soft and of low tension.

The tension of the pulse is dependent upon the blood pressure. In conditions associated with high blood pressure the pulse is of high tension. In cardiac weakness, shock, fainting attacks and Addison's disease, in which the blood pressure is low, the pulse is soft and of low tension.

(c) The **state of the artery**. In health the artery is a soft elastic structure which, when the pulse is stopped by the pressure of the upper and lower fingers, can hardly be felt. In arteriosclerosis lime salts are deposited in its walls and it becomes hard and tortuous.

The normal pulse beat consists of a wave of expansion in the artery which is felt to pass beneath the examining fingers. If this wave is carefully analysed, it will be noticed to consist of 3 parts. The pulse first strikes the finger rather abruptly, this is followed by a brief period during which the tension is at a maximum, and lastly the wave passes away rather more slowly than it arrived. This may be represented diagrammatically. (See Fig. 13.)

In some instances during the third period a small secondary wave may be felt. This is known as the dicrotic pulse and may occur in certain febrile conditions when the tension of the pulse is low, e.g. typhoid fever.

The Waterhammer pulse. This is a remarkable type of pulse occurring in the variety of valvular disease known as aortic regurgitation. It is best felt, not with the finger-tips, but with the palmar surface of the fingers placed across the front of the patient's wrist, his arm being raised above the level of his chest.

This type of pulse beat takes its name from an old-fashioned toy called a 'Waterhammer' which consists of a glass tube half filled with water, from which the air has been exhausted. When it is tilted, the water falls with a peculiar, sharp slap to the other end of the tube.

The waterhammer pulse, unlike the normal pulse, consists of a very abrupt thrust and a rapid falling away of the beat. This shock-like sensation accompanied by the quick recoil of the artery may be felt in the ulnar artery at the same time. Once this condition has been demonstrated to the nurse and she has familiarized herself with the sensation, she should have no difficulty in recognizing the typical pulse of aortic regurgitation.

Patients with a waterhammer pulse have excessive *visible* pulsation of arteries, especially obvious in the neck, and this abnormal visible pulsation is sometimes named after Corrigan, the Dublin physician who first described it.

III. Estimation of the blood pressure

The pressure of blood in the arteries depends on four main factors:

1. The force of the heart beat.
2. Resistance to the blood flow in the peripheral arteries.
3. The elasticity of the arteries.
4. The total amount of circulating blood.

If the force of ventricular contraction is diminished the blood pressure will fall, because the pumping action is weakened.

If the arteries lose their elasticity or become narrowed, the blood pressure may be raised permanently. (See Hypertension p. 143). It may rise temporarily in circumstances of severe emotional and physical stress.

The blood pressure falls in cases of shock and severe haemorrhage.

In a young adult the pressure of blood in the arteries during ventricular systole is sufficient to raise a column of mercury 120 millimetres. As age advances, the blood pressure normally tends to rise and, at the age of 50, a systolic pressure of 140 to 150 millimetres of mercury (mm Hg) is not unusual.

When the blood pressure is below normal the condition is called hypotension. If it is above normal the term hypertension is used (page 143).

The scale of measurement by which blood pressure is estimated is the height, in millimetres, to which a column of mercury is raised when pressure corresponding to that in the arteries is applied to it.

The instrument employed for estimating blood pressure is called a sphygmomanometer. This consists of a rubber cuff which is placed round the arm and which can be inflated by a pump. The interior of the cuff is connected by a rubber tube to a mercury manometer or to a graduated pressure-gauge. When the pressure in the cuff equals the pressure in the artery, the latter is compressed flat and the local circulation is temporarily arrested. The pulse, therefore, disappears from the wrist. The reading on the pressure gauge or manometer, at the moment the pulse disappears, corresponds to the systolic blood pressure. The moment at which the artery becomes completely collapsed can also be determined by listening with a stethoscope over the brachial artery at the bend of the elbow.

The pressure of blood in the arteries is highest at the end of ventricular systole and lowest at the end of diastole. Hence it is customary to record both the systolic and diastolic pressures. The systolic pressure is recorded by inflating the cuff until the pulse has been obliterated at the wrist and all sounds over the brachial artery have disappeared. The pressure is then lowered gradually until distinct beats are heard over the artery. This point registers the systolic pressure. The cuff is then deflated until the loud clear sounds abruptly disappear or give way to dull and muffled sounds synchronous with the heart beat. This is the diastolic pressure. The difference between the systolic and diastolic pressures is called the pulse pressure, e.g.:

$$systolic\ pressure = 120\ mm\ Hg$$
$$diastolic\ pressure = 70\ mm\ Hg$$
$$pulse\ pressure = 50\ mm\ Hg$$

In atrial fibrillation the pulse is irregular in rhythm and force and accurate estimation of the blood pressure becomes impossible as it varies with each beat. Only a rough average can, therefore, be estimated. It may be important to note whether the blood pressure is taken in the sitting or lying down position. This is especially important in patients taking hypotensive drugs.

IV. Response of the heart to exercise

The patient is made to perform exercises such as sitting up and lying down in bed, stepping on and off a chair, or walking up a number of stairs, the exact form depending on the state of the patient. The pulse rate is taken before and after the exercise and the time taken for the rate to return to normal is noted. This test of cardiac efficiency must only be used in patients well enough to tolerate it.

V. Special methods

The size, shape and position of the heart and great vessels can be determined by means of x-ray examination.

An **electrocardiogram** (ECG) is a record of the electrical changes taking place in the heart muscle during the cardiac cycle, and is obtained by connecting the patient to an instrument known as the electrocardiograph. It is of value to the physician in making a diagnosis in certain cases of heart disease (p. 169).

Cardiac catheterization. As a special method of investigation a long catheter can be inserted into one of the veins at the bend of the elbow or in the groin and pushed onwards so that its tip is made to enter the right side of the heart. Its actual position is checked by x-rays. The pressure of blood within the respective chambers can be measured and specimens of blood obtained for analysis. An electrode catheter can be inserted into the right ventricle and used as an artificial pacemaker in cases of heart block.

The left side of the heart can be investigated by introducing a catheter into an artery (brachial or femoral), manoeuvring it into and around the aorta and manipulating it across the aortic valve into the left ventricle. A special coronary artery catheter may similarly be introduced via the brachial or femoral artery. When the catheter tip is lodged in the mouth of a coronary artery the injection of a contrast medium will outline the vessel (coronary arteriogram), revealing irregularities and sites of narrowing.

Angiocardiography. Injection of a radio-opaque substance (70% diodone), using a special x-ray technique, will outline the chambers of the heart and the great vessels.

General consideration of cardiovascular disease

In the first instance the heart must be considered as a pump giving an output of blood under pressure through the arteries and arterioles which, by means of the capillaries, distributes it to all the tissues of the body. Through the walls of the capillaries all the various functions of the blood are carried out. The blood is then returned to the heart by the veins.

It must be remembered, however, that the heart is not a single pump but a double pump supplying both the systemic and pulmonary circulations and that the force of contraction of the left and right ventricles is so balanced that, in health, the output and venous return of both circuits is evenly balanced so that there is no congestion in either of the two systems. In disease, however, disorders may occur in various parts of the heart and circulatory system; this will result in this balance being upset and will affect the blood supply to the body tissues.

It has already been seen that structurally the heart consists of three parts, the pericardium, myocardium and endocardium.

These parts may be involved in disease processes separately or in combination with each other, but it is of the utmost importance to remember that disease either of the pericardium or the endo-cardium may cause an increased strain to fall on the heart muscle.

The myocardium is the structure which performs all the physical work necessary to maintain the circulation of blood and, therefore, all disease of the cardiovascular system must ultimately be regarded from the point of view of their effect upon the myocardium. Valvular disease, it is true, causes an increased strain upon the myocardium, but if the muscle is strong and healthy, it will, for a time, be able to deal with the increased amount of work which it is called upon to perform and no serious symptoms will result.

If, on the other hand, the heart muscle be weak or injured, and, therefore, unable to respond to the increased demands placed upon it, the efficiency of the circulation will be impaired and the train of symptoms known as heart failure will appear.

The main types of heart disease are due to:

1. Congenital abnormalities (congenital heart disease).
2. Acute rheumatism. Patients with chronic rheumatic heart disease may recall attacks of rheumatic fever, with joint pains or may give a history of chorea in childhood.
3. Hypertension (hypertensive heart disease).
4. Disease of the coronary arteries (ischaemic heart disease).
5. Chronic lung disease, e.g. chronic bronchitis and emphysema (pulmonary heart disease or cor pulmonale).
6. Thyrotoxicosis.
7. Syphilis.
8. Other primary disorders of the myocardium often of obscure origin (cardiomyopathy).

Rheumatic heart disease, congenital abnormalities and some cases of thyrotoxicosis account for most of those cases of heart disease which are seen before the age of 40 years. The other conditions are more common in the latter half of life.

All of them may, at some stage of their development, manifest disorders of cardiac rhythm including atrial fibrillation. Likewise, as has already been pointed out, they may ultimately terminate in chronic heart failure when the myocardium can no longer maintain an adequate circulation because of the diminished power of its pumping action.

Disorders of cardiac rhythm

There are three important disorders of cardiac rhythm and one normal variation which can be detected by feeling the pulse in the radial artery or listening to the apex beat. They result from disturbances of the normal automatic rhythm of the cardiac impulse.

1. The premature beat or extra-systole (ectopic beat).
2. Atrial fibrillation (auricular fibrillation).

3. Atrial flutter (auricular flutter).
4. Sinus arrhythmia.

The premature beat or extra-systole (ectopic beat)

Although the normal impulse starts at the sino-atrial node, any part of the heart muscle in the atria or ventricles may, under special circumstances, become abnormally excitable. If this occurs in the atrium, an impulse will spread from the abnormally excitable spot and cause the atrium to contract. The impulse then reaches the atrio-ventricular node, passes along the bundle of His and causes ventricular contraction. The fact that this excitable area is not so far away from the bundle of His as the sino-atrial node means that the abnormal impulse has a shorter distance to travel than the normal one and, therefore, arrives first.

The ventricle responds to the abnormal impulse and contracts. This contraction therefore occurs earlier than it would have done, had the ventricle waited for the normal impulse from the sino-atrial node.

It follows from this that the two beats in rapid succession will be felt in the radial pulse. The second beat will be smaller in volume than the first because the ventricle has contracted before it has had time to fill completely and, therefore, has expelled a smaller quantity of blood into the aorta.

The next point to consider is, what happens to the normal impulse? The normal impulse, starting from the pace-maker, spreads over the atrium and reaches the bundle of His immediately after the abnormal impulse. The bundle, having just conveyed an impulse, is in the refractory state and cannot function. The normal impulse is stopped and fails to produce a ventricular contraction. There is, therefore, no further ventricular beat until the next impulse arrives from the pace-maker. This results in an abnormally long pause in the radial pulse between the extra-systole and the next normal best.

The sequence of events, as felt in the radial pulse, will be: a normal beat, quickly followed by a premature extra-systolic beat of small volume, a long pause and, lastly, a normal beat.

The extra-systole may be so small that it fails to produce a beat at the wrist. What is then felt, is a normal beat, an abnormally long pause, then another normal beat. This is why the condition is sometimes referred to as a 'dropped beat'.

Extra-systoles are common, and are not necessarily a dangerous symptom.

(a) Minor causes include dyspepsia, excessive smoking, excessive tea or coffee consumption and anxiety states.

(b) Among major or more serious causes are thyrotoxicosis, digitalis overdosage and acute myocardial damage in rheumatic fever and coronary thrombosis.

Not infrequently patients are conscious of extra-systoles. They feel the heart missing a beat, or else, a fluttering sensation in the cardiac region. It is important, therefore, for them to be reassured that the condition is not, in itself, dangerous but if troublesome a tranquillizer may help.

Atrial fibrillation (auricular fibrillation)

In certain cases when the muscle of the atrium (auricle) is damaged or has been subjected to prolonged strain, it loses its power to contract in a regular, wave-like manner, and contraction of the chamber, as a whole, never takes place. Instead, very rapid, irregular contractions occur all over the atrium, quite independently of each other, at the rate of about 400 per minute.

A large number of these contractions produce impulses which reach the bundle of His which is, therefore, literally bombarded with irregular stimuli. Owing to the refractory period only a certain number of these impulses are able to pass along the bundle and stimulate ventricular contraction at a rate of 100–180 beats per minute unless controlled by digitalis.

Ventricular contraction is rapid in rate and irregular in rhythm. Since the atrium is not contracting regularly, blood will not reach the ventricle in a steady stream and, therefore, the ventricle never contains a constant amount of blood. The quantity of blood expelled by the ventricle varies with each contraction, and it follows that the volume of the pulse will also vary with each beat. Consequently, the pulse in atrial fibrillation is completely irregular both in rhythm and volume and the efficiency of the heart is diminished.

Causes of atrial fibrillation. Atrial fibrillation is a common condition and is frequently accompanied by heart failure. Common causes are:

1. Mitral stenosis due to rheumatic heart disease.
2. Coronary artery thrombosis and ischaemic heart disease.
3. Hypertensive heart disease.
4. Thyrotoxicosis (p. 454).

Treatment of atrial fibrillation. The drug of greatest value in the treatment of atrial fibrillation is **digitalis**. It is convenient here to explain how the drug acts (see also p. 129).

In addition to stimulating the myocardium to contract more strongly, digitalis acts on the conducting tissues of the heart including the bundle of His, and renders them less sensitive to impulses. In atrial fibrillation, fewer of the irregular impulses bombarding the bundle are allowed to pass and, therefore, the ventricle contracts less often. This slowing of the ventricular rate allows adequate filling of the ventricle with blood from the atrium so that, when the ventricle does contract, it forces a larger quantity of blood into the aorta, and the general circulation is improved. In addition, the ventricle obtains a longer period of rest between each beat. It does not, however, restore normal rhythm.

Quinidine, a drug allied to quinine, has been used in the treatment of fibrillation and, by its action, the normal rhythm of the heart could sometimes be restored. Its use, however, is not without danger.

In some specially selected cases normal rhythm can be restored by one or more high-energy (100–300 Joules) electric shocks applied to the chest wall.

Atrial flutter is a rare condition, detectable on the electro-cardiogram, in which the atrial rate is between 200 and 300 beats per minute. It differs from atrial fibrillation by the fact that the beats are regular in rhythm. As a rule only half the beats get through to the ventricle. Digitalis is used in treatment and if successful first converts the flutter into fibrillation. After a few days digitalis is stopped and normal rhythm is restored. A low-energy electric shock will usually convert flutter to normal sinus rhythm.

Sinus arrhythmia. This is an irregularity of the heart beat which varies with respiration and is probably due to variation in vagal tone. The strength of the beat is unaffected, but the rate of the pulse increases with inspiration and decreases with expiration. It is quite common in children and during convalescence from febrile conditions. It is not in any way abnormal and does not indicate heart disease.

Ventricular fibrillation, which clearly shows on an electrocardiogram, is a very dangerous condition in which the normal spread of impulses over the ventricles is completely disorganized. It may result from conditions such as cardiac infarction, digitalis overdosage, chloroform anaesthesia, particularly if adrenaline has been given, during cardiac surgery and electrocution.

Cardiac massage, artificial respiration and the use of the electric defibrillator may save life if promptly applied.

Other conditions in which the defibrillator may be used in selected cases include ventricular tachycardia, atrial flutter, atrial fibrillation and paroxysmal atrial tachycardia.

Disorders of cardiac rate

Four abnormalities of cardiac rhythm have been described; abnormalities of rate also occur.

Tachycardia is a term used somewhat loosely to describe increased rapidity of the heart beat. This may be due to disease of the heart or to conditions such as haemorrhage, fever, tuberculosis, thyrotoxicosis, dyspepsia and nervousness.

Paroxysmal tachycardia is a condition in which there is the abrupt onset and often equally abrupt termination of rapidity of the heart beat, often without obvious cause, but may be due either to a decrease of vagal tone or increase of sympathetic impulses. It may last only a few seconds or may be prolonged for some hours or even days. The patient may complain of palpitation and dyspnoea. If the attack is prolonged signs of cardiac failure may develop.

An electrocardiogram may show that the suspected condition is due to multiple ectopic beats (extra-systoles) arising from an abnormal focus in either the atria or ventricles or to temporary atrial fibrillation or flutter, with a return to normal rhythm when the paroxysm ceases.

Sometimes careful pressure on the vagus nerve in the neck may cut short an attack. Digitalis, procaine–amide or electrical therapy may be used in treatment.

The patient is often conscious of the heart thumping in tachycardia and this consciousness of the heart beat is known as **palpitation.**

Bradycardia. This is a term used to denote undue slowness of the heart beat (30–50 beats per minute). The condition may occur normally in athletes, in disease of the brain, where there is increased intracranial pressure (meningitis, tumour, cerebral haemorrhage, depressed fracture of the skull), in jaundice, in myxoedema and in poisoning by digitalis.

Sinus bradycardia is probably due to increase in vagal tone.

Propranolol is a drug which may induce a beneficial reduction in heart rate.

Heart block. Bradycardia is also present in a serious heart lesion known as heart block, which is due to damage to the bundle of His or its main branches. Temporary block may occur as a result of toxaemia in acute infections such as acute rheumatism, diphtheria and in overdosage with digitalis. Persistent atrio-ventricular block is often due to fibrosis of the bundle without obvious cause or to disease of the coronary arteries and myocardial infarction. Rarely the condition may be congenital.

If the bundle of His is damaged, impulses from the atria are unable to reach the ventricles. In these circumstances the ventricles, however, have the power to contract on their own, at approximately half the normal atrial rate. In complete heart block the atria and ventricles contract independently of each other, the former at the rate of 72 beats per minute, and the latter at approximately 36 beats per minute. This may be clearly demonstrated by an electrocardiogram (p. 179).

Although heart block does not necessarily cause any special symptoms the condition is sometimes associated with attacks of faintness, loss of consciousness and sometimes convulsions due to lack of blood supply to the brain, known as the **Adams-Stokes syndrome.** During the period of unconsciousness the patient has a death-like pallor but becomes flushed as consciousness returns. Isoprenaline (long acting 'Saventrine' is particularly useful) may help to prevent attacks.

Some cases require the insertion of an 'artificial pace-maker' which gives regular electric shocks to the myocardium causing it to contract.

The pacing box (pulse-generator) is buried under the skin of the abdomen or axilla if permanent pacing is required. The electrode, which conveys the electrical stimuli, may be either endocardial (in the right ventricle) or epicardial (embedded in the muscle of the outer surface of the heart).

Pericarditis

Definition. Inflammation of the pericardium.

Aetiology. This condition usually occurs as a complication of other diseases. Organisms may reach the pericardium either by means of the blood stream or as a result of direct spread of inflammation from neighbouring parts. Among the causes are:

(*a*) Acute rheumatism and chorea.
(*b*) Infectious diseases such as scarlet fever, typhoid, pneumonia and sometimes tuberculosis.
(*c*) Septicaemia and pyaemia.
(*d*) Myocardial infarction.
(*e*) As a terminal condition in chronic nephritis and cancer.
(*f*) Virus infections causing a relatively benign type.

Types of pericarditis

1. Acute—(a) Dry.
   (b) With effusion (either serous or purulent).
2. Chronic (constrictive pericarditis).

(These types of disease are common to inflammation of all serous membranes. Pleurisy, for example, may be dry or with an effusion which may be either serous or purulent, and adhesions of adjacent surfaces of the pleura may follow acute inflammation.)

Symptoms. The onset of acute dry pericarditis is generally abrupt. The patient complains of precordial pain, especially when pressure is applied to the sternum, cough and shortness of breath, and marked facial pallor may be observed. The temperature is raised and the pulse rapid.

The inflammation causes the smooth surfaces of the pericardium to become roughened and covered with flakes of lymph so that, instead of gliding noiselessly over each other, a friction sound or rub is produced, which can be heard with the stethoscope. Occasionally pericarditis occurs without symptoms and its presence is only detected by examination.

Pericarditis with effusion develops as a sequel to the dry variety. If a sufficient quantity of fluid be formed, it will separate the two surfaces of the pericardium and the friction sound may disappear. As much as 2 or 3 pints of fluid may accumulate.

If the germs present are pus-producing organisms, the fluid will become purulent (pyo-pericardium) and a high, remittent temperature with rigors will occur.

Chronic or **constrictive pericarditis** may follow the acute variety but many cases are tuberculous in origin. The two surfaces of the pericardium become adherent as a result of caseation or the formation of scar tissue between them and are unable to glide over each other. The thickened pericardium may become calcified, making it visible on chest x-rays. In addition, adhesions may occur between the outer surface of the pericardium and the adjacent pleura and structures in the mediastinum.

Constrictive pericarditis may be mistaken for heart failure.

Prognosis. The prognosis in acute pericarditis is largely dependent on the cause of the condition. The occurrence of pericarditis as a complication always makes the original disease more serious. As a rule, acute pericarditis subsides, but when constrictive pericarditis supervenes, the life of the patient is shortened unless the constriction is relieved by surgery.

Treatment. In every case of acute rheumatic pericarditis rest in bed is of the utmost importance; excitement and worry must be avoided. The comfort of the patient, so that all unnecessary movement and restlessness on his part are avoided, is more important than the actual position in which he is nursed and he will usually choose the one which is physiologically best for him.

The patient may be kept in bed for several weeks, and only be

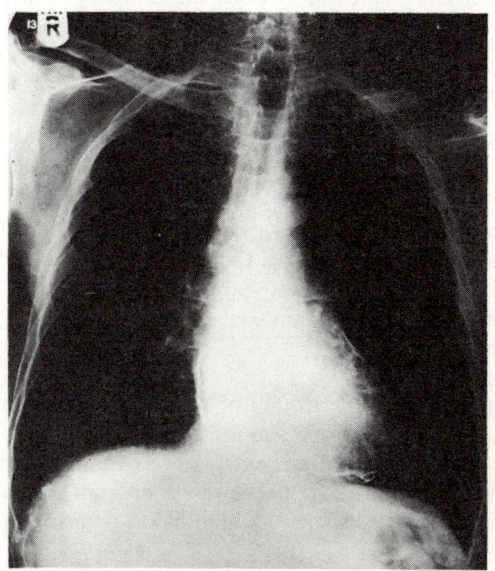

Fig. 14 Constrictive pericarditis.

allowed to get up by degrees after this period. Subsequently some weeks of convalescence may be required in rheumatic cases.

Pericarditis occurring as a complication of coronary thrombosis does not as a rule require any special treatment.

In addition to the treatment of the cause of the condition, special local treatment may be required.

For the relief of pain a kaolin poultice may be applied to the precordium. If this fails, the continuous application of an ice-bag may be of service. (The ice-bag is suspended over the patient so that it produces no pressure on the chest.)

Restlessness and insomnia are treated with sedatives and analgesic drugs. Pethidine or morphine may be necessary.

Occasionally a large effusion may cause distress or signs suggestive of heart failure, and it may be necessary to draw off the excess of fluid by inserting an aspirating needle into the pericardium, using local anaesthesia. This procedure is called paracentesis, or tapping of the pericardium.

If pus be present an operation for drainage of the pericardium may be performed, and penicillin or other antibiotics given. Tuberculous pericarditis is treated with streptomycin and allied drugs.

Operation (pericardectomy) is required to free the heart from constriction in cases of constrictive pericarditis.

Diseases of the myocardium

In order that a clear idea of the mechanism and causes of heart failure may be obtained, the affections of the heart muscle may be considered under the following headings:

1. Hypertrophy and dilatation.
2. Inflammation.
3. Degeneration.

1. Hypertrophy. Hypertrophy of the heart means an increase in the size and amount of heart muscle, which is Nature's response when the heart has to perform extra work over a prolonged period. This may result from damage to the valves or from some abnormality in the general circulation such as high blood pressure or pulmonary disease.

Whatever the cause may be, the heart is called upon to work at a mechanical disadvantage, and is unable to keep up a circulation adequate for the needs of the body. In order to compensate for this disadvantage, it is necessary that a larger and stronger pump be provided. Nature provides this compensation by the process of hypertrophy.

The condition in itself produces no special symptoms but, on examination, the heart is found to be enlarged, the apex beat being displaced outwards and downwards towards the axilla.

Enlargement of the heart may also be demonstrated by x-rays.

Dilatation. Provided the heart muscle is in a healthy state and the extra demands made upon it are not excessive, the process of hypertrophy enables an adequate circulation to be maintained.

If the demand for further work continues, the heart commences to fail. The first stage in this process is dilatation of the chambers of the heart, which become distended with blood, because the force of contraction is not sufficient to empty them completely at each beat.

The reason that the force of contraction is insufficient is that, when the heart becomes dilated, the individual muscle fibres are stretched beyond their normal limits: when thus overstretched they are unable to contract down to their normal size, and the strength of the contraction of the chamber as a whole is therefore reduced.

If, with the onset of failure, further hypertrophy occurs which enables the chamber once again to empty properly, the fibres, which have been overstretched, regain their power.

This process of overcoming dilatation and stretching of the muscle fibres by means of hypertrophy is known as compensation.

If, however, the nutrition of the heart be impaired and the additional hypertrophy does not take place, heart failure continues and the state of **decompensation** or circulatory failure is present.

2. Inflammation (myocarditis). It will be found that the terms myocarditis and cardiomyopathy are in general use both for acute and chronic diseases of the heart. In most chronic affections, however, the actual inflammation has long since subsided and the condition found in the heart muscle is one of fibrous or fatty degeneration. In the present description, the term myocarditis will be applied only to acute inflammation of the myocardium, while chronic conditions, which may be the result of such inflammation, will be referred to as myocardial degeneration or myocardial fibrosis.

Acute myocarditis may occur in the following conditions:

(*a*) In acute rheumatism and chorea.

(*b*) Acute fevers, e.g. diphtheria, typhoid, pneumonia, influenza and infectious mononucleosis.

(*c*) In association with acute pericarditis.

The main symptoms of acute damage to the heart muscle are those of increasing heart failure—including shortness of breath, fainting attacks, dropsy and albuminuria. The pulse is rapid, regular or irregular in rhythm, of poor volume and low tension.

An essential point in treatment is adequate rest. (For details see treatment of heart failure, p. 127.)

3. Myocardial degeneration. Chronic disease of the heart muscle may follow acute myocarditis. It consists of replacement of muscle fibres by fibrous tissue which is unable to contract and, therefore, takes no part in the pumping action of the heart. It also occurs if the nutrition of the heart is impaired as a result of disease of the coronary arteries which reduces its blood supply (myocardial ischaemia). The other causes are included in the following list:

(a) Previous acute myocarditis (e.g. acute rheumatism).

(b) Disease of coronary arteries and coronary thrombosis.

(c) Arteriosclerosis and hypertension.

(d) Syphilis.

(e) Thyrotoxicosis (p. 454).

(f) Chronic pulmonary disease.

(g) Idiopathic cardiomyopathy of obscure origin which may include virus infection, toxins and alcoholism.

Symptoms. The progress of the disease is slow and, therefore, the condition may be present for some time before it becomes manifest. The occurrence of some other illness, such as bronchitis, may determine the onset of symptoms. Occasionally sudden death may occur.

As a rule, the symptoms are those of chronic heart failure, the first being shortness of breath. Later, cough, precordial pain, dyspepsia, albuminuria and oedema develop, and may be associated with disorders of cardiac rhythm, such as atrial fibrillation. (Treatment, see p. 127.)

Endocarditis

By endocarditis is meant inflammation of the lining membrane of the heart. In the majority of cases this is limited to the valves. Those most commonly affected are situated on the left side of the heart, viz. the mitral and the aortic valves.

The disease may be acute or chronic. The chronic variety is, as a rule, the result of previous acute endocarditis and consists of scarring of the valves with the production of an excess of fibrous tissue, rather than an active process of inflammation. The term **chronic valvular disease** is therefore preferable (cf. acute myocarditis and myocardial fibrosis). The commonest cause of acute endocarditis is acute rheumatism.

There is another type of valvular inflammation known as infective, or bacterial endocarditis which requires separate description (see p. 134).

Symptoms. There is often a complete absence of symptoms in acute endocarditis and the condition is then only detected by examination. Palpitation and dyspnoea may be complained of and are accompanied by a rapid pulse. When the condition occurs during an attack of acute rheumatism, there is frequently an associated rise in temperature without any aggravation of the joint symptoms,

It is important to realize that there is usually some degree of acute myocarditis present at the same time, and any symptoms which occur are really the result of the damage to the heart muscle rather than to the valves themselves.

The treatment of the condition is therefore the same as that of acute myocarditis, namely, strict rest until all evidence of acute inflammation has subsided.

Chronic valvular disease

Chronic valvular disease is usually the result of previous acute inflammation, due to acute rheumatism. It may also occur as a result of syphilis, arteriosclerosis or old age.

The mitral valve is affected more frequently than the aortic; less commonly, both valves are involved at the same time. Disease of the tricuspid and pulmonary valves, on the right side of the heart, occurs less frequently. Syphilis is liable to injure the aortic valve, and the disease process may extend into the aorta itself.

Morbid anatomy of endocarditis. The process of acute inflammation causes the formation of small outgrowths on the surface of the valve, rather like warts. These excrescences are known as vegetations and consist of fibrin, blood platelets and leucocytes.

When the condition becomes chronic the vegetations may be absorbed. Fibrous scar tissue appears in their place and in the surrounding portions of the valve. This fibrous tissue has the tendency to behave like scar tissue elsewhere in the body and to contract. The result of this is deformity of the valve associated, in the case of the mitral valve, with shortening of the chordae tendinae.

In the normal heart, when the valves are open, their orifice is sufficiently large to allow the blood to leave the chamber which they guard without any difficulty, and when closed, they prevent any backward flow of blood.

For purposes of example, the mitral valve will be considered. When the left atrium is full of blood, the mitral valve opens and blood flows. Contraction of the atrium aids the flow into the left ventricle. The left ventricle contracts in its turn and all the blood passes into the aorta. This is possible only if the mitral valve is functioning normally, for when the ventricle contracts the cusps of the mitral valve come together and prevent blood from flowing back into the atrium.

As a result of valvular disease, the cusps of the valve may be so damaged that they fail to close completely and, when the left ventricle contracts, only part of its contained blood enters the aorta, the remainder passing backwards into the left atrium. This backward flow of blood into the chamber which it has just left is called **regurgitation**, and the valve is said to be incompetent.

The process of scarring and fibrosis, which has already been mentioned, may also narrow the mitral valve, so that, when the left atrium contracts blood no longer flows easily into the ventricle.

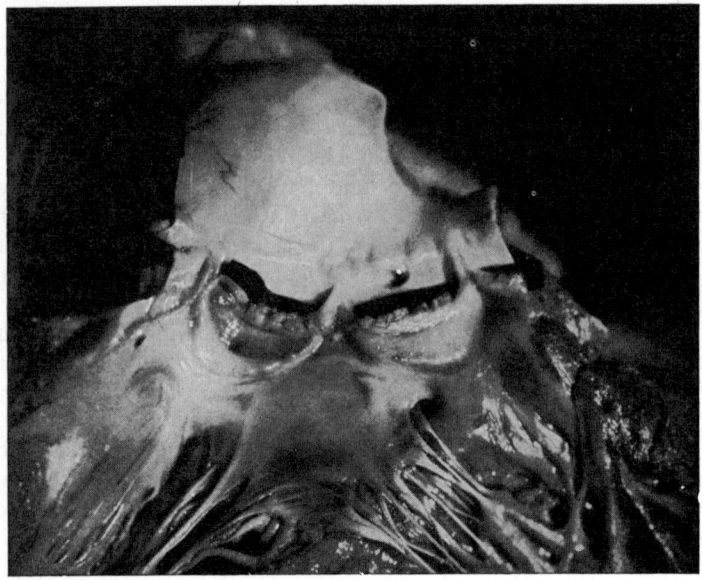

Fig. 15 Showing warty vegetations along the margins of the cusps of the aortic valves in rheumatic heart disease.

This narrowing of the valve is called **mitral stenosis**. Exactly the same state of affairs may exist in connection with the aortic valve.

The actual lesions which may occur in chronic valvular disease are (in order of frequency):

Mitral stenosis and mitral regurgitation (incompetence).

Aortic regurgitation (incompetence).

Aortic stenosis.

It must be realized that a narrowed valve may also fail to close properly, so that both stenosis and regurgitation may be present at the same time.

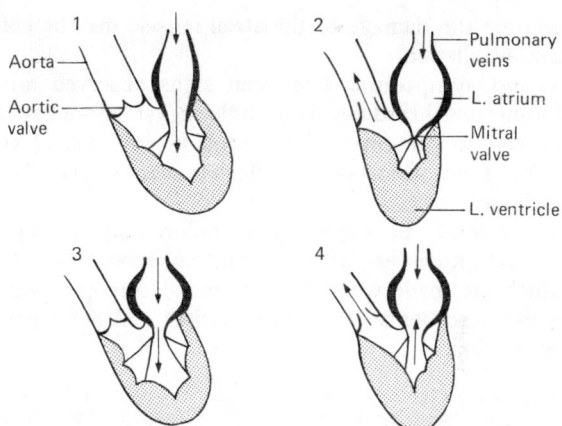

Fig. 16 1. Normal diastole. Mitral valve open. 2. Normal systole. Mitral valve closed, aortic valve open. 3. Mitral stenosis. Hypertrophied left atrium forcing blood through narrowed mitral valve. 4. Mitral regurgitation. Ventricular systole forcing blood into aorta, with regurgitation into left atrium owing to inadequate closure of mitral valve.

Mitral stenosis

Mitral stenosis is nearly always rheumatic in origin. It may develop within 2 or 3 years of an attack of rheumatic fever in childhood. On the other hand, many cases are not detected until the ages of 30 to 40 when it is not always possible to obtain a reliable history of juvenile rheumatism.

Pathology. The scarring which results from the rheumatic endocarditis affecting the mitral valve causes the following effects:

1. The two cusps of the valve become adherent at both ends, producing a slit-like or buttonhole opening instead of the normal circular one.
2. The cusps become thickened by an excess of fibrous tissue. Later this may become calcified.
3. The chordae tendinae are often thickened and shortened.

The effect on the heart is to throw added strain on the left atrium in its attempt to force blood through the narrow opening. After some initial hypertrophy of the atrial muscle there is, later, dilatation of the cavity. Congestion in the pulmonary circulation and hypertrophy of the right ventricle follows and, finally, general congestive heart failure.

At any time the damage to the atrial muscle may be sufficient to cause atrial fibrillation.

Signs and symptoms. The main signs observed are the presence of a murmur heard during diastole or just before systole. Mitral stenosis may be present without causing any special symptoms. There is, however, often a peculiar flush (malar flush) in the skin over the cheek-bones.

Eventually slowly progressive heart failure may develop, in which pulmonary symptoms are predominant, e.g. shortness of breath and cough which are made worse by exertion. Haemoptysis may occur. Later, cyanosis, oedema of the legs, ascites and enlargement of the liver may develop.

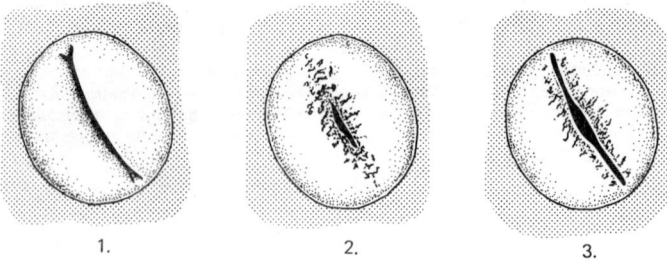

Fig. 17 1. Normal mitral valve (from above). 2. Scarred valve in mitral stenosis. 3. Mitral valve after valvotomy.

Complications

1. Haemoptysis.
2. Atrial fibrillation.
3. Embolism.

As a result of the congestion of blood in the atrium thrombosis may occur especially in that part of the chamber known as the atrial appendix. A portion of this clot may become detached and form an embolus which will be carried in the general circulation, possibly to the brain causing hemiplegia, or to one of the limbs or other organs. (See p. 160.)

Treatment. Apart from care not to exceed the limits of the heart's strength and the routine treatment of symptoms (oxygen for cyanosis; restricted fluid intake, low salt diet and diuretics for oedema; digitalis for atrial fibrillation), many cases of mitral stenosis can be treated surgically. The operation of mitral valvotomy is performed. This consists of approaching the heart through the left side of the chest. The surgeon excises the tip of the left atrial appendage, through which he then introduces his finger into the left atrium. His finger enables him to assess the condition of the mitral valve orifice and to guide a dilator into it. The dilator is inserted through a small incision in the left ventricle and is opened slowly when in position in the mitral valve orifice. This splits the com- misures—the lines of adhesion between the valve cusps.

It is now more usual to make a direct visual approach through the left ventricle.

In suitable cases an artificial valve may be implanted. (See Fig. 18.)

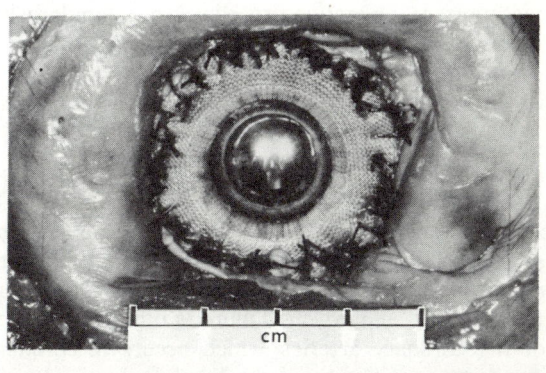

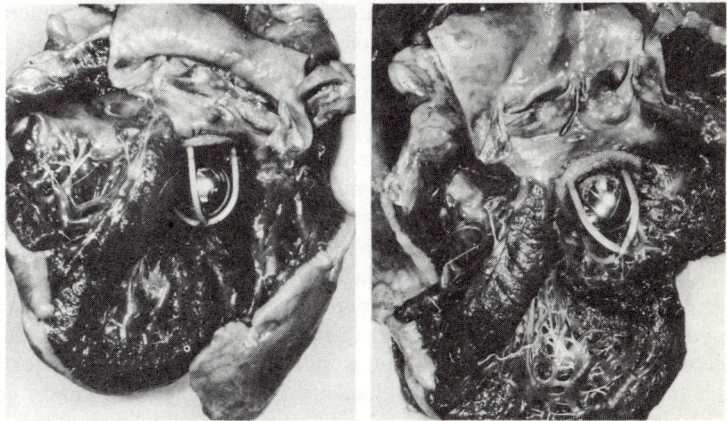

Fig. 18 Starr-Edwards valve. Used to replace regurgitant mitral valve. *Top picture* shows valve from above (left atrium). *Left hand picture* shows ball-valve open; *right hand picture* shows it closed. A similar valve is used for aortic valve replacement.

Operations are usually performed on adults after the risk of further rheumatic infection has passed. Neither advancing age, e.g. 50 years, nor atrial fibrillation are contra-indications to operation which has a relatively low mortality in carefully selected cases. If necessary the operation may be performed during pregnancy.

Aortic valvular disease

In some cases of aortic regurgitation the defective valve may be replaced by an artificial valve or a human tissue graft of a valve obtained post mortem. Operative procedures may similarly be helpful in aortic stenosis. In both instances an efficient myocardium is important.

Heart failure (acute and chronic)

In **acute heart failure** the onset of the symptoms is rapid. There is sudden collapse of the patient, with dyspnoea, cyanosis, and fall in blood pressure accompanied by a rapid, weak pulse. Death is not uncommon and may be almost instantaneous, or may occur in the course of a few hours. Acute heart failure is often due to the sudden blockage of the coronary arteries which occurs in coronary artery thrombosis, whereby a portion of the heart is deprived of its blood supply; it occurs also in acute infections such as diphtheria where there is acute myocarditis, and sometimes from extra-cardiac causes, e.g. during anaesthesia and surgical operations (See also Causes of Sudden Death, p. 500.)

Having considered the diseases of the myocardium and the valves, it is now possible to describe the process of heart failure, which is the inability of the heart to maintain an efficient circulation. It must be pointed out, however, that almost all forms of heart disease may be present for many years before any evidence of failure develops.

Chronic (congestive) heart failure is a gradual process and its development is almost entirely dependent on the inability of the myocardium to perform the work necessary to maintain the normal circulation, i.e. the cardiac output is inadequate to meet the needs of the individual. There are two elements in cardiac failure either, or both, of which may be present and account for individual symptoms.

(i) Excessive pressure in the heart and great vessels causing congestive failure ('Back pressure').

(ii) Insufficient cardiac output ('Forward failure').

This failure may occur as the result of two factors:

(a) The muscle is so badly damaged by disease and is of such poor quality that it is unable to do its *normal* work.

(b) The muscle is not perfectly healthy and when called upon to do *extra* work is unable to respond to the demands made upon it, i.e. the cardiac reserve is diminished.

The heart is a complicated two-sided pump maintaining both the general systemic circulation by the contraction of the left ventricle and the pulmonary circulation by means of the right ventricle. Depending on the cause, either the left side or the right side of the heart may start to fail first. Eventually the failure will become general and involve both sides more or less equally.

It is customary, therefore, to refer to:

(a) Left-sided heart failure.

(b) Right-sided heart failure.

Left-sided heart failure. Strain on the left ventricle occurs particularly as a result of:

(a) Hypertension,

(b) Disease of the aortic valve,

(c) Disease of the coronary arteries.

Since the left ventricle fails to pump adequately blood which it receives from the lungs while at the same time the right side continues to work efficiently, blood accumulates in the pulmonary circulation and the lungs become congested. The main symptoms produced are:

(a) Dyspnoea on exertion,

(b) Sudden attacks of dyspnoea at night (cardiac asthma),

(c) Cyanosis.

Ultimately this state of affairs will put a strain on the right side of the heart, as the next stage of the argument will show.

For purposes of illustration, **the mechanism of heart failure** resulting from stenosis of the mitral valve will be considered. It must be clearly understood, however, that while reference is being made to the muscle of one chamber of the heart, the rest of the heart muscle is to some extent damaged and the actual process of failure involves the heart as a whole and is a gradual one.

Reference to the diagram (Fig. 19) will make the steps in the following argument clear.

If the mitral valve is narrowed, a strain will fall upon the left atrium, which will have to pump harder at each beat in order to force its contained blood into the left ventricle. In order to supply this extra force, the muscle of the atrium hypertrophies. So long as

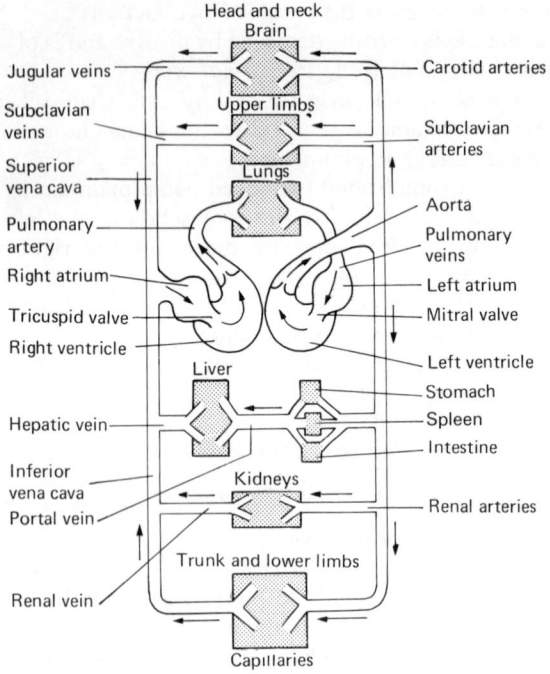

Fig. 19

the hypertrophy provides sufficient power to overcome the obstruction, the circulation will be maintained. If the obstruction increases or the hypertrophy is inadequate, the atrium will be unable to empty all its contained blood at each beat. In order to hold the retained blood it must dilate and the individual muscle fibres are over-stretched.

If the mechanism of compensation by means of hypertrophy fails, the pulmonary veins will be unable to empty properly into the left atrium and so a process of congestion or 'back pressure' is set up in the pulmonary circulation and the lungs become congested with blood. This is sometimes called left-heart failure, and is characterized by dyspnoea and sometimes attacks of cardiac asthma (p. 123).

In an endeavour to empty the lungs and in order to force its contained blood into the congested pulmonary circulation additional strain falls on the right ventricle. The same mechanism of hypertrophy followed by dilatation occurs and affects the tricuspid valve and the right atrium.

When failure of the right side of the heart is present, congestion or 'back pressure' will be found in the superior and inferior venae cavae, with the result that the blood from the veins in the rest of the body will have difficulty in returning to the heart. If reference is made to the diagram, it will be seen that 'back pressure' will produce venous congestion of the brain, the liver and portal circulation (see p. 254 and Fig. 51), the kidneys and the veins of the limbs and body wall.

If the principle involved in this mechanism of chronic heart failure as a result of congestion is fully understood, the reason for many of the symptoms of chronic heart failure can be explained. It can also be understood why failure of the right side of the heart is so common in chronic pulmonary disease. In this condition there is obstruction in the pulmonary circulation and additional strain is placed on the right side. If hypertrophy of this side is insufficient to overcome the dilatation the process of congestion in the veins of the general systemic circulation will occur.

If the whole of the myocardium of both sides of the heart is so weakened by disease that the chambers are not efficiently emptied by each cardiac contraction, the systemic veins will have the same difficulty in emptying their blood into the right atrium and general venous congestion will follow.

The above argument may be summarized briefly.

Failure of any one chamber of the heart, as a result of working against the mechanical disadvantage of a damaged valve or against increased resistance, or as a result of injury to the heart muscle, will cause congestion in that part of the heart, lungs or general venous system, whichever happens to be immediately behind that chamber. It follows from this that congestive symptoms will occur earlier in mitral disease than in aortic lesions.

Right-sided heart failure. From what has already been stated it should be clear that this may ultimately result from left-sided failure and from mitral stenosis and that it is characterized by general venous congestion. It can also arise from diseases of the lung affecting the pulmonary circulation (pulmonary hypertension), while the left side of the heart is functioning efficiently. This state is sometimes referred to as pulmonary heart disease.

Pulmonary heart disease (cor pulmonale)

Cor pulmonale may be defined as hypertrophy and eventual failure of the right ventricle resulting from chronic disease of the lungs and disorders of the pulmonary circulation.

In chronic lung disease, particularly emphysema and fibrosis of the lungs, the number of capillaries in the lungs is reduced and an added strain falls on the right ventricle in its attempt to force blood through the obstructed pulmonary circulation.

In the early stages cyanosis, cough, occasional haemoptysis and obvious distension of the jugular veins may be present. Later, fully developed congestive heart failure with enlargement and tenderness of the liver and oedema occurs.

Morphine should be avoided in this condition as it may produce a serious depressing effect on the respiratory centre.

Symptoms of chronic heart disease

1. Chronic valvular disease

Valvular disease of the heart may exist for a long time without producing any symptoms, provided the myocardium is intact and able to maintain the circulation while the patient is at rest and when taking exercise.

The first symptoms of chronic heart disease are noticed during exertion and these general manifestations are of more importance than the actual valvular lesion present. There are, however, some broad distinctions which separate cases of aortic disease from those of mitral disease in their general symptomatology. Owing to the fact that congestive changes occur relatively early in mitral disease, the associated symptoms are at first those of pulmonary congestion and later of general venous congestion. The first effects of aortic disease are to cause difficulty for the left ventricle to expel the normal quantity of blood into the aorta at each beat, therefore, the symptoms produced are mainly the result of defective arterial supply and general emptiness of the arterial system.

The following table compares the main symptoms:

Aortic Valve Disease	Mitral Valve Disease
Pallor.	Cyanosis.
Precordial pain common.	Palpitation more common.
Dyspeptic symptoms rare.	Dyspeptic symptoms common.
Oedema late.	Oedema frequent and early.
Dyspnoea common.	Dyspnoea common.
Cerebral symptoms common.	Pulmonary symptoms common.
Embolism uncommon.	Embolism common.

Embolism (see p. 160). An embolus consists of a clot of blood or other abnormal substance carried by the bloodstream from its site of origin and lodged in a smaller vessel so as to obstruct its lumen.

Owing to the stagnation of blood in one of the chambers of the heart as a result of valvular disease, e.g. in the left atrium in cases of mitral stenosis and atrial fibrillation, a clot may be formed. If this gets into the bloodstream, it constitutes an embolus and causes symptoms depending on the situation in which it finally lodges.

2. Chronic heart failure (For causes, see p. 112.)

It has been seen that the symptoms of heart disease are almost entirely due to the inability of the heart muscle to maintain the normal circulation.

Chronic cardiac failure, or congestive heart failure as it is sometimes called, commonly occurs in:

1. The later stages of valvular disease and in atrial fibrillation.
2. Hypertension (Hypertensive heart disease.)
3. Chronic pulmonary disease. (Cor pulmonale.)
4. Myocardial degeneration.

A. GENERAL SYMPTOMS

(1) Dyspnoea. Shortness of breath on exertion is one of the earliest and most important symptoms. As the disease progresses, dyspnoea is induced by less and less effort until, in the later stages, it may become continuous. When so severe that the patient is forced to remain sitting up it is known as **orthopnoea.**

A peciliar form of breathlessness termed **paroxymal nocturnal dyspnoea** may occur in heart disease with left-sided heart failure. It is due to pulmonary congestion caused by the patient lying flat or slipping down in bed. This may be associated with reflex spasm of the bronchioles ('cardiac asthma'). It is characterized by paroxysms of dyspnoea, wheeziness and a sense of suffocation, of sudden onset, which usually occur at night. It must be distinguished from bronchial asthma and dyspnoea due to renal disease. Unless spontaneous relief occurs on sitting up the condition may be treated with oxygen inhalations and injections of aminophylline, morphine and frusemide. Some cases require digitalis. The patient should be propped up.

(2) Palpitation and tachycardia. This may result from anxiety but is also common in heart disease and thyrotoxicosis.

(3) Pain. Pain in heart disease is variable, but occurs in coronary artery disease, aortic stenosis and syphilis. It is frequently brought on by exertion and may consist of a dull ache in the precordium, general tightness of the chest, or acute pain spreading from the precordium into the neck and arms (angina pectoris).

(4) Cerebral symptoms. These may be due to congestion of the brain, or may occur as a result of defective arterial (oxygen) supply. The term cerebral anoxia is often used. They include sleeplessness, loss of memory, mental changes, and delirium. Fainting attacks (syncope) are also due to temporary lack of blood supply to the brain, but do not necessarily indicate heart disease, e.g. vaso-vagal syncope.

(5) Cyanosis. Blueness of the lips, cheeks, ears and extremities indicates deficient oxygenation of the blood. This may be due to disorder of the pulmonary circulation, whereby the blood fails to acquire sufficient oxygen during its passage through the lungs, or to stagnation of venous blood in the peripheral parts of the circulation, caused by back pressure and resulting in delay in return of venous blood to the heart. Cyanosis is common in mitral disease, when both these factors may be operative. It is also frequently encountered in lung diseases such as pneumonia and bronchitis.

B. SYMPTOMS DUE TO CONGESTION

It has been seen that failure of the heart to empty completely at each beat results in general congestion of the whole venous system. All parts of the body, therefore, become engorged with blood, a condition which accounts for many symptoms of cardiac failure. The jugular veins in the neck may be observed to be distended.

(1) Congestion of the lungs. Is especially common in mitral stenosis and in atrial fibrillation. Cough, dyspnoea and haemoptysis occur.

(2) Digestive disturbances. The liver may become congested and consequently organs such as the stomach, whose blood passes to the liver by the portal vein, are also affected. The liver becomes enlarged and tender and the patient complains of epigastric discomfort, flatulence and vomiting.

(3) Oedema (or dropsy). The results of congestion of the veins are to interfere with the proper absorption of tissue fluids and to allow fluid to escape from the blood into the tissue spaces. This accumulation of fluid in the subcutaneous tissues is called oedema. It can be recognized by applying pressure with the finger-tips, when 'pitting' of the part will occur.

Oedema in heart disease usually commences in the most dependent part of the body, namely the ankles. When the patient is sitting in bed the sacral region is also involved. As the condition increases, oedema spreads, involving the whole of the legs. Later, fluid collects in the peritoneal cavity (ascites) and in the pleural cavities (pleural effusion or hydrothorax). When the oedema is widespread, the condition is called general anasarca. Other causes of oedema of the legs include nephritis, cirrhosis of the liver, malnutrition, pressure on the inferior vena cava and iliac veins, and varicose veins. Local oedema occurs in inflammation (see p. 10).

Pulmonary oedema. This may be acute or insidious in onset and at post mortem the lungs appear heavy and waterlogged. Their cut surfaces exudes a frothy, often blood-stained albuminous fluid pouring out from the bronchioles and alveoli.

The main symptoms are cough with pink, frothy sputum, orthopnoea and cyanosis. X-ray shows diffuse fluffy shadows throughout the lung fields. The condition is likely to occur in left-sided heart failure (see cardiac asthma, p. 123), inflammatory conditions of the lungs (broncho-pneumonia, tracheobronchitis), inhalation of irritating vapours (chlorine, war gases) and in comatose patients.

Treatment includes oxygen therapy, digitalis in cardiac cases who have not recently taken it, aminophylline, prompt diuretic therapy (e.g. intravenous frusemide) and venesection if necessary.

(4) Urinary symptoms. Congestion of the kidneys will result in alteration of their function. Consequently, albuminuria and diminished secretion of urine are common.

These **symptoms of chronic heart disease** may also be classified briefly in the following way:

(*i*) *Cardiovascular.* Pallor or cyanosis, tachycardia, precordial pain, syncope.

(*ii*) *Respiratory.* Dyspnoea, cough, pulmonary congestion, haemoptysis.

(*iii*) *Alimentary.* Loss of appetite, dyspepsia, flatulence, constipation, congestion with pain, fulness and tenderness of the liver.

(*iv*) *Nervous.* Insomnia, loss of memory, mental changes and delusions, delirium.

(*v*) *Renal.* Diminished urinary output, albuminuria.

(*vi*) *General.* Oedema, ascites, pleural effusion.

The treatment of heart disease

The treatment and general management of cases of heart disease is of utmost importance and, in many instances, prompt therapeutic measures may prolong life for many years or, at least, save patients from much suffering.

It has been seen that the onset of symptoms occurs when the

heart is unable to maintain an adequate circulation, as a result of failure of the heart muscle to withstand additional strain.

The essential element in the treatment of all cardiac affections irrespective of the cause, therefore, is to see that the patient's life is so regulated that he never exceeds the limits of the heart's strength. This principle applies not only to physical exertion but also to mental activity. Excitement, anxiety, mental fatigue and emotional strain should, as far as possible, be avoided. This can often be attained more easily by impressing the relatives and business associates than by constantly insisting to the patient that he should not worry.

In view of the varying degree of damage which may occur to the heart and the differences in compensation which may be present in individual cases, the treatment of heart disease will be considered under the following headings:

(1) Slight lesions with good compensation.

(2) Cardiac failure (acute and chronic).

(3) Special conditions and symptoms.

(1) Slight lesions with good compensation

In these cases there is little special medical treatment or nursing required. The patient must carry out the instructions given to him and endeavour to lead a quiet, well-regulated life.

No hard-or-fast rules can be laid down, and each case must be judged on its own merits. Some degree of exercise is beneficial and this is best taken in the form of walking. All sudden and violent physical strains, in particular such actions as hurrying after a bus or train, running upstairs and energetic games, must be avoided. The amount of exercise allowed can, to some extent, be gauged by ensuring that breathlessness, palpitation, tightness of the chest and fatigue, are never produced.

Adequate rest is of cardinal importance. Eight to 10 hours in bed are advised, and it is wise to insist on rest for half to one hour after meals and after exercise.

A well-balanced diet, preferably taken as a number of small meals rather than one or two large ones, is advised. Obesity should be avoided and if present should be treated with a reducing diet.

In some cases, the daily amount of fluid should not exceed 1·5 litres (60 ounces). Alcohol and tobacco are best avoided and should only be taken in amounts permitted by the doctor.

Constipation and straining at stool must not occur. The bowels should be kept regular by a diet of high fibre content or, if necessary, the use of a laxative.

Cold and very hot baths are to be avoided. No special drugs are required and digitalis is of no value in this stage of heart disease except for the treatment of disorders of rhythm. Suitable cases of mitral stenosis can be treated surgically before serious symptoms develop.

(2) Cardiac failure

In **acute** heart failure, the onset of which is often rapid and unexpected, prompt measures must be adopted. In all such cases the nurse should summon medical aid, at the same time carrying out any instructions which she may have received if the emergency has been anticipated.

She must be prepared for the administration of such drugs as morphine, aminophylline, frusemide ('Lasix') and digoxin. The latter drug may sometimes be given intravenously.

Oxygen should be at hand and may be given at once, by the nurse. In some cases, especially those with marked cyanosis, a venesection may be performed.

The patient should be disturbed as little as possible and placed in the position which produces the least distress.

If the heart has stopped beating cardiac massage combined with mouth-to-mouth respiration may be life-saving.

In **chronic** heart failure, or failure of gradual onset, rest in bed is necessary in the first instance. Lying flat may be impossible on account of the dyspnoea present, and the patient should be propped up in bed by using pillows or a back-rest. In some instances the patient is more comfortable when sitting forward; he should then be provided with a bed table covered with a pillow, upon which he can support his arms and head. In very severe cases with gross oedema, the patient may prefer to remain continuously in a chair and should be allowed to do so. This attitude permits fluid to drain from the upper parts of the body into the legs, thereby allowing the heart and lungs to work more easily. A special 'cardiac bed' may be available.

The patient must be spared from exertion. He must not talk too much and all movements must be accomplished without excessive effort on his part. He should be lifted on to the bed-pan or preferably placed on a commode and when the bed is made, must be maintained in the position in which he is being nursed (usually propped up).

On the other hand, especially in elderly patients, some degree of ambulation may be permitted. This may hasten convalescence and reduce the risk of venous thrombosis associated with prolonged bed rest.

Diet. A light, easily digested diet is essential. In very severe cases it will consist mainly of toast and butter, milk, diluted if necessary, Benger's food, junket, fruit juice, custard and a little fish.

In other cases eggs, chicken, vegetables and stewed fruit are allowed. Meat may be added later.

When oedema is present, it may be necessary to restrict the patient's salt intake and, occasionally, also his or her fluid intake. On no account must food be forced on the patient, excessive feeding will not save him, whereas a quiet stomach, free from flatulence and tolerant of medicine, will help to do so.

Bowels. Attention to the bowels is important and they should be kept comfortably open. This is necessary in order to avoid abdominal distension and straining at stool. Enemata or suppositories may be given and aperients such as salines (Epsom salts) or 'Senokot' may be ordered. Liquid paraffin is sometimes sufficient.

Urine. The quantity of urine passed during each 24 hours must be measured carefully and tested, especially for albumin. A fluid intake and output chart should be kept.

Oedema. The presence of oedema is often a source of considerable discomfort to the patient and, if ascites and pleural effusion occur, the action of the heart may be seriously embarrassed.

In addition to a low salt diet and restriction of fluid intake, certain drugs (**diuretics**) acting by increasing the amount of urine passed, are of great value. The most effective oral diuretics include frusemide, ethacrynic acid and the thiazides (e.g. chlorothiazide). These may increase urinary potassium loss so that potassium salts (e.g. 'Slow K') should be administered at the same time. Spironolactone may be useful in patients who become resistant to other diuretics. This and two other diuretics, amiloride and triamterine, have a useful potassium-conserving action. These diuretics are used together with the potassium-losing ones and may make potassium supplements unnecessary (or even dangerous).

If these measures fail, fluid may be withdrawn from the pleural or peritoneal cavities by paracentesis. Fluid from the lower limbs was, in former times, removed by inserting a fine silver tube (Southey's tube) into the subcutaneous tissues. By attaching a piece of fine rubber tubing, the fluid was collected in a bowl of antiseptic lotion placed under the bed.

Another method of allowing fluid to escape is to make an incision (1·25 cm long) on the dorsum of each foot. Strict aseptic precautions must be taken, and the limbs wrapped in sterile dressings, as infection occurs easily in the distended tissues but is minimized by the use of antibiotics.

In addition to keeping an intake and output chart, regular weighing of the patient is of great importance. A steady loss of weight indicates that the fluid retention in the tissues is diminishing.

Digitalis therapy. It has been pointed out that atrial fibrillation, a condition which is frequently a sequel to mitral stenosis, is often associated with heart failure and the mode of action of digitalis has been explained (p. 104).

Digitalis is also given in cases of heart failure other than those with atrial fibrillation because it increases the strength of cardiac contraction and increases the cardiac output. It, thereby, improves especially the circulation to the kidneys, which are enabled to excrete more fluid when oedema is present.

Continued use of the drug or the administration of large doses may produce **toxic symptoms**, which it is important for the nurse to recognize. In the presence of such symptoms, she should not administer a further dose of the drug until she has ascertained the wishes of the doctor. The symptoms of digitalis poisoning are headache, loss of appetite, nausea, vomiting and diarrhoea. Psychological disturbances may occur especially in the elderly. In addition, there may be undue slowness of the pulse or the development of pulsus bigeminus (p. 96), in which the beats are coupled and occur in pairs. Either of these two groups of symptoms may be manifest before the other or they may occur together. They are specially likely to occur when the blood potassium is low and this may happen if diuretics are being given at the same time.

If the cardiac rate, as heard with the stethoscope at the apex, falls to 70 beats per minute the drug must either be stopped or its dose reduced.

Digitalis is given in the form of digoxin, 0·25 mg, digit oxin, 0·1 mg or digitalis folia, 60 mg. See also p. 508.

N.B.— Digoxin (0·75–1·0 mg) may be given intravenously in cases of acute failure provided the patient is known not to have been taking the drug until then. Intravenous ouabain (0·25 mg) also has a rapid action.

Dyspnoea, cyanosis and general venous congestion

The administration of oxygen

The administration of oxygen may be necessary in a number of conditions including certain types of heart disease, notably 'blue babies' with congenital heart disease and adults suffering from cor pulmonale.

Since the task of supervising this type of therapy usually falls to the nurse, a proper understanding of the reasons for giving oxygen, the methods available and the occasional dangers involved, is very important.

The aim of oxygen therapy is the correction of anoxia or hypoxia. This is said to be present when the tissues are not getting sufficient oxygen to meet their metabolic needs. Its presence may often, but not always, be suspected by blueness or cyanosis of the parts involved. If this blueness is limited to the extremities and if these parts are cold to the touch the term peripheral cyanosis is used, and the condition is usually the result of slow circulation of the blood rather than deficient oxygenation in the lungs. When the affected parts are warmer and the cyanosis also affects the lips, mouth and ears the term central cyanosis is used. This implies that the blood is not saturated with oxygen when it leaves the heart.

Peripheral cyanosis may result from blocking or temporary spasm of the blood vessels or from failure of the heart to pump the blood fast enough, for example, in aortic or mitral stenosis.

Central cyanosis occurs when there is impaired ventilation of the lungs such as may be present when the respiratory muscles are paralysed or the respiratory centre in the medulla is depressed, e.g. by drug overdosage and asphyxia from any cause. Impaired interchange of gases between the inspired air and the blood in the lungs also occurs in pulmonary oedema, bronchitis and fibrosis of the lungs. In some cases of congenital heart disease blood may be 'shunted' from the right side of the heart to the left so that a considerable portion never passes through the lungs.

In some cases of heart failure both central and peripheral cyanosis may be present at the same time.

Since cyanosis depends on the amount of haemoglobin which is not oxygenated it is possible for a severely anaemic patient to be seriously anoxic without being cyanosed.

Methods of oxygen administration

The method used depends upon whether a high or a low concentration of oxygen is required.

(1) High concentrations of oxygen (40–80%) are administered in acute conditions such as severe myocardial infarction, haemorrhagic shock and carbon monoxide poisoning. High oxygen concentrations are provided by certain masks which fit closely to the face and to which oxygen is delivered at high flow rates (6–10 litres per minute). These masks are equipped with a reservoir bag to conserve

oxygen during the expiratory phases of a patient's breathing. The bag may permit rebreathing of expired air (as with the **Polymask** and the **Pneumask**) or a non-return valve may prevent rebreathing (as in the Portogen mask). A properly fitting MC mask will produce a high oxygen concentration up to 60%.

(2) Low concentrations of oxygen (25–40%). In normal subjects, changes in the arterial concentration of carbon dioxide cause changes in the depth and rate of breathing. If carbon dioxide accumulates in the lungs, the arterial partial pressure of carbon dioxide (Pa_{CO_2}) rises and the respiratory centre is stimulated. The stimulation causes an increased depth and rate of breathing which tends to restore the Pa_{CO_2} to its normal value (about 40 mm Hg). In chronic respiratory diseases such as chronic bronchitis and emphysema, however, the patient may be accustomed to retention of carbon dioxide and the respiratory centre may no longer be sensitive to its action. The patient now relies largely upon oxygen lack (hypoxaemia) to stimulate his breathing. If high concentrations of oxygen are administered to such a patient, serious depression of respiration may occur and carbon dioxide retention may increase, giving rise to **carbon dioxide narcosis** with coma and probably death. High concentrations of oxygen are therefore contra-indicated in patients with chronic diffuse airways obstruction. Low concentrations of oxygen may, however, be very beneficial or, indeed, vital and may be provided by a mask, a nasal catheter, or an oxygen tent.

Suitable masks are the **Ventimask** and the **Edinburgh mask.** The former provides an almost constant concentration of oxygen (28%) and alternative face masks are available if other constant concentrations (24%, 35% and 40%) are required.

These masks do not have rebreathing bags, which would contribute to the production of carbon dioxide narcosis. A perfect fit of the mask is not required and oxygen loss at the low flow rates used is not of major importance.

Plastic **nasal catheters** and cannulae are surprisingly comfortable and may be preferred by patients. Oxygen flow rates of 1–2 litres/min are delivered via twin nasal catheters and give an inspired oxygen concentration of 25 to 30%. Masks may cause discomfort over the bridge of the nose, become hot and sweaty, obscure vision, or cause an uncomfortable flow of gas into the eyes. With nasal catheters, patients may eat, talk comfortably and eject sputum easily. In addition, many patients like to feel that they can get to their faces. Oxygen given by nasal catheter should be humidified to prevent dryness of the upper respiratory tract.

Oxygen tents enclose the patient, making him less accessible for diagnostic observations and treatment procedures, and have to be carefully tucked in to prevent serious leakage. They are less often used now that more efficient and more convenient methods of giving oxygen are available. They are, however, still useful for small children.

The tent is composed mainly of transparent plastic sheeting and has a special sleeve for nursing purposes, which must be kept closed by twisting and applying a clip when not in use. There is an inlet pipe for oxygen and an outlet pipe which is connected with a drum containing soda lime and caustic soda to absorb the carbon dioxide expired by the patient. (This is omitted from some types of tent.)

Fitted into the apparatus is an ice container, which is filled from the outside. There is a rubber tube leading from the bottom of the container to the exterior which is closed by a clip. When this is opened it allows water from the melted ice to be withdrawn. In order to economize in the use of ice this should not be done too frequently, since water only a few degrees above freezing point will be as useful as ice itself. The purpose of the ice-box is to keep the chamber cool and to allow moisture breathed out from the patient's lungs to condense on its cold exterior, so that the atmosphere of the tent does not become too humid.

Two gauges are attached to the oxygen cylinder. (a) The pressure gauge which indicates when the cylinder is becoming empty. (b) The flow meter which can be adjusted so that the flow of oxygen is between 4 and 10 litres per minute.

N.B.—A 100-cubic foot oxygen cylinder with a rate of flow of 4 litres per minute will last about 12 hours.

Important points to remember when using the tent include:
1. The plastic sheeting must be tucked very carefully under the mattress in order to prevent leakage.
2. Under no circumstances must a naked light, cigarette or electrical apparatus, including hand lamps connected to the mains, be brought near the tent. An ordinary electric torch may be used.
3. Periodic inspection of the flow meter and pressure gauge must be carried out and adjustments made when necessary.
4. Sudden removal of the patient from the tent is inadvisable. The rate of flow should be reduced gradually before this is done.

Oxygen (95%) mixed with 5% carbon dioxide is sometimes used in the treatment of carbon monoxide poisoning if hyperbaric oxygen is not available. Carbon dioxide acts as a potent stimulant to the respiratory centre.

Hyperbaric oxygen. This term means the administration of oxygen at more than atmospheric pressure. It is available at special centres or a mobile unit may be obtained. Normally, apart from the oxygen carried by haemoglobin only a small amount is carried in solution by the blood. Under double the atmospheric pressure, however, this quantity can be greatly increased. This method has been used successfully in the treatment of carbon monoxide poisoning and decompression sickness. Its usefulness in acute ischaemia of a limb with threatening gangrene, certain cases of shock, and infections of the gas gangrene type is limited.

Dangers of oxygen administration

1. **In babies,** continuous administration of high concentrations of oxygen to a premature infant in an incubator may lead to the condition of retrolental fibroplasia which is a cause of blindness.

2. **In adults,** prolonged administration of high concentrations of oxygen may lead to collapse of the lungs, and sometimes to mental disturbances and even fits.

3. Patients with a long history of chronic bronchitis are specially at risk from oxygen. Although it is often essential in acute exacerbations these patients, if given oxygen in high concentration, may cease to ventilate their lungs at a sufficient rate to eliminate carbon dioxide. This, therefore, accumulates in the blood and in the lungs where it displaces oxygen. The condition of 'carbon dioxide narcosis' may develop. It is characterized by confusion, drowsiness, hot hands and a bounding pulse together with small pupils and muscular twitchings or tremor. Finally there may be loss of consciousness. It is in this group of patients that the Ventimask is indicated as the concentration of oxygen is adequate and the accumulation of carbon dioxide does not occur.

The use of intermittent oxygen to avoid carbon dioxide narcosis is dangerous as during the period without oxygen patients commonly become even more anoxic than before treatment was started.

It should be remembered that the administration of oxygen to a collapsed patient who is not actually breathing is useless. Under these circumstances artificial respiration is indicated in the first place.

Venesection. The practice of venesection or blood-letting is a very ancient one and was largely employed by the old barber-surgeons. It still occasionally plays a part in medical treatment.

In some patients who have an excessive amount of blood (polycythaemia, p. 187), and in cases of haemochromatosis (in which there is iron overload) regular venesection is often beneficial.

The indications for venesection may be summed up as:

(1) Some cases of heart failure, especially those associated with acute oedema of the lungs or severe pulmonary congestion.

(2) Polycythaemia (p. 187).
(3) Haemochromatosis.

In heart failure a similar effect but more transient than venesection can be obtained by causing the venous blood to be retained temporarily in the limbs. This is done by placing the legs in a dependent position and applying tourniquets or sphygmomanometer cuffs around the proximal parts of all four limbs and adjusting the pressure so that the venous return is stopped without impeding the arterial blood flow.

Sleeplessness and cerebral symptoms, etc. If a patient with cardiac disease does not get sufficient sleep his progress will not be satisfactory. The ventilation of the room must be adequate and, while the patient should be kept warm, the bedclothes must not be too heavy. If attention to the general comfort of the patient is insufficient to promote sleep, drugs such as nitrazepam ('Mogadon') or chloral are given. If restlessness is marked and pain severe, morphine or similar analgesic may be used.

Haemoptysis in cardiac disease is rarely a serious symptom and, by relieving congestion in the pulmonary circulation, may actually be beneficial. A linctus may be required for cough.

Convalescence after heart failure must obviously be slow and carefully supervised so that the patient in his activities never exceeds the limits of his heart's strength. A room on the ground floor is advantageous but should be so placed that visits to the lavatory and bathroom do not necessitate climbing stairs.

Gradually increasing exercises should be given before the patient starts to get up. Provided breathlessness, palpitation and precordial pain do not occur, increasing exercise is the best way to reassure the subject of cardiac disease.

Infective endocarditis
(Bacterial endocarditis)

This disease is a variety of endocarditis, which is of importance on account of its gravity and often fatal termination, rather than of its frequency.

There are two types of infective (bacterial) endocarditis
1. acute (malignant or ulcerative)
2. subacute.

The difference between these two types depends on the virulence of the organism which infects the valve. In the acute type large soft vegetations develop on the affected valves and lead to their progressive ulceration and destruction. This is much less marked in the subacute type. Both types differ from acute simple (non-infective) endocarditis, such as occurs in rheumatic fever, where the vegetations are small and wart-like and the inflammation results in scarring and contraction of the valves rather than their actual destruction.

(1) Acute bacterial endocarditis

Cause. The organisms most commonly responsible for the malady are the staphylococcus, streptococcus or pneumococcus. They may attack healthy valves. The source of the septicaemia is usually obvious and may be, for example, osteomyelitis or pneumonia. Infective endocarditis of the tricuspid valve may result from the

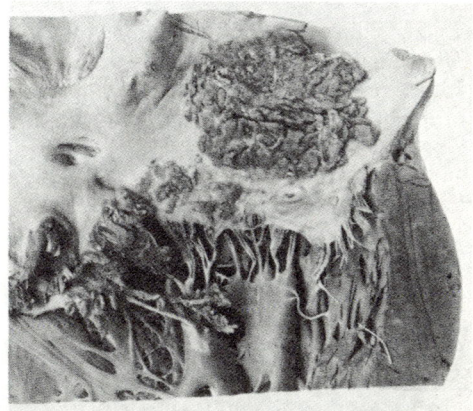

Fig. 20 Bacterial endocarditis of mitral orifice.

self-administered intravenous injection of drugs (e.g. heroin) by drug addicts. Infective endocarditis may, rarely, complicate open heart surgery.

Symptoms. The soft character of the vegetations, containing organisms, is responsible for infected portions becoming detached and entering the bloodstream. The condition is, therefore, a septicaemia, with involvement of the heart. The symptoms are very variable but may best be considered under three headings: septi-caemic, cardiac, embolic.

Septicaemic symptoms. The onset of the condition is sudden. There are high temperature, rigors, profuse sweating and haemor-rhagic rashes.

Cardiac symptoms. Heart failure may occur with rapid pulse, shortness of breath and swelling of the legs, together with the development of murmurs.

Embolic symptoms. Portions of vegetations which break off and enter the general circulation constitute emboli (see p. 160). The symptoms depend upon the site in which they lodge, the common ones being the brain, causing paralysis, and the kidneys, causing pain in the loin and haematuria.

The diagnosis of the condition is often difficult because the main symptoms may be referred to any one of these groups. The appearances may suggest typhoid fever, cerebral disease or may be entirely cardiac in character. It is frequently possible, however, to obtain the causal organism from the bloodstream by means of blood culture.

Treatment. Penicillin or other antibiotics in large doses are required. In every instance it is important to discover the susceptibility of the causal organism to the various antibiotic drugs. Even with the most intensive treatment many patients succumb to the infection.

(2) Subacute Infective (Bacterial) Endocarditis

Cause. The organism is almost always a certain streptococcus, the *Streptococcus viridans*. It almost invariably attacks heart valves and defects which are already abnormal as a result of congenital or rheumatic disease. The focus of infection may be in the teeth or elsewhere in the body. In many cases there is a history of dental sepsis or of recent tooth extraction.

Symptoms. The symptoms tend to be less dramatic than those of acute bacterial endocarditis and may consist merely of vague malaise and mild or intermittent fever. Fatigue, anorexia and joint pains are common symptoms. The spleen is enlarged. Progressive wasting and anaemia are very common. Large emboli are rare but emboli of a size sufficient to block the radial artery are common. Small haemorrhages in the skin and under the nails are frequently seen. Osler's nodes may be seen in the pads of the fingers and toes. They are painful, pink, tender nodules, which may be as large as peas. Clubbing of the fingers is also seen and changing cardiac murmurs are heard. Frank or microscopic haematuria is common and in some cases there is an acute diffuse glomerulonephritis which causes renal failure. The disease may resemble tuberculosis or other disorders causing a low-grade fever. Blood culture enables the diagnosis to be made but the examination may have to be repeated several times before a positive result is obtained. The condition may persist for many months.

Treatment. Penicillin in large doses is required, e.g. 10 to 50 million units daily for 6 weeks or other antibiotic to which the organisms is sensitive. On this regime many patients recover. A destroyed valve, usually the aortic, may be replaced surgically to overcome heart failure.

When dental extraction or surgery is contemplated in cases in which cardiac damage is known to exist it is customary to cover the procedure with a short course of antibiotics.

Congenital heart disease
(Congenital morbus cordis)

The heart develops early in the intra-uterine life of the fetus by a very complicated process from a simple, primitive vascular tube, and any imperfection occurring will result in persistent anatomical changes in the structure of the organ. Some of these abnormalities are so marked that they are incompatible with life and the infant is stillborn or fails to survive for more than a few days. Others are relatively minor in character, such as a small defect in the septum between the right and left atria or ventricles. These may cause no symptoms and may only be detected by careful examination or at post mortem.

An intermediate group of cases occurs in which the individual survives infancy but may not reach adult life. In these the signs and symptoms may be well marked. They vary according to the site and degree of the lesion but may be divided into two main groups:

1. Those without cyanosis (acyanotic).
2. Those with cyanosis (cyanotic).

Dyspnoea on exertion may be a feature of both types, but in the cyanotic variety marked clubbing of the fingers and toes, and delayed growth are often present. (Clubbing consists of a bulbous enlargement of the terminal phalanges.) These features are commonly detected a few weeks after birth (blue babies), but may be delayed for some years. Associated with the cyanosis, which is due to insufficient blood reaching the lungs to become oxygenated, there is usually a considerable increase in the number of red blood corpuscles called polycythaemia (e.g. 6 to 10 million per cubic millimetre instead of 5 million).

The commonest variety of cyanotic congenital heart disease is Fallot's tetralogy which consists of:

(*a*) pulmonary artery stenosis.

(*b*) a defect in the interventricular septum (a 'hole in the heart').

(*c*) hypertrophy of the right ventricle.

(*d*) displacement of the aortic orifice.

Such individuals may die from heart failure or as the result of intercurrent infection. In other cases bacterial (infective) endocarditis may develop.

A serious cyanotic type occurs in the newborn in which the pulmonary artery arises from the left ventricle and the aorta from the right ('Transposition of the great vessels').

Sometimes the heart is reversed in its position in the body so that the apex is situated in the right side of the thorax (*dextrocardia*), a condition which is generally discovered accidentally and produces no symptoms. It is occasionally associated with transposition of the abdominal viscera, e.g. the appendix is situated in the left iliac fossa.

In congenital heart disease diagnostic information is often obtained by cardiac catheterization and angiocardiography (page 101).

The treatment of congenital heart disease is sometimes limited to protecting the patient from cold and infection and preventing over-exertion. Certain cases are, however, suitable for surgical operation. This may consist of joining a large systemic artery (the subclavian) to the pulmonary artery, thus allowing additional blood to reach the lungs, or division of a narrowed pulmonary valve by the passage of a suitable cutting instrument through the walls of the right ventricle. With modern surgical technique and anaesthetic methods this procedure is not unduly dangerous. In successful cases cyanosis becomes less or disappears, the exercise tolerance increases and those children who habitually adopt a squatting attitude are able to get about.

Operations are also performed to close atrial and ventricular septal defects.

Total correction of Fallot's tetralogy is now possible in either one or two stages, using the heart–lung bypass technique.

The more usual types of acyanotic congenital heart defects which may be treated surgically include:

1. Patent interatrial or interventricular septa.

2. Patent ductus arteriosus.

3. Pulmonary stenosis.

4. Coarctation of the aorta.

Disease of the arteries

Considerable confusion exists in the description of arterial disease and it is quite common for any chronic disease of the arteries to be called arterio-

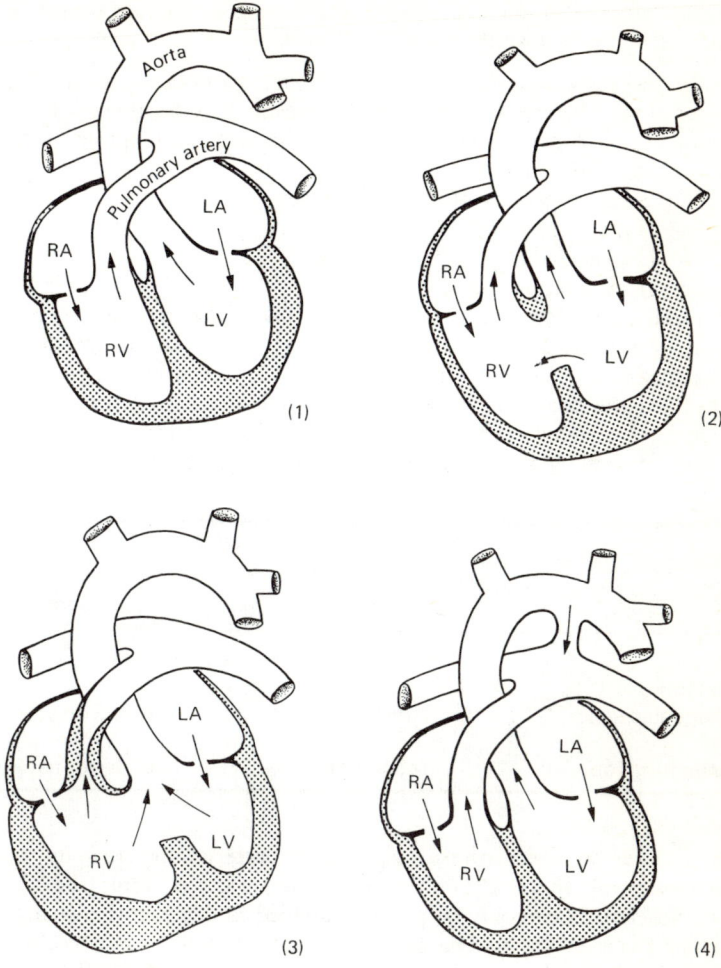

Fig. 21 Diagram illustrating: (1) Normal heart. (2) Patent interventricular septum. (3) Fallot's tetralogy. (4) Patent ductus arteriosus.

sclerosis—a term meaning hardening of the arteries, without any reference to the pathological process which may be responsible for the condition.

The structure of the arteries is essentially the same as that of the heart. There is an outer fibrous coat (adventitia) which may be taken as corresponding with the pericardium. A middle layer containing elastic tissue and muscle fibres is known as the media. The inner layer or intima is the lining membrane and is analogous to the endocardium.

In the present account the outer lining requires no further consideration. The media and intima, however, may be affected by the same types of pathological process as the heart although the actual causes are different.

The main affections of the arteries are:

(*a*) Hypertrophy and dilatation.

(*b*) Degeneration.

(*c*) Inflammation (acute or chronic).

We may, therefore, speak of arterial hypertrophy, arterial degeneration or arterial inflammation (arteritis). If the inflammation affects the media the term mesarteritis is used. If the intima is primarily involved the condition is referred to as endarteritis. Arterial dilatation is considered separately in connection with aneurysm.

The following plan may help to classify these conditions:

	Involvement of:	
	Media	Intima
Hypertrophy	Arterial hypertrophy	
Dilatation	Aneurysm	
Degeneration	Arteriosclerosis	Arteriosclerosis (Atheroma)
Inflammation	Mesarteritis	Endarteritis

It should be clear from this, that in arterial hypertrophy and aneurysm all the coats of the artery are affected, while the term arteriosclerosis can only be properly applied to degenerative changes taking place in the middle and inner coats. It will be noticed, also, that the term atheroma is used when degeneration only affects the inner coat.

With the exception of acute arteritis the diseases are chronic.

Arterial hypertrophy. This condition occurs in association with high blood pressure.

Arteriosclerosis. The hardening of the arteries is due to the deposit of lime salts, especially in the middle coat. It is a form of degeneration which, in addition to occurring alone, may also affect arteries subject to hypertrophy. It is for this reason that arteriosclerosis and high blood pressure are so often referred to together.

Atheroma. Degeneration occurs primarily in the intima. This affects particularly the aorta and coronary arteries and tends to increase with advancing age. It consists of the deposit of lime salts in patches or plaques, which may break down to form ulcers. In addition, part of a plaque may become detached and, being in the bloodstream, constitute an embolus.

Atheroma is associated in some cases with a high blood cholesterol and the intake of an excess of animal fats.

The term **atherosclerosis** is sometimes used to describe atheromatous degeneration.

Arteriosclerosis and atheroma may be generalized or may be especially marked in certain arteries.

In cerebral atherosclerosis, when the arteries of the brain are affected, the main symptoms are giddiness, loss of memory, and mental changes. These may be followed by cerebral thrombosis and haemorrhage.

Involvement of the renal vessels occurs in hypertensive renal disease (page 341).

The coronary arteries which supply the heart may also be affected. Clotting of blood may also occur in these arteries producing the condition known as coronary thrombosis.

Mesarteritis. When inflammation of the middle wall of the artery is due to *syphilis*, the aorta and arteries of the brain are most likely to be affected. In *polyarteritis nodosa*, in which there are multiple nodules on the small arteries, sometimes a finding in hypertension.

Endarteritis. The process of chronic inflammation of the intima produces a generalized thickening of this membrane in the part affected. This results in narrowing of the lumen of the artery so that the quantity of blood which can pass through it is diminished.

Thrombo-angiitis obliterans (Buerger's disease)

In this condition, diseased sections of arteries are separated by normal sections. The intima is thickened and thrombus forms in the lumen. Inflammatory cells infiltrate all three coats of the artery. In addition to arterial changes, the veins are also affected. The main symptoms are coldness and numbness in the extremities and the development of **intermittent claudication,** that is pain and cramps in the muscles on exertion which subsides with rest. It may lead to gangrene which may require amputation. Excessive tobacco consumption appears to be a causative factor.

Giant-cell arteritis (cranial arteritis, temporal arteritis) is a disease of elderly people. All layers of the affected arterial walls are inflamed and there are giant cells in the media. Severe headache is often the main symptom and the temporal arteries may be palpably thickened and tender. Thrombosis of the central retinal artery may occur, resulting in permanent blindness; the early administration of corticosteroids may prevent this.

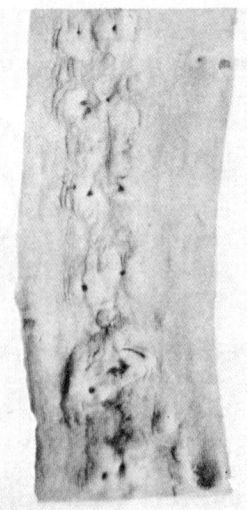

Fig. 22 Atheroma of the aorta.

Clinically, the effect of arterial disease may be summarized thus.

Main Vessels Involved	Results
Cerebral vessels	Apoplexy or stroke (cerebral thrombosis or haemorrhage).
Cardiac vessels (coronary arteries)	Coronary thrombosis, myocardial degeneration often leading to heart failure.
Kidney vessels	Renal failure and uraemia.
Peripheral vessels	Gangrene.

Hypertension (high blood pressure)

This condition is also spoken of as hypertension or hyperpiesis. It is relatively common and cases may be divided into 2 groups:

1. Essential hypertension.
2. Secondary hypertension.

Either type may be *benign* or *malignant*.

1. The term essential hypertension is used because the causes are not fully understood and may possibly vary in different cases. Heredity plays a major part in its development and there is frequently a family history of high blood pressure, strokes or coronary thrombosis.

In the early stages there is some general spasm of the arteries; later actual degenerative changes take place in their walls and arteriosclerosis occurs. Eventually the prolonged hypertension causes a strain on the heart which has to pump harder in order to maintain an adequate circulation against the resistance of the narrowed arteries. The heart tends to hypertrophy, especially the left ventricle, but ultimately may not be able to stand up to the strain so that, following the development of **hypertensive heart disease**, congestive heart failure may ensue.

2. By secondary hypertension is meant that there is an underlying condition. A temporary rise in blood pressure occurs in acute nephritis. This usually falls to normal as recovery takes place, but may become permanent in some cases of chronic nephritis and other types of kidney disease, including pyelonephritis and chronic obstruction to the urinary outflow caused by enlargement of the prostate gland. The blood pressure is also raised in toxaemia of pregnancy, when albuminuria also indicates that the kidneys are affected. This hypertension may persist after delivery. Hypertension may also occur when the intracranial pressure is raised, e.g. cerebral tumour or haemorrhage within the skull. This is a compensatory mechanism whereby the heart by raising the blood pressure endeavours to maintain the circulation to the vital centres in the brain.

There are also a number of causes of secondary hypertension which may be relieved by surgery. These include coarctation of the aorta, renal artery stenosis, unilateral chronic pyelonephritis, tumours of the adrenal cortex (Cushing's syndrome and Conn's syndrome) and a tumour of the adrenal medulla (phaeochromocytoma).

Malignant hypertension is an advanced phase of hypertension characterized by a high diastolic blood pressure (usually over 130 mm Hg) and papilloedema. Untreated it runs a rapid and progressive course usually leading to death within 1 year. There are degenerative changes in the retina which lead to failure of vision. Albuminuria is present. There is often severe headache and cerebral attacks with convulsions or paralysis may occur. The urgent use of hypotensive drugs is indicated.

In hypertension both the systolic and diastolic pressures are raised and readings between 180/100 and 250/150 millimetres of mercury are not uncommon.

The seriousness of hypertension is generally assessed by considering the diastolic pressure rather than the systolic.

Symptoms. The symptoms of essential hypertension are variable. They may be entirely absent and the individual may live to old age without being aware that the blood pressure is raised. In many cases, therefore, it may not be wise to let patients know too much about their blood pressure lest they worry about it and become overanxious and introspective. Others, however, suffer from a sensation of fullness and throbbing in the head, headache, giddiness, insomnia and palpitation.

The effects of high blood pressure and the associated arterial degeneration are, however, very important. In addition to the possible development of hypertensive heart disease and failure already mentioned, cerebral thrombosis or cerebral haemorrhage leading to hemiplegia or death may occur. In some cases there may be hypertensive cerebral attacks which are associated with loss of consciousness, convulsions and temporary paralysis. There may be evidence of chronic kidney disease with albuminuria and, finally, renal failure. In these cases it is sometimes difficult to say whether the hypertension has caused the renal disease or whether it is due to the presence of pre-existing chronic nephritis, i.e. secondary hypertension.

Treatment. 1. *General.* It has been pointed out that great care should be taken not to over-emphasize or even comment on the presence of hypertension, in order to avoid causing the patient anxiety and mental tension which, in themselves, are contributory causes. Further, in many cases, high blood pressure may persist for a long time without producing symptoms or complications, or any interference with an individual's normal activity.

The key-note of case management is moderation in all things, with adequate rest and freedom from mental strain. Provided there is no serious heart trouble, moderate exercise is beneficial.

2. *Diet*. In the past, considerable emphasis was placed on dietetic restrictions but, provided the patient is not obese and does not over-eat, an ordinary diet can be taken in most cases. There is, however, some advantage in giving a low salt, reducing diet to those who are grossly over-weight until they have resumed normal proportions. The consumption of alcohol and tobacco should be strictly moderate. The bowels should be kept regular with simple aperients or liquid paraffin, if necessary, and straining at stool should be avoided.

3. *Drugs*. There are no drugs which can be regarded as curative.

(*a*) A tranquillizer may be all that is required in mild cases.

(*b*) *Rauwolfia* and its alkaloid reserpine ('Serpasil'—0·5 mg daily in divided doses) has a relatively mild hypotensive effect. It appears to act on the centres in the brain which control blood pressure but it is little used now because of its tendency to cause suicidal depression.

(*c*) *Diuretics* such as chlorothiazide, chlorthalidone ('Hygroton') and clorexolone ('Nefrolan') alone reduce blood pressure to acceptable levels in some cases. Provided a potassium supplement is given, these drugs are usually free from harmful effects which are liable to occur with more potent antihypertensive agents. A thiazide combined with a potassium salt (e.g. 'Navidrex-K', 'Neo-Naclex-K') is commonly used.

(*d*) *Ganglion-blocking agents*. These drugs are very powerful and their use is limited to selected cases. They act on the ganglia of the autonomic nervous system and block the nervous impulses to the arterioles which cause vasoconstriction. The consequent dilatation reduces peripheral resistance and thus lowers the blood pressure. Other nerve impulses transmitted through the ganglia may also be affected so that side effects may occur. These include dry mouth, blurred vision, constipation and possibly, with high dosage, paralytic ileus which is a dangerous condition the risk of which can be avoided if regular aperients are taken. In some cases difficulty in micturition or even impotence may occur. When adjusting the dosage for individual patients frequent blood pressure readings are necessary. They should be made while the patient is standing up, which affords a lower reading than when they are lying down. If the recumbent reading is relied on the patient may have a syncopal attack on rising (postural hypotension).

Examples of oral forms of these drugs are mecamylamine ('Inversine'), bretylium ('Darenthin') and pempidine ('Perolysen'). Ganglion-blocking agents are now used mainly for their rapid and powerful effect in hypertensive emergencies. For this purpose, pentolinium ('Ansolysen') or trimetaphan ('Arfonad') is given by injection.

(*e*) *Adrenergic-blocking agents,* i.e. drugs which interfere with nerve impulses in the fibres which supply the arterioles, e.g. guanethidine ('Ismelin'), guanoxan ('Envacar'), bethanidine ('Esbatal') and debrisoquine ('Declinax'). Postural hypotension is often the most troublesome unwanted effect and necessitates reduction of dosage.

(*f*) *Methyldopa* ('Aldomet') which has a complex action but is very effective and useful.

(*g*) *Clonidine* ('Catapres') acts both centrally and peripherally. In lesser dosage it is also used to prevent attacks of migraine.

(*h*) *Beta-receptor blocking agents* such as propranolol ('Inderal') and oxprenolol ('Trasicor 80 mg') sometimes produce useful falls of blood pressure without notable side-effects. They are, however, contraindicated in patients with bronchial asthma or heart failure, which they tend to make worse.

(*i*) *Diazoxide* ('Eudemine') is useful by intravenous injection for the rapid reduction of blood pressure. It may also be given as a tablet for maintenance therapy but may cause hyperglycaemia.

It is important to remember that diuretics such as chlorothiazide increase considerably the effect of hypotensive drugs, the dose of which may have to be halved when they are given together.

Summary

Blood pressure is maintained by:
1. The force of the heart beat.
2. Resistance to the blood flow in the peripheral arteries.
3. The elasticity of the arteries.
4. The total amount of circulating blood.

High blood pressure, e.g. 180/100 to 250/150 mm of mercury.

Types: 1. Essential hypertension.

Causes: (*a*) Heredity.

(*b*) Prolonged anxiety or mental strain.

(*c*) Arterial degeneration.

2. Secondary hypertension.

Causes: (*a*) Chronic renal disease,

e.g., nephritis,

prostatic obstruction.

(*b*) Raised intracranial pressure,

e.g., cerebral haemorrhage,

cerebral tumour.

(c) Metabolic or endocrine diseases,
e.g., Cushing's syndrome,
phaeochromocytoma.
(d) Toxaemia of pregnancy.
3. Physiological or temporary rise in blood pressure due to excitement or emotion.

Results of hypertension:
1. Arterial degeneration.
2. Hypertensive heart disease:
    (a) atrial fibrillation,
    (b) congestive heart failure,
    (c) myocardial infarction ('coronary thrombosis').
3. Hypertensive cerebral attacks.
4. Cerebral haemorrhage and thrombosis.
5. Chronic renal damage (hypertensive renal disease).

Treatment:
1. Moderation in diet and exercise.
2. Reducing, low-salt diet for the obese.
3. Hypotensive drugs including diuretics.

Low blood pressure (hypotension)

This is a manifestation of some underlying condition and not, in itself, a disease.

It may be due to damage to the heart muscle whereby the force of cardiac contraction is weakened, e.g. acute myocarditis and toxic conditions such as enteric fever, diphtheria and pneumonia, in which acute poisoning of the heart muscle takes place, and in chronic myocardial degeneration, coronary thrombosis and some cases of valvular diseases. It is seen in certain disorders of the ductless glands, in particular, a disease of the suprarenals known as Addison's disease (p. 462). General disturbances of the circulation by severe haemorrhage, surgical shock, dehydration, and drug overdosage, are also temporarily associated with low blood pressure. Diseases (such as diabetes mellitus and neurosyphilis) affecting the autonomic nervous system may cause postural hypotension.

The main symptoms are general weakness, faintness, especially on adopting the upright posture, giddiness and mental depression, which can largely be accounted for by a deficiency of the blood supply to the brain.

In acute hypotension the patient should be placed in the supine position and it may help if the foot of the bed is elevated. If there is hypovolaemia (an abnormally low blood volume), intravenous fluids should be given. High doses of corticosteroids (e.g. hydrocortisone) may be required, especially if there is evidence of adrenal failure.

Acute hypotensive states may require treatment with a slow intravenous drip containing noradrenaline or by injections of mephentermine ('Mephine') or metaraminol ('Aramine'). These are contra-indicated in the presence of haemorrhage in which event blood transfusion is the treatment of choice.

Disease of the coronary arteries
(Ischaemic heart disease)

The heart muscle receives its blood supply from the coronary arteries (left and right) which are the first branches of the aorta. As age advances, these arteries, like the other arteries of the body, are liable to be affected by atheroma or arteriosclerosis so that the walls become thickened and the lumen narrowed. This results in a diminished blood supply and lack of oxygen to the heart muscle which may lead to myocardial degeneration and, finally, to congestive heart failure. In addition, two other important conditions may occur as a result of coronary artery disease, viz.:

1. Angina pectoris.
2. Coronary artery thrombosis (myocardial infarction).

Angina pectoris

Angina pectoris is a symptom characterized by sudden attacks of severe pain behind the sternum and perhaps in the left arm, some-times associated with a sensation of impending death.

It occurs mostly in men over the age of 40. Important factors in its production are heredity, hypertension, diabetes mellitus, gout, hyper-lipoproteinaemia (an excess of fat in the blood), smoking, lack of exercise and obesity. These conditions may be described as **predisposing causes.**

The actual factors which determine the onset of an attack, the **exciting causes,** are sudden exertion or emotion or chilling. For example, an individual subject to the condition is liable to have an attack if he hurries to catch a train after a heavy meal, or walks rapidly uphill against a cold wind. The sight of a serious accident or an outburst of temper may also precipitate an attack. It is therefore referred to as *angina of effort*, although in severe cases it does not require much activity to bring on the pain.

The actual pain is caused by inability of the coronary arteries to convey blood to meet the extra requirements of the heart resulting from the sudden effort. In other words there is a discrepancy between the work of the myocardium and the available supply of oxygen. Something of the nature of a cramp occurs in the temporarily exhausted heart muscle, which results in pain. It is situated behind the sternum and frequently radiates into the left side of the neck, the left shoulder and may extend down the left arm. Occasionally, it spreads to the right side. It is accompanied by a feeling of tightness in the chest and a sense of suffocation.

The patient stops and rests until the pain passes off, which it usually does in a few minutes.

Treatment. During an attack the patient should be allowed to remain at rest.

The drug which is generally used is glyceryl trinitrate (trinitrin). It is given in the form of tablets (0·5 mg, gr $\frac{1}{130}$), but it is essential for these to be retained under the tongue or chewed slowly and retained in the mouth, for the absorption of the drug takes place from the mucous membrane of the mouth. It is without effect if it is swallowed. It is, therefore, very important that the nurse should instruct the patient accordingly. Long-acting types of glyceryl trinitrate which may be swallowed include 'Sustac' but these are for prevention of attacks and not for treatment of an attack of angina. A more rapidly acting remedy preferred by a few patients is amyl nitrite; 0·3 ml are contained in a small glass capsule covered with linen. The glass is crushed between the fingers and the vapour inhaled. The effect is usually immediate but of short duration. Several capsules may be required.

These drugs dilate the blood vessels and their administration may be followed by flushing of the face and throbbing of the arteries.

It is advisable, therefore, for all patients who suffer from angina pectoris to carry a supply of tablets of glyceryl trinitrate or amyl nitrite capsules with them wherever they go.

Between attacks, the general health must receive attention and any anaemia should be treated. Weight reduction may be desirable and smoking should be curtailed. The patient should be instructed to avoid sudden effort and to regulate his life within the limits of the heart's strength.

Regular administration of a beta-blocking agent benefits many patients. It prevents angina by slowing the heart rate and by increasing the efficiency with which the heart uses oxygen. Available agents include propranolol ('Inderal'), practolol ('Eraldin') and oxprenolol ('Trasicor'). Beta-blockade may make bronchial asthma and heart failure worse. An alternative drug is prenylamine ('Synadrin 60'), 60 mg 3 times a day, but this too may be contra-indicated in patients with severe heart failure.

Intractable angina may be treated by inserting vein grafts between the aorta and one or more of the coronary arteries, bypassing the narrowed portions. A length of the patient's long saphenous vein is usually used for the purpose.

A condition known as false angina (**pseudo-angina**) is more common in women and is associated with flatulent dyspepsia, effort not being a factor in its production. There is some pain in the region of the heart, palpitation and a feeling of faintness. The pain is not severe. There is no cardiac damage nor risk of death. The patient, as a rule, is agitated and active and of a neurotic temperament. She must be reassured after investigation to exclude an organic lesion. Hot water, peppermint or some other carminative are useful during the attack.

Myocardial infarction (coronary thrombosis)

The myocardium receives its blood supply from the coronary arteries. Coronary thrombosis means that a blood clot has developed in one of the branches of a coronary artery, the walls of which are roughened by disease or degeneration. When this happens the lumen of the artery becomes blocked and an area of heart muscle will be deprived of its normal blood supply and will undergo degenerative changes; finally, if the patient recovers from the acute attack, a fibrous scar will be formed in the affected area.

Myocardial infarction is a fairly common condition, especially in males over the age of 40, and occurs as a result of atheroma of the walls of the artery. The victim may or may not have previously suffered from angina pectoris.

Retrosternal pain characteristically starts at rest and may be very severe. It may spread to the neck, arms and epigastrium, when it may resemble gall-bladder disease or other abdominal conditions. The pain usually lasts much longer than angina. Dyspnoea, cyanosis, sweating, vomiting and irregularities of the pulse, e.g. ventricular premature beats, atrial fibrillation may be present. The blood pressure may fall and in some cases the degree of shock is severe and the patient may become unconscious. A rise in temperature is commonly seen for a few days and pericardial friction may develop. Changes in the electro-cardiogram help to confirm the diagnosis. The serum transaminase

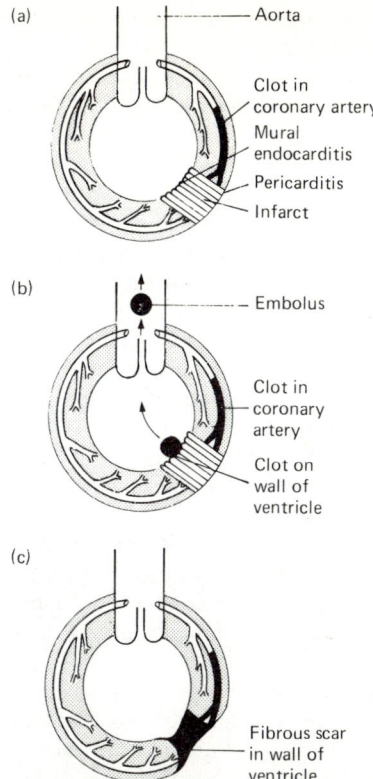

(a) Aorta

Clot in
coronary artery

Mural
endocarditis

Pericarditis

Infarct

(b) Embolus

Clot in
coronary
artery

Clot on
wall of
ventricle

(c)

Fibrous scar
in wall of
ventricle

Fig. 23 Diagram illustrating coronary artery thrombosis. (*a*) Formation of infarct;
(*b*) formation of mural clot and embolus; (*c*) formation of scar in wall of ventricle.

(SGOT) and sedimentation rate (ESR) are raised and there may be a
leucocytosis during the first few days.

Progress and complications

1. Sometimes very mild attacks occur which may be overlooked
and only detected later when an electrocardiogram has been taken.
    Painless infarction is not uncommon in the elderly.

2. A very extensive or critically placed thrombosis may lead to
sudden death.

3. Congestive heart failure may develop and may be associated
with atrial fibrillation. Other disorders of cardiac rhythm, including
ventricular fibrillation, may occur, especially during the first 48 hours.

4. If the infarct involves the whole thickness of the wall of the

heart this may later rupture and sudden death occur with haemorrhage into the pericardial sac.

5. An infarct involving the inner part of the heart muscle may cause roughening of the endocardium. A further clot may then develop on the wall of one of the chambers of the heart (mural clot). This clot may subsequently become detached, pass along in the general circulation forming an embolus which, if derived from the left side of the heart, may lodge in the cerebral arteries causing a stroke with hemiplegia, or in a vessel in one of the limbs which may cause gangrene. If such a clot comes from the right side of the heart it will produce pulmonary embolism. Pulmonary emboli may also have their origin in the leg veins as a result of immobilization.

Death may occur very rapidly or else, after gradual convalescence, the patient may recover. Recurrences are not uncommon but may be delayed for many years.

Treatment. The majority of acute cases are best treated in the first instance in a coronary care unit in which the cardiac rhythm can be monitored on an ECG oscilloscope.

The patient is placed in bed in a comfortable position. Strenuous exertion and anxiety must be avoided. A light but nutritious diet is given and the bowels are kept comfortably open to avoid straining. (**N.B.**—A bedside commode has advantages over the bedpan if the patient is not hypotensive.

In an uncomplicated case, the patient may start to sit out in a chair after 24 hours and may be discharged home ambulant within 2 weeks. Severe hypotension, serious arrhythmias or cardiac failure necessitate a longer period in bed and in hospital.

The main aspects of treatment are:

1. Morphine or similar analgesic for pain, oxygen for cyanosis and dyspnoea.

2. Shock: Intravenous nor-adrenaline or metaraminol ('Aramine') or intramuscular mephentermine ('Mephine'). However, these drugs may be positively harmful and should be generally avoided. They raise blood pressure by constricting the arterioles and the distressed heart is made to work harder in order to overcome the resistance in the constricted vessels.

3. Arrhythmias: Lignocaine or direct current electric shock may be required. Heart block is treated preferably with an artificial pacemaker.

4. Prevention of deep venous thrombosis and subsequent embolism, especially from leg veins, by early mobilization or the use of anticoagulants.

Anticoagulant drugs, i.e. heparin, phenindione ('Dindevan'), warfarin sodium ('Marevan') or similar drugs, are used in some cases to prevent extension of the clotting and to minimize the risk of embolism. The administration and dosage of 'Dindevan' is controlled by estimation of the prothrombin level. Some patients are given 'long-term anticoagulant therapy' for many months or even years with a view to preventing a further thrombosis. Some authorities, however, are not in favour of using anticoagulants partly because these drugs may themselves cause serious symptoms from over-dosage and partly because many cases do very well without them.

N.B.—Trinitrin and amyl nitrite generally have no effect on the pain in this condition because the artery is already completely blocked by clot and a vasodilator drug will not increase the blood supply to the damaged muscle. Digitalis should only be used with great care in recent cardiac infarction for fear of inducing ventricular premature beats and ventricular fibrillation.

5. Rest: as indicated above. Convalescence should be slow and the average patient should be off work for 3 months.

The following table illustrates the main points of difference between coronary thrombosis and angina pectoris, but the diagnosis is usually confirmed by the electrocardiogram.

	Angina Pectoris	Coronary Thrombosis
Onset	With effort	At rest.
Character of pain	Paroxysmal.	Continuous.
Duration of attack	Seconds or minutes.	Hours or days.
Patient	Remains still.	Often restless.
Blood pressure	Rises.	Falls.
Pulse	Regular.	Sometimes irregular.
Vomiting	Uncommon.	Common.
SGOT and ESR	Normal.	Raised.
Treatment	Amyl nitrite, or Glyceryl trinitrate.	Morphine. Anticoagulants. Amyl nitrite has no effect.

Aneurysm

An aneurysm is a localized and persistent dilatation of an artery resulting from disease or injury to its wall. A common cause of aneurysm used to be syphilis, which has already been described as producing inflammation of the middle coat of arteries (mesarteritis). However, as syphilis is now less common and more efficiently treated, arteriosclerosis is the most frequent cause. The elastic tissue and the muscle fibres of the middle coat being damaged, the wall of the artery is unable to support the pressure of blood within it, and progressive dilatation takes place in the diseased area. In this way a tumour, pulsating with each beat of the heart, is formed.

Aneurysms are divided according to their shape into two types:

The fusiform type consists of a uniform dilatation of the whole circumference of the vessel; the saccular forming a globular projection from one side of the artery and connected to it by a constricted portion or neck.

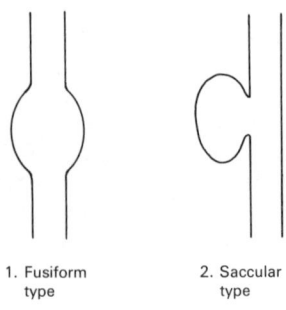

1. Fusiform
type

2. Saccular
type

The commonest position for an aneurysm to develop is the thoracic aorta where it may be demonstrated by means of x-rays. Other sites are the abdominal aorta, the innominate, carotid, popliteal and subclavian arteries, and arteries of the brain (congenital intracranial aneurysm, which is responsible for subarachnoid haemorrhage, p. 401).

Aneurysm of the aorta. Aneurysm of the thoracic aorta may develop in the ascending aorta, the arch or in the descending portion and is an important medical condition.

From the point of view of symptoms the condition must be regarded as a tumour occurring in the thorax which produces its effects as a result of pressure on surrounding structures.

(1) Pressure on the thoracic walls. An aneurysm occurring in the posterior part of the thorax will exert continuous pressure on the vertebrae, which eventually results in the wearing away of the bone. If situated anteriorly, the sternum and ribs are eroded, and a pulsating swelling appears on the front of the chest (Fig. 24).

(2) Pressure on the thoracic contents. The important structures within the thorax which may be compressed by an

aneurysm are the trachea and bronchi and the oesophagus. Pressure on the former produces dyspnoea and a harsh, noisy (brassy) cough; on the latter, difficulty in swallowing.

(3) Pressure on the nerves. This produces pain.

The common symptoms of thoracic aneurysm may therefore be summarized as:

Pain in the chest or back; brassy cough and dyspnoea; difficulty in swallowing; the formation of a pulsating swelling in the later stages.

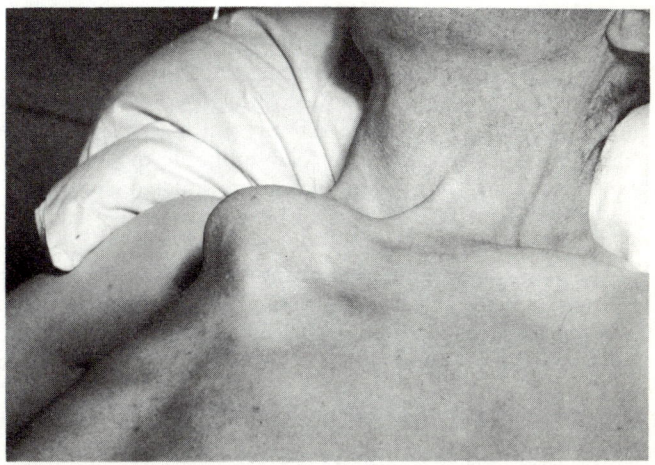

Fig. 24 Aortic aneurysm eroding the sternum.

Results. In rare cases clotting occurs in the sac and the aneurysm undergoes spontaneous cure. Sometimes the walls of the aneurysm eventually rupture and sudden, fatal haemorrhage takes place into the oesophagus, the trachea, pericardium or pleural cavity.

Treatment. A Wasserman test is performed. If the aneurysm is due to syphilis this condition must be treated by a course of penicillin. The risk of a serious (Herxheimer) reaction is small.

Aneurysms occurring in the arteries of the limbs produce pulsating swellings. They are treated by surgical means; if possible, the vessel being ligatured above and below the aneurysm.

It is sometimes possible to excise an aneurysm and to restore the lumen of the vessel by bridging the defect with a graft of either living or synthetic material, e.g. Dacron.

Syphilis of the circulatory system

The principal effects of syphilis on the heart and blood vessels are: disease of the aortic valves, disease of the mouths of the coronary arteries, disease of the bundle of His producing heart block, and aneurysm.

Diseases of the veins

Varicose veins

This condition is most often seen in the leg veins, which become dilated and tortuous. It is probably due to a congenital deficiency of the valves and muscular tissue in the walls of the veins and may be aggravated by any conditions interfering with proper venous return (tight garters, tumours, pregnancy and prolonged standing).

The chronic congestion of the skin present may result in pigmentation and in the formation of a scaly eruption known as varicose eczema. In long-standing cases ulceration situated just above the ankle is common. Such ulcers may be very extensive and encircle the whole limb.

Varicose veins may rupture, causing severe haemorrhage which, as a rule, is easily controlled by pressure on the bleeding point or by simple elevation of the limb until a pressure pad and bandage can be applied to the bleeding point. They are frequently the seat of phlebitis and thrombosis.

Treatment. In mild cases, relief may be obtained by wearing elastic stockings and by avoiding long standing.

A common method of treatment is to inject the vein with a preparation such as ethanolamine, which causes the blood to clot in the vessel, thereby producing an artificial thrombosis which obliterates completely its lumen. Modern injection therapy (sclerotherapy) aims to obliterate some of the communicating veins which are transmitting high pressure from the deep veins to the superficial veins. After injection, a pressure pad of sponge rubber is applied over the injection site and the leg is firmly bandaged and clothed in an elastic stocking. The patient is instructed to walk at least 3 miles a day with the bandages and stockings on. The treatment is known as *injection-compression sclerotherapy*. Excision or ligature of varicose veins by surgical means is often performed.

Varicose (gravitational) ulcers are best treated initially by bed rest so that the knee is higher than the heart. Infection may be treated with antibiotics either locally or by systemic administration after identification of the organism. Local dressings are necessary

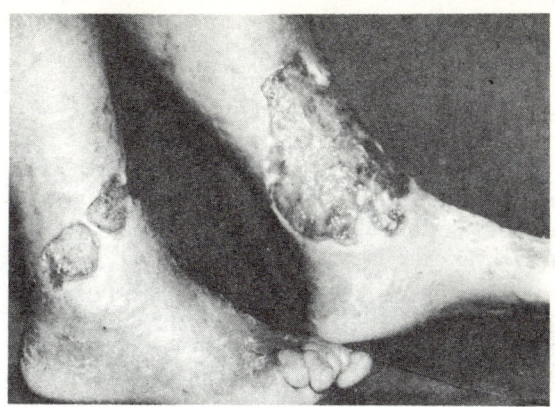

Fig. 25 Varicose (gravitational) ulcers.

and may be supported by firm rubberized bandages, which permit ambulation. Skin grafting may subsequently be possible in some cases.

Phlebitis is inflammation of a vein. Although it can occur elsewhere, it is most common in the legs and may affect either the superficial veins under the skin or the deep veins of the part. Varicose veins are often the site of phlebitis, or it may arise as a result of infection or minor injury. The vein, if accessible, is felt as a hard, tender cord over which the skin is hot and dusky in appearance.

The inflammation causes roughening of the inner lining or intima of the vein at the site of which the blood may commence to clot and thus the process of thrombophlebitis develops.

Thrombosis

Thrombosis is the term applied to clotting of blood within the heart, veins or arteries; the resulting clot being called a thrombus.

Sites. Any part of the cardiovascular system may be affected by thrombosis, but the more common sites are:

Heart	The left atrium in mitral stenosis and atrial fibrillation.
Arteries	Coronary (coronary artery thrombosis, p. 150). Cerebral thrombosis (p. 399).
Veins	Superficial varicose veins of the leg.
	Deep veins of the calf of the leg especially in patients who are confined to bed.

Femoral and iliac veins in pregnancy, typhoid fever and
after abdominal or pelvic operations.
Thrombosis of the portal vein.
Lateral sinus, following mastoiditis.
Cavernous sinus, following sepsis of the face.

Causes. There are a number of factors which either predispose
to or actually cause thrombosis:

1. Damage to the vessel wall and its lining membrane,
phlebitis, injury, bruising or infection, prolonged pressure.

2. Diminished rate of blood flow. This may occur in serious and
debilitating illnesses such as typhoid; prolonged rest in bed with lack
of muscular movement particularly after operations; pressure on the
muscles surrounding the calf vein when lying in bed, especially if
these are flabby and toneless; during pregnancy, when pressure of the
uterus on the pelvic veins may interfere to some extent with the
venous return from the legs.

3. Increased coagulability of the blood, which may result from the
loss of fluid and dehydration associated with diarrhoea, vomiting or
severe haemorrhage.

4. Oral contraceptives containing oestrogens cause changes in
the blood and a significantly increased incidence of thrombo-
embolic disease.

Some examples of these causes have already been mentioned,
including slowing of the circulation of blood in the heart which may
occur in mitral stenosis and atrial fibrillation with the formation of
clots in the left atrium. Disease of the intima of the coronary arteries
(atheroma) is responsible for coronary artery thrombosis.

Symptoms and signs. When thrombosis occurs in the superficial veins of the leg the signs and symptoms are similar to those
of superficial phlebitis, namely pain, tenderness and a thickening of
the vein, together with redness of the skin.

If the deep calf veins are affected, the symptoms are variable. In
some instances the condition may be unsuspected and the first
indication of its occurrence may be a sudden and serious pulmonary
embolism. In others, there may be a slight unexplained rise in
temperature for a few days. Possibly the patient may complain of a
slight or even severe aching in the back of the calf and tenderness
may be elicited on deep palpation. In such instances full dorsiflexion
of the foot may produce pain (Homan's sign).

Progress. Provided the thrombosis does not spread, these
symptoms gradually subside, although sometimes a little oedema of

the ankle may be present. If the thrombosis extends and involves the femoral vein the whole leg may become oedematous ('white leg') and it may be some months before the oedema clears up.

Some clots are firmly adherent to the walls of the vein while others are easily dislodged either in pieces or as a whole, thus constituting emboli. Eventually the clot in a vein may be partly absorbed and partly converted into connective tissue, so that the lumen of the vein becomes open again and the local circulation is restored.

The symptoms and treatment of thrombosis in other parts of the body depends on the site of the lesion.

Treatment. This may be considered under three headings:

1. Prevention.
2. Local treatment.
3. Anticoagulant drugs.
4. Thrombolytic therapy.
5. Thrombectomy.

1. *Prevention.* A nurse can do a great deal to prevent the development of postoperative thrombosis and thrombosis developing in patients who are confined to bed. Whenever possible, postoperative patients are got out of bed as soon as their condition permits. In all other cases regular exercises should be carried out several times a day. Simple massage of the calf muscles is also helpful. Care must be taken not to tuck the bedclothes in so tightly that the patient cannot move his legs easily, and in many cases a bed cradle is useful. A hard bolster under the knees should be avoided as this may cause pressure on the legs and impede the venous return. Breathing exercises are important because the respiratory movements help to maintain the venous return to the heart, thus preventing congestion and diminished blood flow in the peripheral venous circulation. Plenty of fluids should be given, especially if there is any dehydration from diarrhoea or vomiting.

2. *Local treatment.* It is doubtful whether any local treatment influences venous thrombosis. Applications of glycerin of ichthammol may help to relieve pain in superficial thrombophlebitis. Phenylbutazone orally has both an analgesic and anti-inflammatory action.

Sometimes ligation of the vein above a thrombus may be indicated to prevent its spread or embolus formation.

3. *Anticoagulant drugs.* The purpose of these drugs is to prevent further clotting from taking place and thus limiting the spread of the area of thrombosis. They do not 'dissolve' the clot once it has formed.

Heparin is an anticoagulant drug which acts rapidly and is soon eliminated from the system. It is therefore usually given by intravenous injection, 5,000 to 10,000 units every 6 hours. In order to facilitate this a special needle with a non-leaking diaphragm may be left in a vein if desired. Alternatively 1,000 units per hour is given in a saline drip.

If the administration is prolonged the dosage is controlled by estimating the clotting time of the blood. The antidote to overdosage is the intravenous injection of protamine sulphate, 50 mg of which will neutralize the effect of 5,000 units of heparin.

Phenindione ('Dindevan') or similar drugs are given by mouth.

Because there is some delay before these drugs become effective, heparin may be given at the same time for the first 36 hours. Treatment may be continued for several weeks or months.

In anticoagulant therapy the exact daily dosage is controlled by estimations of the prothrombin time. Overdosage with these drugs results in bleeding into the skin and mucous membranes (purpura), the presence of red cells in the urine, vaginal haemorrhage, etc. The treatment is to stop the drug at once and to give blood transfusion and intravenous vitamin K_1 (p. 432).

Anticoagulants may be used in thrombosis of veins of the limbs, and coronary thrombosis, but not usually in cerebral thrombosis.

4. Thrombolytic therapy. This is expensive and hazardous but may result in rapid dissolution of thrombus in veins and of thrombotic emboli in pulmonary arteries. Streptokinase or urokinase is used.

5. Thromboectomy. A thrombus may in some cases be removed surgically by incising the vessel and inserting a special balloon-catheter (Fogarty catheter) which, after inflation, is pulled back together with the thrombus.

Embolism

An embolus is a clot or other abnormal body carried by the blood stream from one situation and forced into another blood vessel so as to obstruct the circulation.

It has been seen how a clot of blood, forming in the heart, may be carried to some other part of the body. In the same way thrombi occurring in other situations such as the femoral vein or deep veins in the calf may become detached from the vessel wall and become emboli. A thrombus is the commonest type of embolus.

Vegetations from diseased valves, especially in bacterial endo-carditis, may break off and enter the circulating blood. Air entering large veins as a result of injury or during operations, and fat particles liberated as the result of fracture of a bone may also act as emboli.

An embolus passing along the blood vessel will eventually come to a place where the channel is too small to allow it to proceed any farther. It will therefore become lodged in this position and will block the vessel, so that no more blood can pass. This results in the cutting off of the blood supply to the affected part which will undergo degenerative changes because its nutrition is disturbed. The lesion thus produced is called an **infarct.**

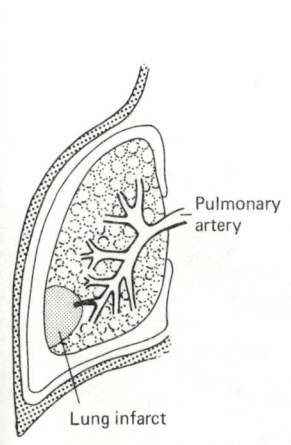

Fig. 26 A small pulmonary embolus has blocked a branch of the pulmonary artery.

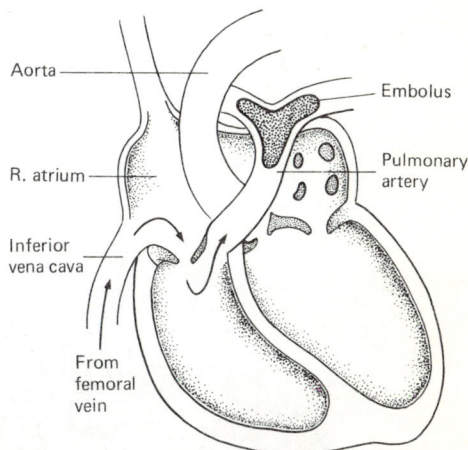

Fig. 27 The main pulmonary artery is blocked by a large clot which has travelled from the leg.

If reference is made to the diagram on p. 120 it will be evident that an embolus starting from the veins of the limbs will reach the right side of the heart and thence pass, via the pulmonary artery, into the lungs (a pulmonary embolism causing an infarct of the lung). On the other hand, an embolus resulting from a clot in the left atrium or a vegetation from the mitral or aortic valve will enter the general arterial system and eventually reach the brain, an artery of the limbs, the kidney, spleen or some other part.

Symptoms. The symptoms of embolism are dependent upon the situation in which the embolus is finally arrested, and are abrupt in onset.

Embolism from the veins and right side of heart

Pulmonary embolism is an important and serious condition. It occurs when an embolus reaches one of the pulmonary arteries or its branches in the lung, either from the general venous circulation, particularly from thrombosis in the deep veins of the calf, or occasionally from the right atrium in atrial fibrillation.

If an embolus is small it will cause no embarrassment to the general circulation but may result in pulmonary infarction. This causes pleuritic pain, which is sharp and is exacerbated by deep

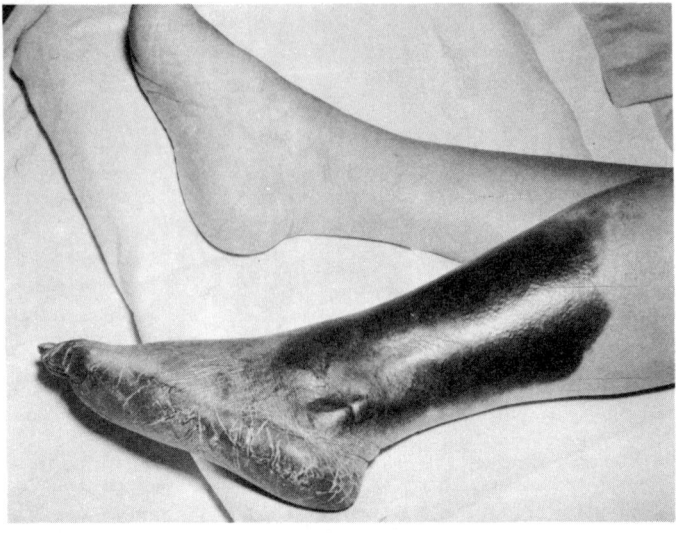

Fig. 28 Spreading gangrene of the foot following embolism of the popliteal artery.

breathing, and often haemoptysis. The chest x-ray usually shows a wedge-shaped opacity, with the base of the wedge at the pleural surface of the lung.

Massive pulmonary embolism is a cause of sudden death, immediately prior to which the patient may experience an urgent desire to defaecate. Classically, the patient asks for a bedpan and falls back dead. Such a sequence is not peculiar to pulmonary embolism, however, and occurs in cases of sudden death due to other causes (p. 500).

Some patients with massive pulmonary embolism survive for several hours and some make a full recovery. The patient experiences the sudden onset of intense dyspnoea and may have central chest pain. The pulse rate rises and the blood pressure falls. The jugular venous pressure rises and a gallop rhythm can be heard on auscultation of the heart. Chest x-rays often show no definite abnormality but an electrocardiogram may indicate right ventricular strain. Lung scanning, using a radioactive tracer, may provide support for the diagnosis but pulmonary arteriography is required for complete confirmation and for precise assessment of the sites and sizes of the embolic fragments.

Pulmonary infarction is treated with analgesics and anticoagulants are administered to prevent further emboli. Massive pulmonary embolism demands treatment with high concentrations of oxygen and sometimes with metaraminol to counteract hypotension. The patient may rapidly deteriorate and die unless pulmonary embolectomy, under cardiopulmonary bypass, is performed. Other patients, whilst having major pulmonary emboli, are less ill and do not require emergency embolectomy. In such patients treatment with streptokinase or urokinase intravenously, or via a catheter in the pulmonary artery, may successfully dissolve the thrombus. Anticoagulants are subsequently administered to prevent further thrombus formation.

Embolism from the left side of the heart

Cerebral embolism. This will result in the sudden onset of paralysis of some part of the body, depending on the area of brain affected, sometimes associated with loss of consciousness (a form of apoplexy). (See also p. 399).

Embolism of a large artery to a limb. Sudden pain in the limb occurs, followed by numbness and loss of power. The pulse below the seat of the embolism disappears and the affected part of the limb becomes cold to the touch. It may be pale at first but later becomes bluish in appearance. The upper limit of discoloration may be clearly defined. Unless the circulation is re-established or the thrombus is removed surgically within a few hours **gangrene** may result.

If the **spleen** is affected there will be pain in the left side associated with enlargement of the organ. Embolism involving a **kidney** is followed by pain in the loin and haematuria. If the emboli are septic and contain micro-organisms, abscesses will be produced where they lodge (a form of pyaemia).

Anticoagulant drugs may be given in some cases in order to prevent further thrombosis.

Types of emboli

Blood clot (thrombus).	Air.
Detached vegetations.	Fat cells.
Atheromatous plaques.	Tumour cells.

Acute rheumatism
(Rheumatic Fever)

Acute rheumatism and chorea may be studied in connection with heart disease because of the frequency with which acute cardiac inflammation and chronic valvular disease supervene in these disorders. In addition, the nursing of these conditions is very largely determined by their liability to cardiac complications.

Definition. Rheumatic fever may be defined as an acute febrile disease characterized by inflammation of joints (multiple or polyarthritis), and a special tendency to endocarditis.

Cause. A full explanation of the cause of the disease is not possible. The joint symptoms are probably an allergic reaction or 'hypersensitivity response' to the antigens of haemolytic streptococci in susceptible individuals, following an infection of the throat. In most instances there has been a recent attack of tonsillitis. It is essentially a disease of children and young adults between the ages of 3 and 20 years and recurrences are not uncommon.

The frequency of its incidence and severity have diminished in recent years.

Symptoms. The onset is usually abrupt with pyrexia and pain in one or more joints, the knees and ankles being the commonest. There is a marked tendency for the pain to wander from joint to joint, the inflammation subsiding in one as it increases in another. The joints are hot, red, swollen and exquisitely painful when touched or moved. Effusion of fluid into the joint occurs but is never followed by suppuration.

The tongue is coated, the pulse rapid and sweating profuse, the sweat having a peculiar 'acid' odour. Occasionally hard, painful, fibrous nodules (rheumatic nodules) may be felt around the joints and over the bony ridges. With treatment, the joint pains and temperature subside, but the liability to complications is not prevented. The blood sedimentation rate (ESR) and antibody (anti-streptolysin O or ASO) titre is raised.

Complications. Nearly half the cases develop some form of heart trouble and this may usually be demonstrated by ECG. Although described as a complication it may be considered as part of the disease. Acute pericarditis, with or without effusion; endocarditis, especially affecting the mitral and aortic valves, and myocarditis may occur after the first week, the onset being accompanied by a further rise in temperature.

The importance of these conditions cannot be over-emphasized as they are responsible for so much chronic heart disease with its crippling effects and ultimate mortality. Other complications include pleurisy, skin eruptions, and, very rarely, hyperpyrexia and delirium which may be fatal.

Rheumatic fever in children. Although the acute type of disease just described affects children as well as adults, the condition is frequently insidious in its onset during childhood and the joint lesions may be slight or overlooked. Some people are found with

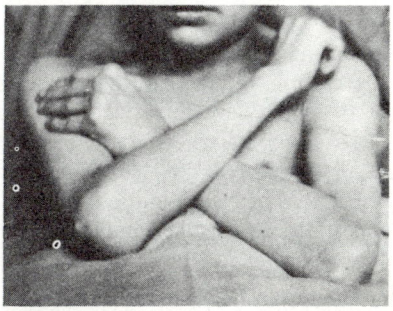

Fig. 29 Rheumatic nodules on both elbows.

obvious cardiac disease of rheumatic origin, in whom there is no history of fever accompanied by swollen joints. The only symptoms which can be remembered may be vague discomfort in the limbs which has been attributed to 'growing pains'.

Since the heart lesions occurring in what may be described as 'sub-acute rheumatism' are just as serious as those produced by acute rheumatic fever, its recognition is of importance. The term 'growing pains' is a very unfortunate one and a misnomer, because growing is not painful. Vague pains are quite common in children and have nothing to do with rheumatism but may be associated with fatigue and postural defects.

The diagnosis of acute rheumatism is usually clear, but occasionally acute osteomyelitis and other conditions may be confused with it. The ultimate prognosis is almost entirely dependent upon the severity of the cardiac lesions. Death during the first attack is very uncommon.

Treatment

The aim of treatment in this condition is twofold:

1. To prevent or limit the extent of the cardiac damage.
2. To relieve the fever and joint pains.

The patient is put to bed in the position of maximum comfort, usually sitting up with pillows and back-rest. Rest in bed is continued until temperature, sleeping pulse rate and blood sedimentation rate have returned to normal.

The affected joints should be placed and supported in the most comfortable position. They may be wrapped in cotton-wool or methyl salicylate liniment may be applied on lint, and the weight of the bed-clothes supported by a cradle.

While the acute symptoms remain a light diet, with milk as a basis, is given. This is gradually increased.

Aperients are given as required. The drugs universally employed in the treatment of rheumatic fever are **salicylates** (either sodium salicylate or aspirin). These have the effect of reducing pyrexia and, if given in adequate doses, of relieving the joint symptoms within 48 hours. So markedly specific is their action that, if a patient suffering from acute arthritis with fever is not considerably improved after this period, the condition is almost certainly not rheumatic fever. The dosage is regulated according to the age of the patient and the administration evenly distributed throughout the 24 hours. In a few instances the drugs produce toxic symptoms which it is important for the nurse to recognize and report to the medical attendant. These include headache, deafness, tinnitus (ringing noises in the head), general depression or mild delirium and occasionally vomiting, with an increase in temperature while the joint pains are subsiding. (See also page 529.)

The administration of salicylate is generally continued in reduced doses for some weeks after the subsidence of fever and joint pains, in order to prevent their recurrence. It is unlikely that the drug diminishes the cardiac complications.

The general management of cases with cardiac complications has been discussed in dealing with the treatment of acute endocarditis and pericarditis (pp. 112, 108), the essential point being prolonged rest. Hyperpyrexia is treated by cold sponging. Penicillin is given to destroy streptococci in the nose and throat.

Small daily doses of sulphonamide or oral penicillin should be given with a view to preventing relapses for periods of several (e.g. 5) years.

The acute stages of the disease are influenced by steroid drugs and although they do not appear to affect the incidence of cardiac complications, they are sometimes used in severe cases.

Convalescence is generally slow and may be completed in the country or seaside, under supervision to prevent excessive activity. In view of the lengthy nature of the illness it is of importance for children to be transferred to special units where educational facilities are available.

The necessity of adequate and prolonged rest can be explained to adults. Children, as a rule, remain contented but must never be subject to disappointment resulting from foolish remarks such as 'perhaps the doctor will let you get up next week' made by their attendants or thoughtless visitors. It is the duty of the nurse to see that this is avoided.

Blood sedimentation rate. A fixed volume of blood, well mixed with sodium citrate to prevent clotting, is allowed to stand in an upright graduated glass tube. The red cells, being heavier than plasma, gradually sediment to the bottom of the tube. The level of the red cells is read in millimetres at the end of an hour. [Normal = up to 15 mm fall in the first hour.]

In many diseases including active acute rheumatism, tuberculosis, and in the later stages of pregnancy, the rate of sedimentation is increased. The normal results tend to be slightly higher in women than in men and also over the age of 50.

The test is most useful in assessing the progress of a disease and repeated readings showing a gradual return to normal often help to indicate that its activity is declining or has ceased. For example, this test may be of value in helping to decide when a patient with acute rheumatism may be allowed to get up.

N.B.—The abbreviation ESR (erythrocyte sedimentation rate) is often used.

Chorea

Chorea or St. Vitus' Dance is really a disease of the nervous system, but it is allied to acute rheumatism and is sometimes associated with identical heart lesions. Like rheumatic fever the incidence and severity are less marked at the present time.

Cause. The condition is due to the same general cause as acute rheumatism (a reaction to streptococcal infection) which produces a mild inflammation of part of the brain, i.e. it may be regarded as a form of 'rheumatic encephalitis'. It is essentially a disease of childhood, the common age incidence being between 5 and 15 years; females are more often affected than males. It is especially obvious in highly-strung, clever children and may be made worse by any emotional disturbance or overwork at school. Very occasionally it occurs in pregnancy and may be serious.

Symptoms. The onset as a rule is gradual. The child becomes nervous and irritable, laughing and crying without any obvious cause. Movements are clumsy, objects are dropped or knocked over and, at the same time, irregular spasmodic movements occur in the limbs. These are of a jerky, fidgeting type and quite purposeless. Such movements as opening and closing the hands, rotating the arms and wrists, grimacing by screwing up the eyes, pulling down the corners of the mouth and thrusting the tongue into the cheek, are common, and if once seen are easily recognized. They may be confined to one limb, or one half of the body or the whole body may be affected. The movements, which disappear during sleep, vary from mild twitchings to those of such violent degree that the writhing of the trunk and throwing about of the limbs render it difficult to prevent the patient from falling out of bed. They are often accompanied by difficulty in speaking.

• Chorea may last from 6 weeks to 6 months, but relapses are common. The cardiac complications are identical with those occurring in rheumatic fever but are probably less common.

Treatment

The essentials of treatment are rest and quietness. The patient may need to be kept in bed for several weeks. If cardiac complications occur, the period of rest in bed is prolonged and the general management of the case is then based on that of acute rheumatism. A light room, an interesting companion and various forms of quiet amusement are beneficial in mild cases.

The child must be prevented from causing itself injury. This may be affected by padding the cot side with pillows and bandaging the bony points such as the wrists, elbows and knees with cotton-wool. In very severe but rare cases in which it is difficult to prevent the patient falling out of bed, a mattress may be placed on the floor. Such cases require the attention of a nurse day and night. No mechanical restraint is ever justifiable.

A woollen nightgown should be worn as the movements are liable to dislodge the bedclothes and leave the patient uncovered. A liberal diet is essential, for choreic children are often thin and undernourished. Milk and eggs should be given freely. In severe cases, when swallowing is difficult, nasal feeding is employed. In all cases, care must be taken that the child does not drink out of thin glass or china vessels which may easily be broken by movements of the jaw and a portion swallowed. Fluids may be given with a spoon or out of a feeding-bottle with a teat and long tube.

Many drugs have been used in the treatment of chorea, among them are aspirin and phenobarbitone but there is no specific treatment.

During convalescence, massage and exercises are of value; later, games requiring skilled control of the muscles, such as building with bricks and knitting, may be employed.

THE ELECTROCARDIOGRAM

An electrocardiogram is a record of the electrical changes taking place in the heart muscle when it contracts. Although it is not the duty of a nurse to interpret these records, many features of the normal electrocardiogram can be understood by her in the light of what she learns in anatomy and physiology.

Physiology of the heart beat (p. 93 and Fig. 30)

1. The impulse causing the atria to contract starts at the sino-atrial node and spreads over the atria. This is represented on the ECG by a wave labelled P.

2. The impulse reaches the atrio-ventricular node and passes down the bundle of His before the ventricle starts to contract. This period is called the PR interval and is represented by a short horizontal line between P and Q.

3. The ventricles consist of a big mass of muscle. Their contraction is therefore slower and longer than that of the atria and in consequence the wave produced on the ECG is larger, longer and more complicated than that caused by the contraction of the atria. It is labelled, from its commencement to its end, by the letters QRS and T, R being the main upward deflection and T a well-marked wave at the end which is followed by a horizontal line representing the diastole before the next atrial beat (P).

N.B.—One standard lead only is illustrated in the examples shown.

The abnormal electrocardiogram

Atrial fibrillation (p. 104 and Fig. 31). In this condition the atria fail to contract as a whole in a regular wave-like manner. Instead

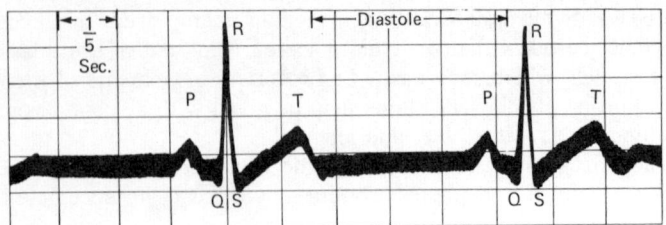

Fig. 30 Normal electrocardiogram with two complete heart beats. P = atrial systole. QRST = ventricular systole.

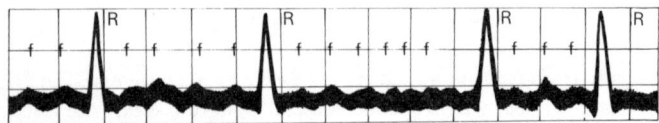

Fig. 31 Atrial fibrillation. Note the irregular spacing of the ventricular complexes (R) and the numerous fibrillation waves 'f' occurring irregularly, in this instance, at the rate of about 360 per minute. T wave is obscured by 'f' waves.

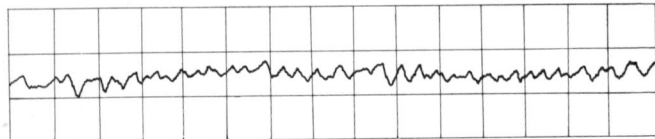

Fig. 32 Ventricular fibrillation. Note the complete absence of normal pattern.

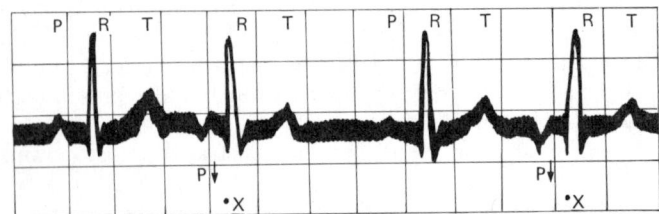

Fig. 33 Electrocardiogram showing two extra-systoles arising in the AV junction and two normal beats. P ↓ = AV junctional extra-systole (P wave inverted). X = the point exactly half-way between two normal P waves at which another normal P wave would have appeared if the premature beat had not occurred.

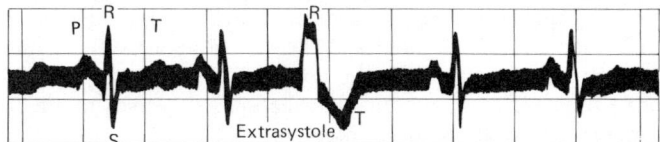

Fig. 34 A ventricular extra-systole occurring in the middle of four normal ventricular beats. Note its abnormal form with exaggerated R and inverted T wave. Also observe that it is placed nearer to the beat preceding it on the left than to the one on the right. In other words it is premature and takes the place of a normal beat which had it occurred would have been situated exactly half-way between the other two ventricular beats. The notch on the top of R is a superimposed P wave.

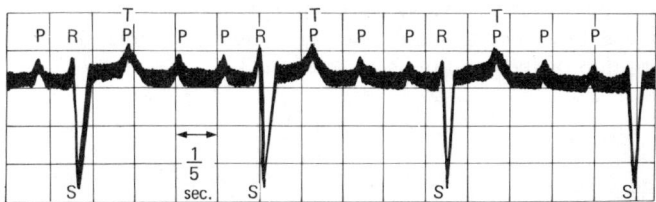

Fig. 35 Atrial flutter. Note the flutter waves (P) occurring approximately every $\frac{1}{5}$ second or 300 per minute. A P wave is lost in each QRS complex and one is superimposed on each T wave.

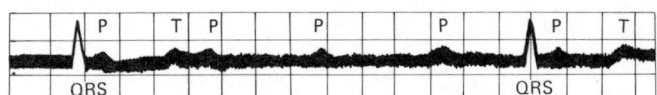

Fig. 36 Complete heart block. Note the P waves occurring at regular intervals quite independently of the ventricular complexes (QRS).

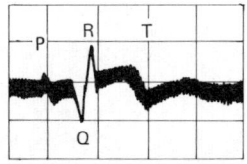

Fig. 37 Coronary artery thrombosis (acute myocardial infarction). Note the high 'take off' of ST with inversion of T.

very rapid irregular contractions occur all over the atria and bombard the AV node and bundle of His at the rate of about 400 per minute.

It follows that in the ECG the normal P waves disappear and are replaced by a series of irregular fibrillation ('f') waves to which the ventricle responds at irregular intervals.

Atrial and ventricular extra-systoles (p. 103, Figs. 33 and 34)

Atrial flutter (p. 105, Fig. 35)

Heart block (p. 106, Fig. 36)

Coronary artery thrombosis (acute myocardial infarction). (p. 150, Fig. 37). Because an area of heart muscle is damaged by the cutting off of its blood supply the piece of muscle is electrically abnormal and therefore the ECG will be distorted in various ways according to the actual area affected. A typical example is shown in Fig. 37 but other variations are commonly observed.

These brief notes should be followed in conjunction with the description of the conditions in the text.

4 Diseases of the Blood

The composition and formation of the blood

When human blood is examined under the microscope it is seen to consist of two kinds of corpuscles floating in a pale yellow fluid, the blood plasma.

The red corpuscles or erythrocytes are more numerous than the second variety, the white corpuscles or leucocytes. In addition, other small bodies known as blood platelets are found and are concerned in the process of clotting.

Normal blood contains approximately:

Red cells (Erythrocytes)	5,000,000	per cubic millimetre
White cells (Leucocytes)	6,000 ,, ,, ,,
Platelets (Thrombocytes)	250,000 ,, ,, ,,

The red cells contain haemoglobin which carries oxygen to the tissues. The amount of haemoglobin present in the corpuscles is expressed as a percentage. The normal content is described as 100% or 14·8 grams per 100 ml of blood, any deficiency being indicated by a lower percentage. Estimation of the haemoglobin, and enumeration of the number of red and white cells is referred to as a blood count.

Diseases affecting the red cells

Anaemia may be defined as a reduction in the normal amount of either red cells or haemoglobin or both. The result of this is diminution in the capacity of the blood to combine with and transport oxygen to the tissues.

The formation of red cells. To understand the commoner diseases of the blood, it is necessary to have some knowledge of the process by which blood is formed in the body.

The red cells are produced in the bone marrow from large nucleated cells called proerythroblasts (Greek: erythros = red). The next stage in development is the formation of smaller nucleated cells known as normoblasts. In order that this step may take place vitamin B_{12} (cyanocobalamin) and folic acid are required. Folic acid (see p. 180) is present in the diet and is normally readily absorbed. Vitamin B_{12}, however, can only be absorbed in the presence of a substance secreted in normal gastric juice (intrinsic factor). Vitamin B_{12} is then stored in the liver and is available to the bone marrow for its part in the development of the red cells.

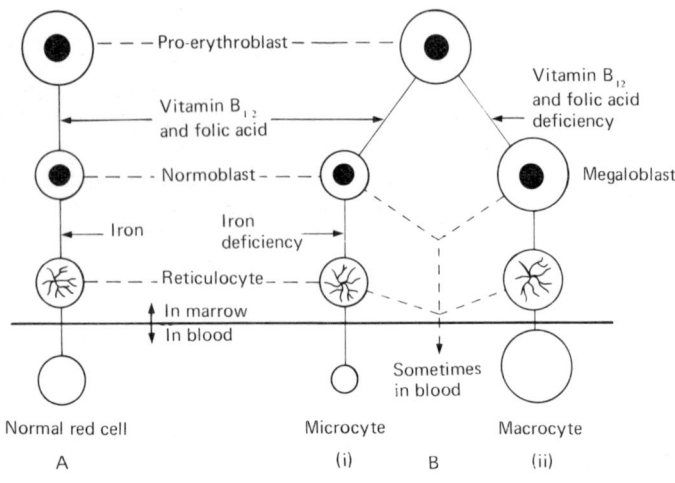

Fig. 38 Diagram Illustrating A. Development of normal red cell from proerythroblast. B. Development of red cell in (i) iron deficiency, (ii) B_{12} and folic acid deficiency.

The final stage is the transition from the nucleated normoblasts into the non-nucleated red cells or erythrocytes. The red cells are filled with haemoglobin and this process requires an adequate amount of iron which is essential for the manufacture of haemoglobin. Mature red cells finally leave the bone marrow and enter the blood stream. Immature red cells are seen in the blood stream in certain conditions. In them the nuclear material has not completely disappeared and on staining has a fine net-like appearance. Such immature red cells are called reticulocytes.

Two types of deficiency anaemia may exist. The first is due to lack of vitamin B_{12} or folic acid. The proerythroblasts do not develop into normoblasts but into larger cells known as megaloblasts (Greek: megas = large). In their turn the megaloblasts develop into non-nucleated red cells which are larger than normal and which are called macrocytes (Greek: macros = large). The second type of deficiency anaemia is due to lack of iron. Development proceeds until the final stage when the red cells contain less haemoglobin than normal and may also be smaller than normal when they are known as microcytes (Greek: micros = small). Cells of normal size are termed normocytic.

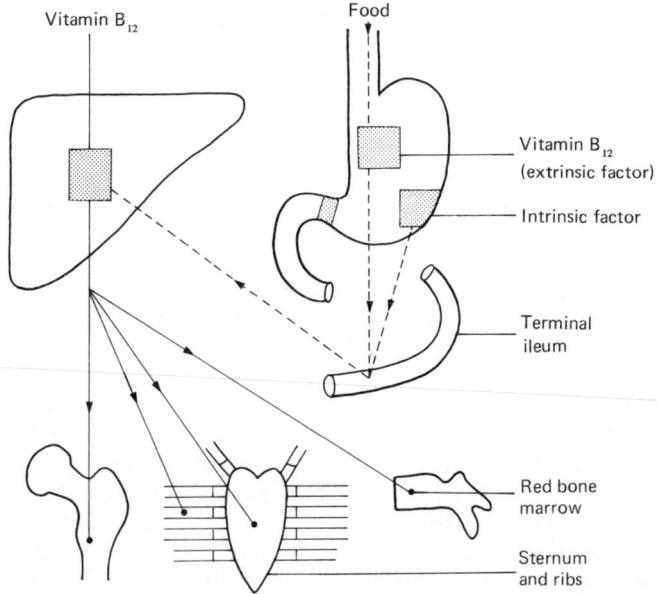

Fig. 39 The absorption of vitamin B_{12}, its storage in the liver, distribution to red bone marrow.

These normal and abnormal stages are illustrated in the accompanying diagram.

The intensity in colour of the red cells is dependent upon the amount of haemoglobin they contain. If a red cell contains a normal amount of haemoglobin it is fully coloured (normochromic), but, if there is a diminished quantity, it is paler than normal.

In those varieties of anaemia in which the process of blood formation is interrupted at the erythroblastic stage, each cell contains a relatively large amount of haemoglobin. This type of anaemia is, sometimes, referred to as hyperchromic (Greek: *hyper* = over, *chroma* = colour).

In the types associated with iron deficiency there is a reduced amount of haemoglobin in each red cell and they are called hypochromic (Greek: *hypo* = under).

There are, therefore, three main classes of anaemia:

1. Macrocytic anaemia (often hyperchromic).
2. Microcytic, hypochromic anaemia.
3. Normocytic, normochromic anaemia.

Symptoms of anaemia. Certain features are common to all cases of severe anaemia, irrespective of the cause of the condition.

The skin is pallid and waxy-looking. The mucous membrane of the lips, gums and conjunctiva is seen to be pale. The superficial veins on the back of the hand and feet have a pink, rather than a bluish appearance. The patient is weak and languid; he complains of headache, giddiness, and, occasionally, fainting attacks. There is breathlessness on exertion, palpitation, loss of appetite and sometimes oedema of the feet. The pulse rate is usually increased.

Generally speaking, the more severe the anaemia and the acuter the onset, the more intense will the symptoms be. In fact, quite a severe degree of anaemia may develop slowly before any very marked symptoms are complained of by the patient.

It has been seen that anaemia may be due to defective blood formation. It may also result from loss of blood and from excessive blood destruction and may be of the hyperchromic or hypochromic type, depending upon whether the maximum deficiency is in the number of red cells or in their haemoglobin content.

The following account deals with the more common types of anaemia and has been simplified accordingly; other rarer types will sometimes be seen. (See also p. 184.)

1. Anaemia due to loss of blood

Haemorrhage may occur either as a rapid loss of a large amount of blood, or repeated losses of smaller quantities. The former type occurs as a result of injury, from gastric, duodenal or typhoid ulcers, post-partum haemorrhage, abortion, ruptured ectopic gestation, and haemoptysis. The latter in conditions such as haemorrhoids, menorrhagia, chronic peptic ulcer, carcinoma of the stomach, colon or rectum and ulcerative colitis.

A pint (0·5 l) of blood may be lost rapidly by the healthy adult without producing symptoms. A loss of two pints (1 litre) must be regarded as serious haemorrhage while, if the amount exceeds four pints (2 litres), the result is frequently fatal.

In anaemia due to loss of blood, the body replaces the red cells more rapidly than the haemoglobin, and it will therefore be of the hypochromic type.

Treatment. After arresting the haemorrhage, the subsequent anaemia is treated by blood transfusion (p. 185) in very severe cases, or by full doses of iron in others. Sudden loss of blood is always associated with depletion in amount of the body fluids which may be relieved by intravenous saline and dextran or plasma whilst blood is being cross-matched.

In most cases of severe haemorrhage the foot of the bed should be raised on blocks in order to increase the blood supply to the brain.

Morphine is sometimes ordered to stop restlessness and to check the tendency to further bleeding.

2. Anaemia due to deficient blood formation

There are two main types of anaemia resulting from deficient blood formation:

(a) The macrocytic (hyperchromic) type due to deficiency of vitamin B_{12} (cyanocobalamin) or folic acid.

(b) The microcytic (hypochromic) type due to iron deficiency.

The most important condition of the first type is pernicious anaemia. Examples of the second type are simple achlorhydric anaemia: together with anaemia due to chronic infection, cancer, other debilitating conditions and malnutrition.

A. Anaemia due to deficiency of 'intrinsic factor'

Pernicious anaemia (Addison's anaemia)

Although it was about 100 years ago that Addison first described this type of anaemia, it was not until Minot and Murphy in 1926 showed that it could be cured by giving liver that its cause began to be understood. Ten years later Castle showed that a special blood-forming or anti-anaemic factor was necessary for the development of the pro-erythroblast into the normoblast and suggested that this factor was formed by the interaction of two substances, namely, an extrinsic factor in the food and an intrinsic factor present in the gastric juice, i.e. anti-anaemic factor = intrinsic factor + extrinsic factor.

Intrinsic factor. It is well known that the gastric mucous membrane is abnormal in pernicious anaemia. It appears pale and atrophic when seen with a gastroscope and it fails to secrete hydrochloric acid (achlorhydria). The underlying cause of pernicious anaemia is, therefore, the failure of special cells in the cardia and fundus of the stomach to produce intrinsic factor. Its exact nature is not known but it appears to be a muco-protein.

Extrinsic factor. The fact that liver cures pernicious anaemia proves that it contains an anti-anaemic substance. In 1948 it was found that from over a ton of liver about 1 gram of minute red crystals could be obtained which had the same effect as the whole liver. Later it was discovered that this substance could be prepared commercially by other methods and it was identified as vitamin B_{12} (Cyanocobalamin) and shown to contain traces of the metal cobalt.

Erythrocyte-maturing factor. It is known that the intrinsic factor is necessary for the utilization of extrinsic factor from the alimentary tract. It is probable that the two substances do not actually combine, as suggested by Castle, but that the intrinsic factor acts by aiding the absorption of the extrinsic factor (cyanocobalamin—vitamin B_{12}), i.e. deficiency of intrinsic factor is the basic cause of pernicious anaemia.

It is clear, however, that in pernicious anaemia the absence of intrinsic factor from the gastric juice leads to failure of vitamin B_{12}, which is present in meat and other animal products, to be absorbed and stored in the liver. In turn, this results in defective formation of the red cells in the bone marrow and the proerythroblasts fail to develop into normoblasts but become large abnormal cells called megaloblasts which appear in the circulating blood as macrocytes after the nucleus has disappeared so that a macrocytic (hyperchromic) anaemia results. At the same time the total number of red cells is considerably reduced, often to between 1,000,000 and 2,000,000 per cu mm, while the haemoglobin content of each cell remains relatively high.

Pernicious anaemia which is most common in middle and later ages, and which sometimes has a familial tendency, has a gradual onset and the symptoms are those of increasing weakness, pallor and shortness of breath. The pallor is accompanied by a peculiar and characteristic lemon-yellow coloration of the skin. Frequently the patients complain of soreness of the tongue which is seen to be much smoother than usual and almost devoid of papillae.

The spleen is sometimes enlarged. A pentagastrin test meal or a Diagnex Test on the urine reveals the absense of hydrochloric acid from the gastric juice (achlorhydria).

The most common complication is degeneration of certain tracts in the spinal cord, known as *subacute combined degeneration of the cord*. The symptoms produced by this condition are numbness and tingling in the legs, followed by difficulty in walking (ataxia), in fact, the word 'combined' implies a mixture of sensory and motor symptoms. Mental changes sometimes occur in pernicious anaemia.

Before the introduction of liver treatment pernicious anaemia was regarded as a progressive and fatal malady. At the present time, provided the patient continues treatment permanently, the prognosis is good.

Diagnosis. This is established by:

1. The symptoms and signs including the lemon-yellow skin, smooth tongue and sometimes enlargement of the spleen.
2. The blood picture: a macrocytic, hyperchromic anaemia with leucopoenia which may be confirmed by examination of the bone marrow obtained by sternal puncture.
3. Achlorhydria (achylia) in a pentagastrin test meal or Diagnex Test.
4. A low serum vitamin B_{12} level.
5. *The Schilling Test.* This is done with radioactively labelled vitamin B_{12}. In pernicious anaemia the Schilling test shows that a failure of absorption of the labelled vitamin, unless intrinsic factor is administered with it.

Treatment. The main principle in treatment is to supply the missing anti-anaemic factor in the form of vitamin B_{12}, which enables an adequate supply of normal red cells to be manufactured in the bone marrow and passed into the blood stream.

Vitamin B_{12} (Cyanocobalamin, 'Cytamen'). This is given by intramuscular injection in doses of 100 to 1,000 micrograms. Hydroxocobalamin ('Neocytamen') is effective in smaller doses given at longer intervals. Oral preparations and snuff are also available but they are not always as reliable as the injection and are not generally suitable for routine treatment. Cases in which the nervous system is involved require very large doses of B_{12}.

The treatment of pernicious anaemia may be considered in two stages.

I. The *therapeutic* stage, in which relatively large and frequent doses, e.g. up to 1,000 micrograms of Vitamin B_{12}, are employed, until the number of red cells reaches the normal of 5,000,000 per cu mm.

II. The *maintenance* stage, in which a somewhat reduced dose is given at longer intervals and is continued throughout the patient's life, e.g. 250 to 500 micrograms.

In the therapeutic stage, daily injections may be given during the first week, followed by weekly injections until the blood count has reached normal. When the maintenance period is reached, injections are given at intervals of 1 or 2 months, depending on whether cyano-cobalamin or hydroxocobalamin is used. There is no reason why an intelligent patient should not be taught to administer his own intra-muscular injection, in the same way that a diabetic gives his own insulin. The addition of oral iron is useful in some cases.

Blood counts should be performed at regular intervals to ensure that an adequate maintenance dose is being taken and that the number of red cells is being kept up to 5,000,000 per cu mm.

Folic acid deficiency anaemia

Folic acid, a member of the vitamin B complex given by mouth, is present in many foodstuffs such as green vegetables, yeast and liver. Deficiency may be due to dietary lack, impaired absorption or exces-sive alcohol intake. Macrocytic anaemia due to folic acid deficiency occasionally develops in later pregnancy or the early puerperium and is a marked feature of tropical sprue and sometimes also of idio-pathic steatorrhoea.

Folic acid is effective in restoring the blood count to normal in pernicious anaemia but will not prevent the onset of nervous com-plications and is, therefore, not used in this condition.

In order that normal cell division can take place desoxyribonucleic acid (DNA), which is the nucleo-protein molecule of chromosomes, must be doubled. The synthesis of DNA requires the presence of B_{12} and folic acid. If either substance is deficient the manufacture of nucleo-protein is im-paired. The result is that the proerythroblasts fail to divide and develop properly. Further, these immature cells have a shorter span of life than normal cells, hence the development of anaemia of the macrocytic type.

B. Anaemia associated with iron deficiency

In this variety of anaemia there is interference with the proper development of the normoblast into the mature red cell. Haemoglobin contains iron and it is therefore easy to understand that, if there is iron deficiency, the red cells will contain a diminished amount of haemoglobin and the anaemia will be of the hypochromic (microcytic) type.

Iron shortage may be due to three causes:

1. Deficiency of iron in the diet.
2. Imperfect absorption of iron from the alimentary tract.
3. Excessive loss as a result of haemorrhage.

The iron in the average daily diet is only slightly in excess of the body's needs and the body is not able to store iron in any quantity. Any factors, such as hypochlorhydria, which cause diminished absorption, if long-continued, and particularly if the patient is taking a diet poor in iron-contained foodstuffs, tend to produce anaemia. Iron-deficiency anaemia is not uncommon in elderly people who live alone and tend to rely on a cheap, mainly carbohydrate diet.

It is mainly seen:

1. In premature and artificially fed infants.
2. During pregnancy and after delivery.
3. Following loss of blood by haemorrhage (acute and chronic).
4. Dietetic deficiency.

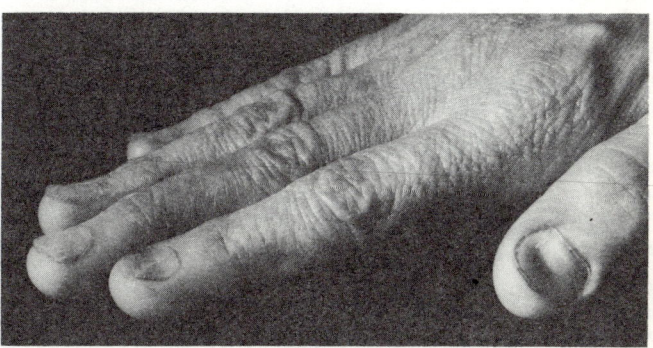

Fig. 40 Spoon-shaped nails (koilonychia).

Simple achlorhydric anaemia is a condition, commonest in women of middle age, associated with absence of hydrochloric acid from the gastric juice, although the intrinsic factor is present. Spoon-shaped nails are often present in this condition (p. 489).

A similar type of anaemia is often present in cases of cancer, nephritis, chronic infective processes, malnutrition and starvation. Anaemia due to haemorrhage is hypochromic, because the bone marrow has less difficulty in replacing the lost red cells than the body has in manufacturing the haemoglobin necessary to fill them.

The **symptoms** of these conditions are essentially those described on p. 176.

The **treatment** consists in the administration of iron by mouth, e.g. ferrous sulphate, 200 mg, ferrous gluconate, 300 mg 3 times a day. Iron should always be given directly after meals in order to obviate any abdominal symptoms which might arise.

Special preparations (e.g. 'Jectofer' and 'Imferon') may be given intramuscularly in repeated doses. Alternatively a large dose of 'Imferon' calculated to supply the necessary amount of iron may be used in an intravenous drip infusion given slowly. Iron by injection is mainly indicated: (*a*) when absorption of oral iron is known to be defective, (*b*) when the patient cannot tolerate oral iron or (*c*) when he cannot be trusted to take it.

Severe cases may required blood transfusion.

Vitamin C is given in some cases.

3. Anaemia due to excessive blood destruction

Blood may be destroyed by the action of various poisons which may be either chemical or bacterial in origin. In addition, these poisons may also have some effect on the bone marrow and so interfere with blood formation, thereby increasing the severity of the anaemia. The common chemical poisons are lead and benzene. Those of bacterial origin include the toxins of the streptococcus, which may be present in a number of septic conditions, bacterial endocarditis and septicaemia. Malaria also causes anaemia as a result of blood destruction.

Anaemia of this type is called **haemolytic**. Because of the excessive destruction of red cells and haemoglobin the condition is often associated with haemolytic jaundice (p. 249).

The causes of haemolytic anaemia so far mentioned are all **acquired** during life. A very severe haemolytic anaemia occurs as the result of incompatible blood transfusion. The red cells are destroyed so rapidly that free haemoglobin may appear in the urine (haemoglobinuria). A condition similar to that of an incompatible blood transfusion may develop in a baby at the time of birth if its blood group is different from that of its mother. This is called **haemolytic disease of the newborn.** Almost all cases are due to incompatibility of the 'rhesus factor'; e.g. the father is rhesus positive, the mother rhesus negative and the baby rhesus positive, and the baby's cells, while it is still in utero, provoke the formation of rhesus antibodies in the mother's serum. The fact that the mother is rhesus negative can easily be detected early in pregnancy. So the doctor is alerted to the possibility of this disease in good time. Late in pregnancy special tests can also be done to find out whether there are rhesus antibodies in the mother's serum and also whether they are increasing. When an affected baby is born he rapidly becomes anaemic and jaundiced and is likely to die. The treatment is to give an exchange blood transfusion: small volumes of blood are alternately withdrawn and replaced by fresh Rh negative donor blood. The umbilical vein is usually used for this. The purpose of doing this is to remove from his blood the rhesus antibodies, breaking down cells and excessive bilirubin. Greatly raised serum bilirubin is dangerous as it causes **kernicterus,** a condition of mental deficiency and spasticity which may develop after several months. In the most severe forms of haemolytic disease of the newborn the fetus dies before birth.

Father	Mother	Infant	
Rh +	Rh +	Rh +	Normal
Rh −	Rh +	Rh +	Normal
Rh −	Rh −	Rh −	Normal
Rh +	Rh −	Rh +	At risk

In some cases intra-uterine death can be prevented by intra-uterine transfusions. Group O rhesus negative packed cells are injected into the baby's peritoneal cavity via a plastic catheter introduced through a long needle which pierces the mother's abdominal wall and uterus.

Haemolytic disease of the newborn is now being prevented by giving mothers at risk an injection of anti-D immunoglobulin. This must be given within 48 hours of delivery of the first child in order to prevent the mother manufacturing rhesus antibody. The next child will not then be affected by haemolytic disease. The first child is not affected unless the mother has at some time received a rhesus incompatible blood transfusion.

Sometimes in adults an acquired haemolytic anaemia develops without any discoverable cause (**idiopathic acquired haemolytic anaemia**). Special tests may be required to detect this type, which often responds well to treatment with steroids. Excessive haemolysis may be caused by a spleen which has enlarged due to a variety of causes and in certain conditions splenectomy may be beneficial. The operation is not without danger, however, and is not often done.

The classification overleaf may be helpful:

Classification of anaemia

1. Due to blood Loss (hypochromic, microcytic)

TYPES: Acute   large haemorrhage.

       Chronic   repeated small haemorrhages.

TREATMENT: Iron. Blood transfusion.

2. Due to deficient blood formation

A. Deficiency of vitamin B_{12}

   e.g. Pernicious anaemia.

   TREATMENT: Vitamin B_{12}.

B. Deficiency of folic acid, e.g. sometimes in pregnancy.

C. Iron deficiency (hypochromic, microcytic)

   e.g. Simple achlorhydric, malnutrition, etc.

   TREATMENT: Iron. Blood transfusion.

3. Due to excessive blood destruction, haemolytic anaemia

e.g. Chemical poisons: drugs, lead, benzene.

    Bacterial poisons: toxins, malaria, parasites, etc.

    Congenital haemolytic anaemia (acholuric jaundice) p. 252).

    TREATMENT: Transfusion, steroids, eradication of cause.

4. Due to defective bone marrow function

There may be absense of blood-forming cells in the bone marrow (aplastic anaemia) or the marrow may be filled with tumour cells or other abnormal cells which can be detected when marrow is obtained by sternal puncture. e.g. Aplastic anaemia due to toxic drugs, x-rays, radium.

The above is a simple classification of the basic causes of anaemia. It should be remembered, however, that anaemia may occur in many general diseases, e.g.

Chronic infective conditions   Liver disease

Cancer of all types   Renal disease

Rheumatoid arthritis   Collagen diseases

Myxoedema (hypothyroidism)   Autoimmune disease

Other rare causes of anaemia include thalassaemia (Mediterranean anaemia: an inherited condition associated with deficient manufacture of haemoglobin) and sickle-cell anaemia (a hereditary tropical disease).

Aplastic Anaemia. This is a rare type of anaemia due to defective blood formation in which red cells, white cells and platelets are diminished in number. It is due to the failure of the bone marrow to produce blood cells. In many instances the cause is unknown. In others it may be due to the action of bacterial toxins, to poisons such as benzol and arsenic, and drugs such as potassium perchlorate and chloramphenicol. Excessive doses of x-rays, radium and the products of atomic fission will produce the same effect. The prognosis is serious and repeated blood transfusion is usually necessary, but the condition may respond to oxymetholone, an anabolic agent.

General nursing of anaemia

The usual routine nursing treatment of a general medical case is employed. In severe cases the patient is confined to bed, and blanket bathing may be required.

If the patient is very ill a light diet with plenty of fluids will be given, in less serious cases an ordinary diet with an adequate amount of green vegetables and fruit is desirable. The pulse, temperature and respiration are taken and charted regularly. A record of actions of the bowels is kept and the urine should be tested at regular intervals. Medicines, iron after meals in particular, must be administered as they are ordered. Adequate ventilation, fresh air and sunshine are desirable. It is often necessary to follow up cases of anaemia with periodic blood counts after they have been discharged from hospital.

Sternal puncture. Much information can be obtained which will assist in the diagnosis of the rarer types of anaemia if the bone marrow is examined under the microscope.

This may be obtained either from the sternum, tibia or iliac crest by puncturing the bone, under local anaesthesia, with a special needle and sucking out a specimen of marrow with a syringe.

A preliminary injection of diazepam may be desirable.

Blood transfusion

The transfusion of blood from one individual to another is a procedure which is frequently carried out, but which should not be used indiscriminately because blood is, in fact, a potentially dangerous, scarce and expensive commodity. The person giving the blood is called the donor, and the patient the recipient.

It has been found that, for purposes of blood transfusion, individuals may be divided into 4 groups, and it is only when they belong to the same group that their bloods will mix properly. If blood from the wrong group is transfused, the red cells in it are destroyed with very serious results such as haemoglobinaemia and suppression of urine which may prove fatal. It is, therefore, most important to discover the group to which the patient belongs and to select a suitable donor, having also tested the Rhesus factor.

There is an exception to this rule concerning what are called group O donors. In most instances, their blood may be given to any patient without causing ill effects and they are, therefore, referred to as universal donors, but even with these donors a preliminary test must be made to ensure compatibility. In every case of blood transfusion, therefore, the donor's cells must be cross-matched against the recipient's serum.

Any nurse handling bottles of blood for transfusion must be particularly careful that they reach the right patient as confusion can occur, especially if more than one transfusion is going on at the same time. Before each bottle of blood is given its group and label should be checked by 2 persons.

Approximately 5% of individuals belong to group AB, 40% to group A, 10% to group B, and 45% to group O.

As a rule, 500 to 1,000 ml (about 1 to 2 pints) or more of blood are given as a single transfusion, but occasionally repeated injections of smaller quantities are employed.

The method of grouping given above is known as the Landsteiner or International method, which has been introduced into scientific work and is used in connection with paternity tests.

International group	Population
AB	5%
A	40%
B	10%
O	45%

A blood transfusion is sometimes followed by a reaction, which usually takes the form of a rigor. Blankets should be applied, and a doctor informed.

The main indications for blood transfusion are:
1. Severe haemorrhage following—
   (a) Accidents.
   (b) Before and after operation.
   (c) Conditions such as haematemesis, abortion, and post-partum haemorrhage.
2. Medical conditions—
   (a) Severe hypochromic anaemia.
   (b) Some cases of septicaemia.

(c) Haemophilia.

(d) Occasionally in pernicious anaemia.

(e) As supportive treatment in leukaemia, whilst awaiting response to antileukaemic drugs.

Concentrated human red blood corpuscles (packed cells). This is a preparation of blood from which some of the plasma has been removed. It follows, therefore, that a greater number of red cells can be given in a smaller volume of fluid, which may be an advantage in certain cases of anaemia when it is considered undesirable to add to the total amount of blood for fear of overloading the circulation.

Marrow transfusion. By inserting a special trocar and cannula, under local anaesthesia, directly into the bone marrow of the sternum or tibia, it is possible to introduce blood directly into the circulation. This is a method of transfusion used for selected cases, especially in infants or when no veins are available. Marrow transplants may be possible. Blood may also be infused into the peritoneal cavity.

Plasma transfusion. Plasma will keep longer than citrated blood containing red cells, and therefore plasma may be withdrawn from citrated blood after the red corpuscles have fallen by sedimentation to the bottom of the collecting bottle, and stored for a long period.

Plasma is of value in restoring the blood volume in cases of shock. It may also be stored in dry form. Dry plasma is rendered suitable for intravenous injection by dissolving 20 grams in 500 ml of sterile 5% dextrose in distilled water and using it at once.

Blood plasma substitutes

Dextran is a polysaccharide containing no protein. It is of value in increasing the blood volume and the osmotic pressure of the blood in cases of burns or shock. It can also be used in haemorrhage when blood is not immediately available and in some cases of chronic nephritis. A special low-molecular weight dextran ('Rheomacrodex') is used to improve capillary blood flow, e.g. in patients with severe burns.

Polycythaemia. This condition is the opposite of anaemia, for the number of red cells is increased and varies between 6 and 12 million per cubic millimetre (Greek: *Poly* = many, *cytos* = cell). The haemoglobin rises to 120% or more.

It is found in persons who live some time at high altitudes, and is then the physiological response of Nature to the diminished oxygen supply in the rarefied atmosphere. It occurs also in some cases of congenital heart disease and chronic pulmonary conditions. In a few instances it is seen in association with enlargement of the spleen and is then described as **polycythaemia vera** or Osler's Disease, a rare malady treated by repeated venesection or radioactive phosphorus (^{32}P). Cytotoxic drugs e.g. busulphan and trenimon are sometimes used.

Diseases affecting the white cells

There are two important varieties of white cell, the polymorphonuclear or granulocyte and the lymphocyte. The former develop in the bone marrow: the latter are mainly produced in the lymphoid tissue of the body, such as the lymph glands and spleen.

The normal number of white cells circulating in the blood is 6,000 to 10,000 per cu mm, of which about 70% are granulocytes and 30% lymphocytes. If the number of white cells is less than 5,000 per cu mm the condition is called **leucopenia,** if more than 10,000 per cu mm, it is called **leucocytosis.**

Leucopenia may occur as a result of certain toxins and drugs circulating in the blood which damage the bone marrow, and is seen in typhoid fever. Leucocytosis is one of the responses of the body to infection and is present in most cases of inflammation, especially if pus formation results.

A special type of white cell, called an eosinophil, is formed in increased numbers in certain skin conditions, in asthma, allergic states and in various diseases due to worms and parasites.

Agranulocytosis

Agranulocytosis, granulocytopenia or neutropenia are terms used when almost all the granulocytes disappear from the blood, i.e. severe leucopenia. The resistance of the body to infection is therefore impaired. It is a serious condition which may prove fatal. It usually follows the administration of certain drugs which poison the bone marrow in those patients who are over-sensitive to them, although most people can take them without danger. The risk is greater in individuals with a previous history of allergic disorders. These drugs include sulphonamides, chloramphenicol, gold and bismuth salts, phenylbutazone ('Butazolidin'), and thiouracil. It has also followed the use of dinitrophenol, benzol and some arsenic preparations. It may be associated with aplastic anaemia.

As a rule, one of the earliest features is the development of a severe sore throat which may become ulcerated. In such a case anyone taking such drugs should stop them at once and have the condition confirmed by a blood count. The essential point in treatment is to give an antibiotic such as penicillin or tetracycline to prevent further infection. Blood transfusion may be necessary.

Leukaemia

A leucocytosis consists in the increase in number of *normal* white cells and it may be stated as a general principle that a leucocytosis accompanies an infection.

Leukaemia, on the other hand, is a **disease** of those portions of the blood-forming tissues which are responsible for the production of the white cells. The main change in the blood occurring in this condition is the presence of a large number of *abnormal* and *immature* white cells, which may be increased in number to 100,000 per cu mm or even more. As a rule the red cells are not seriously affected until later in the disease when anaemia develops.

There appears to have been an increase in the incidence of the disease in recent years, but its cause is not fully understood, although in some cases viruses and external factors such as x-rays, radiation and some chemicals may be associated with it.

It may be considered as a neoplastic disorder of the blood-forming tissues and is, therefore, sometimes called 'cancer of the blood'.

There are two main varieties of leukaemia which depend on the type of abnormal cells present, viz. myeloid and lymphatic leukaemia, although, rarely, other varieties occur, e.g. monocytic leukaemia.

1. Myeloid leukaemia: in this variety abnormal (neoplastic), immature granular leucocytes derived from the bone marrow are increased in number (Greek: *myelos* = marrow).

2. Lymphatic leukaemia: in which abnormal lymphocytes derived from the spleen and lymph glands are increased.

Depending on the rate at which the abnormal cells develop two main clinical types of the disease are seen.

1. The acute leukaemias.
2. The chronic leukaemias.

The acute forms are rapidly fatal, often in a few days or weeks although cytotoxic drugs and steroids may produce remissions lasting several months, up to several years.

Acute lymphatic leukaemia is more common in the younger age group, especially in children about 5 years old. The chronic leukaemias tend to occur among older age groups and patients may survive as long as 5 to 10 years.

Symptoms. Acute leukaemias. These often begin like an ordinary infection with high fever, sore throat and joint pains. Subcutaneous haemorrhages (purpura), bleeding from the gums and elsewhere usually occur and there is often some enlargement of the spleen, liver and lymphatic glands less marked, as a rule, than in the chronic leukaemias. Blood and bone marrow examination confirms the diagnosis.

Treatment. On the whole better results are to be expected in children than in adults. There are no exact rules as the patient may become rapidly refractory to one drug and yet respond to another (or a combination of drugs). Among those used are:

(*a*) Steroids (e.g. prednisolone) which usually produce an immediate improvement in the blood picture and the tendency to bleeding.

(*b*) Cyclophosphamide ('Endoxana').

(*c*) Mercaptopurine.

(*d*) Vincristine ('Oncovin').

(*e*) Methotrexate.

(*f*) Daunorubicin ('Cerubidin').

(*g*) Cytarabine ('Cytosar').

There are always special problems when the acute disease occurs in children and as much care, comfort and happiness should be afforded the child for as long as possible. It is evident that the parents must be warned, that, in spite of temporary, even encouraging, remissions induced by treatment, the ultimate outlook remains grave.

Chronic leukaemias

The main **symptoms** are weakness, lassitude, loss of appetite and weight with moderate anaemia. The liver and spleen are enlarged. The splenic enlargement tends to be more marked in the myeloid type and may appear to fill half the abdominal cavity. In the lymphatic type enlargement of the lymph glands in the neck, axillae and groins is more evident than in the myeloid variety.

Treatment. As in acute leukaemias this will vary from case to case.

Chronic myeloid leukaemia

(*a*) Busulphan ('Myleran'), e.g. 4 mg daily for 8–12 weeks followed if necessary by a smaller maintenance dose.

(*b*) X-rays (e.g. to the spleen) but they are less effective than busulphan.

(*c*) Radioactive phosphorus.
(*d*) Dibromomannitol and mercaptopurine in advanced cases.

Chronic lymphatic leukaemia
(*a*) Chlorambucil ('Leukeran')
(*b*) Cyclophosphamide ('Endoxana')
(*c*) Steroids for complicating haemolytic anaemia.

In both types the dose and duration of treatment is controlled by regular blood counts, so that the white cells remain about 15,000 per cu mm. Severe anaemia may require blood transfusion, and antibiotics are required for intercurrent infections.

Haemorrhagic diseases

Purpura

This is a condition the cause of which is not always clear. It is sometimes associated with changes in the blood such as diminution in the number of platelets (thrombocytopenia), or else some alteration in the walls of the capillaries which permits blood to escape into the surrounding tissues. In some cases the spleen is enlarged. Spontaneous extravasation of blood into the mucous membranes, skin and subcutaneous tissue occur. It is seen either in the form of small purpuric spots (petechiae) or as more extensive bluish-red areas which look like bruises and which change colour in the same way. The following indicates common causes of purpura:

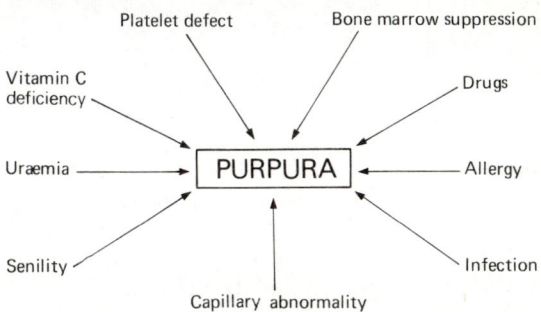

Purpura is a symptom rather than a disease. It occurs in the haemorrhagic types of acute specific fevers (e.g. diphtheria, small-pox). It is seen also in scurvy (vitamin C deficiency), in old age, in cachectic states such as cancer and chronic Bright's disease, and occasionally as a result of the administration of certain drugs, especially over-dosage with anticoagulant drugs in which the level of the blood prothrombin is diminished. In other cases it has an allergic basis, e.g. Henoch-Schönlein purpura.

Thrombocytopoenia may be caused by drugs, e.g. sulphonamides, phenylbutazone and oral antidiabetic drugs (p. 447).

More commonly, however, no explanation can be given for its appearance and it is then called idiopathic purpura or purpura simplex. Steroids may be used in treatment.

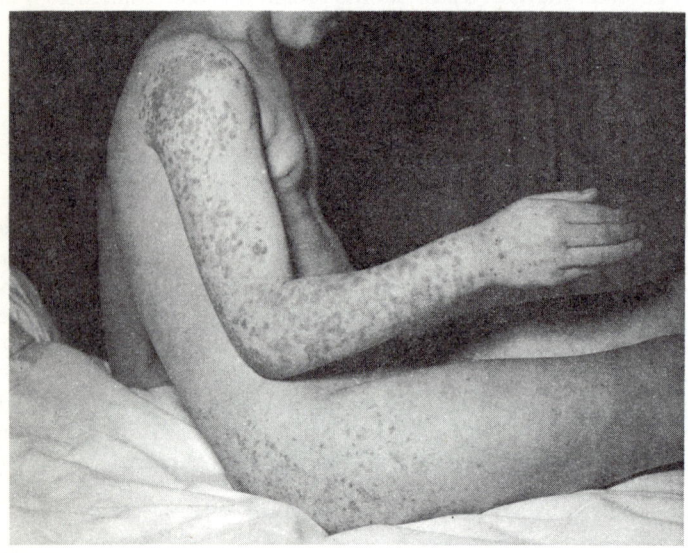

Fig. 41 Purpura.

Haemophilia

This disease consists of the tendency to uncontrollable bleeding at the slightest trauma, and is due to the absence of a special clotting factor in the blood plasma (Factor VIII, AHG). The platelets are normal but their disintegration may be delayed.

It is a hereditary and familial condition associated with an abnormal gene which is transmitted by the females but only affects the males. This means that if a woman from a haemophilic family marries and has children, some of the male children will suffer from the condition, but if they marry a normal woman, their offspring will all be normal. On the other hand, the daughters of the woman from the haemophilic family will not suffer from the condition themselves, but their male children may be affected and their female children may transmit the condition.

Haemorrhage may occur from minor cuts, after tooth-extraction or into joints (haemarthrosis) or muscles as a result of slight injuries for which admission to hospital is essential. The treatment of the condition is mainly prophylactic. A sheltered and careful life is necessary to reduce the risk of trauma. Known sufferers should be in touch with a local Haemophilia Centre. Before and after operations, including the extraction of teeth, a blood product containing factor VIII is given intravenously. This may be **cryoprecipitate** or fresh plasma. Blood lost at operation is replaced by fresh blood. Application of fresh human blood on cotton-wool swabs may check bleeding. **Snake venom** obtained from Russell's Viper also has a very powerful action in producing clotting of blood. When used in suitable dilution (1 in 10,000, e.g. Stypven), it is especially valuable in checking bleeding from local lesions in haemophilia by inducing the blood to clot. For example, a bleeding tooth-socket may be plugged with cotton-wool soaked in snake venom. This may be repeated as often as necessary. Local applications of thrombin powder may also be used. Fibrin foam or oxidized foam may be a useful dressing.

Bleeding episodes should be treated by bed rest and intravenous administration of a factor VIII concentrate. Transfusion with fresh blood may also be required. A haemarthrosis should be treated initially by splinting and light bandaging. Prolonged splinting must be avoided as it may result in fibrous ankylosis (fixation). Cold packs or icebags applied to the joint may give considerable relief from the pain. If an analgesic is required, drugs of addiction and aspirin should be avoided. Aspirin may cause gastric haemorrhage which is likely to be serious in a haemophiliac.

Centres are available throughout the country where the condition may be fully investigated and treated. Females belonging to haemophilic families should probably be advised not to bear children.

DISEASES OF THE SPLEEN

The spleen is an organ, which, although it fulfils a number of important functions, is not essential to life and may be removed by operation, without any serious effect upon the individual.

In some animals the spleen acts as a reservoir for red blood cells, which it discharges from time to time into the general circulation when sudden and increased demands are made upon the oxygen-carrying powers of the blood (e.g. severe haemorrhage, exercise, and exposure to a rarefied atmosphere at high altitudes) but this function is probably of minor importance in man. In fetal life it is actively engaged in the formation of red cells, a function which ceases after birth. It also takes an important part in the destruction of diseased and worn-out red cells (e.g. malaria). In common with lymphoid tissue elsewhere in the body, it produces lymphocytes and, in addition, is an important factor in the defence mechanism of the body in connection with formation of antibodies and the development of immunity.

The spleen is particularly liable to enlargement in disease. Slight increase in size occurs in a number of acute specific fevers, in particular typhoid fever. Enlargement is also found in malaria, glandular fever, bacterial endocarditis, septicaemia, cirrhosis of the liver, Banti's syndrome and Hodgkin's disease. Great increase in size is found in leukaemia. The spleen may be the site of infarcts (p. 161).

Enlargement is sometimes referred to as splenomegaly.

When enlarged, the spleen is peculiarly vulnerable to trauma and even a minor blunt injury may cause rupture of the organ and death from consequent haemorrhage.

Splenic anaemia or Banti's syndrome. This rare condition is a manifestation of portal hypertension and consists of progressive anaemia, associated with enlargement of the spleen. In the later stages the liver sometimes becomes enlarged. The latter is due to an overgrowth of fibrous tissue in its substance, which is called cirrhosis, and which may be followed by the development of ascites. A common complication of the condition is haematemesis.

The duration of the disease varies between 3 and 10 years. In the early stages it may be helped by removal of the spleen (splenectomy) in some cases or a porto-caval anastomosis may be carried out. Iron is given for the associated anaemia.

DISEASES OF THE LYMPHATIC SYSTEM

The lymphatic system consists of a series of channels which convey the tissue fluid or lymph. These channels or lymphatics pass to and from the lymph glands which are situated in various parts of the body. Lymph finally reaches the bloodstream, via the thoracic duct which opens into the left brachiocephalic (innominate) vein.

The most important groups of lymph glands are situated in the neck, the axilla, the thorax, the abdomen and the groin.

There are 3 main types of disease which affect lymph glands:

1. Septic.
2. Tuberculous.
3. Malignant.

1. Septic Adenitis. This occurs as the result of inflammation in the area drained by a group of glands. For example, a septic finger may be followed by swelling of the lymph glands in the axilla (axillary adenitis). If the infection is a severe one an abscess may form in the glands, which will require incision and drainage. Treatment with antibiotics may be indicated.

Inflammation of the lymph channels is called lymphangitis.

2. Tuberculous Adenitis. Lymph glands are sometimes the site of tuberculous disease, especially those situated in the neck and thorax.

3. Malignant Adenitis. Lymph glands draining the site of a malignant tumour frequently become infiltrated with cancer cells. For instance, in cancer of the breast, the axillary glands may be involved.

Lymph glands are also enlarged in leukaemia, in Hodgkin's disease, in the second stage of syphilis, in rubella and in glandular fever.

Glandular fever

Glandular fever **(infectious mononucleosis)** is an acute disease probably due to a virus. It is characterized by fever, general glandular enlargement and an increase in the number of lymphocytes in the blood. These may be abnormal in appearance. Rashes, enlarged spleen and a sore throat with exudate on the tonsils are sometimes present. The infectivity is not high and the disease is rarely fatal although debility and nervous depression may persist for some months. No special treatment is known and it is, therefore, symptomatic but a short course of steroids with antibiotic cover may be helpful in severe cases. The Paul-Bunnell agglutination test is used to confirm the diagnosis and to differentiate the condition from leukaemia. Two to four weeks may elapse before the test becomes positive.

Hodgkin's disease or lymphadenoma

The cause of this disease is unknown. It is characterized by painless enlargement of one or more groups of lymph glands, often associated with increase in size of the spleen and sometimes the liver. The glands in the neck, mediastinum or abdomen may be involved. The intake of alcohol may cause pain, an interesting but unexplained fact.

The disease is a slowly progressive one, the patient becoming weaker and often anaemic in the later stages. Untreated, the average

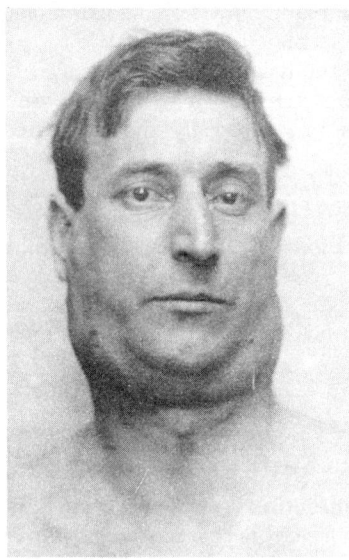

Fig. 42 Hodgkin's disease, with enlargement of cervical glands.

duration of life is about 2 years but the prognosis is greatly improved by modern treatment, which in many cases results in cure of the disease. Bouts of pyrexia are liable to occur during the course of the disease. These may last for several days or weeks and are followed by a period during which the temperature remains normal. (A temperature of this nature is said to be of the Pel-Ebstein type.)

The diagnosis may be confirmed by biopsy of an enlarged gland. Surgery and radiotherapy are the treatment of choice if the disease is localized to one group of lymph nodes. If it is more widespread, cytotoxic drugs are given. These include cyclophosphamide, nitrogen mustard (Mustine, BP), vinblastine ('Velbe') and procarbazine ('Natulan').

Myeloma (multiple myelomatosis)

This is a rare neoplastic type of disease usually affecting the over 40's, the cause of which is unknown. It follows the overgrowth of 'plasma' cells in the bone marrow. Areas of bone destruction and their replacement by the myelomatous cells may occur anywhere in the skeletal system. Fractures of the ribs or long bones or collapse of vertebrae with consequent pressure on the spinal cord are liable to occur. Anaemia and renal failure may be present. The malignancy of the condition leads to death in 2 or 3 years. Prednisone and melphalan or cyclophosphamide are of value in treatment. X-ray therapy may be helpful in relieving pain.

5 Diseases of the Alimentary System

The Alimentary Tract. The following are the main structures through which the food passes during its course down the alimentary canal:

The Mouth, Pharynx, Oesophagus, Stomach.

The small intestine: 1. Duodenum. 2. Jejunum. 3. Ileum.

The large intestine: 1. Caecum. 2. Ascending colon. 3. Transverse colon. 4. Descending colon. 5. Pelvic colon.

The rectum and anus.

Diseases of the mouth, teeth, tongue and salivary glands

Stomatitis, or inflammation of the mouth, is a common condition of which there are several types some of which can be prevented by careful oral hygiene. It is often associated with gingivitis and glossitis.

(a) Acute Stomatitis. This may result from chemical or mechanical irritation (e.g. acids, lysol poisoning, tobacco, etc.) or may be associated with gastrointestinal disturbances in children who are cutting teeth. It is also seen in debilitated patients and in any febrile condition, especially the infectious fevers (e.g. measles). The symptoms consist of swelling and redness of the mucous membrane covering the cheeks, lips and tongue, accompanied by dryness of the mouth and difficulty in mastication. Sometimes small circular grey ulcers, called aphthae, are seen. They tend to be recurrent and are often difficult to treat. These may be associated with emotional stress in some cases.

Inflammation may spread to the parotid gland causing parotitis.

(b) Thrush (parasitic stomatitis). This may be seen in weakly, bottle-fed infants and is associated with lack of cleanliness of the teats and failure to keep the mouth clean. It occurs also in adults who

are seriously ill, in old people who are unable to care for themselves, and sometimes after the administration of broad-spectrum antibiotics by mouth. It is due to a fungus called *Candida albicans*. **(Candidiasis.)** This produces slightly raised milk-white patches surrounded by a thin red margin, which generally start on the tongue and spread to the mucous membrane of the gums, cheeks and palate. In rare cases the infection may spread to the oesophagus, trachea and bronchi. The fungus is sometimes called *Monilia albicans*.

(c) Other forms of stomatitis. These include (1) stomatitis resulting from mercury or bismuth poisoning, which sometimes follows prolonged medicinal administration of these drugs; (2) stomatitis due to vitamin C deficiency; (3) stomatitis due to infection with Vincent's organisms (p. 267).

Treatment. The general treatment of all forms of stomatitis consists of careful toilet of the mouth, which must be cleaned after each feed and all debris removed. Tablets of hydrocortisone ('Corlan') allowed to dissolve slowly in the mouth are helpful in aphthous ulceration. Carbenoxolone ('Bioral gel') or 'Bonjela' may also be applied to ulcers every 4 to 6 hours.

Thrush is treated with nystatin mixture or amphotericin ('Fungilin') lozenges.

The care of the mouth is of great importance in nursing. Any seriously ill patient is liable to develop stomatitis for the following reasons. Firstly, he is unable to attend to his mouth himself and, secondly, the dryness and diminished salivation associated with febrile conditions predispose to the development of infection.

The occurrences of stomatitis during the course of a febrile illness may be a reflection on the efficiency of the nursing, because the condition can usually be prevented if sufficient care and attention are given. It is serious because the infection may spread up the duct of the parotid gland and produce suppurative parotitis (p. 202). The toilet of the mouth should receive attention at least twice daily in every case. In patients who are seriously ill it must be performed after each meal.

False teeth should be removed and cleaned. The natural teeth are cleaned, if possible, with a tooth-brush. The mouth may then be carefully swabbed with mops of cotton-wool moistened with mouth-wash.

Swabs are held in sinus forceps or rolled firmly round the end of a stick, care being taken that the point is well covered. Special attention is given to the space between the gums and the cheek and also to the palate. The patient should afterwards use a mouth-wash.

In infants it is often difficult to use sinus forceps or a stick. The mouth may then be cleaned with a piece of soft linen wrapped round the little finger and dipped in water or normal saline. This method is only suitable when a single infant is being nursed and is not applicable to a children's ward in hospital, on account of the liability of conveying infection from one infant to another. In any case, the nurse must take great care to wash before and after the procedure.

The Teeth

Decay, or caries of the teeth, often commences in childhood and may become very extensive. It is due to two causes. Firstly, soft enamel of poor quality, which is caused by defective formation in childhood. This is frequently a result of deficiency of vitamins in the diet and lack of fluoride in drinking water. Secondly, failure to carry out efficient dental hygiene, thereby permitting the accumulation of food debris between the teeth, especially sweets, and the multiplication of decay-producing bacteria, which act on exposed dentine. Irregularity of the teeth and overcrowding, by making cleaning more difficult, are contributory causes.

It will be seen, therefore, that dental caries is, to a great extent, preventable. All infants should receive an adequate supply of vitamins in the form of orange juice, butter, cod liver oil, etc.; growing children should also have plenty of fruit and the teeth should be cleaned after each meal throughout life. A properly shaped toothbrush must be used and the teeth should be brushed in one direction only, viz. away from the gums.

Regular visits to a dental surgeon are most important in order that minor caries can be detected and treated.

Alveolar abscess. Infection may travel to the root of a tooth producing an abscess in the alveolus of the jaw. This is generally associated with much pain and swelling of the jaw or face, which is relieved when extraction of the tooth permits free drainage of the pus. In some cases, small abscesses develop at the apices of the teeth but remain quiescent. Toxins which produce general ill-health and rheumatic pains may be absorbed from these small collections of pus. **Apical abscesses** can be detected by means of x-rays.

Chronic infection around the teeth is frequently seen and small pockets are formed between them and the gum margin, in which food debris and bacteria collect. The resulting inflammation produces pus —a condition referred to as **pyorrhoea.**

In the early stages, scaling of the teeth, massage of the gums and hydrogen peroxide mouth-washes may prèvent the condition from extending. Later, dental extraction may be necessary.

Inflammation of the gums is called **gingivitis.** Bleeding from the gums may occur in blood disease, leukaemia and purpura; also in vitamin C deficiency (scurvy) and in infection with the organisms causing Vincent's angina (p. 267).

Dental haemorrhage may occur after tooth extraction, not infrequently when a dental surgeon is not available! After cleaning the socket with warm saline the patient should be instructed to bite firmly on a folded gauze swab placed on the site for not less than 10–15 minutes continuously. This is often effective. In other cases packing the socket with ribbon gauze soaked in adrenaline or even suturing may be necessary. It should be remembered that sometimes excessive haemorrhage is associated with an underlying blood disease requiring further investigation.

The tongue

The appearance of the tongue affords a valuable indication of the state of the digestive functions and the progress of febrile or other disorders. Three main points are to be observed; its size or shape, its movements and the condition of its surface. Swelling may occur if the tongue is inflamed **(glossitis)** or when it is the site of new growths. Paralysis of the tongue, or one half of it, may be present in various diseases of the nervous system. The protruded organ is tremulous in chronic alcoholism and in general paralysis of the insane. In chorea, the movements are sudden and jerky.

The amount of salivary secretion combined with the normal movements of mastication are chiefly responsible for the appearance of its surface. These movements cease during sleep and furring is, therefore, more marked in the morning.

The normal tongue is moist and clean, although there is usually a slight collection of fur on the back. Generalized coating of the organ is associated with stomatitis, dental caries, gastritis, constipation and abdominal disease, such as inflammation of the gall-bladder, appendicitis, and intestinal obstruction. It is also seen in any febrile condition including tonsillitis, influenza, pneumonia and the acute specific fevers. A thick dry brownish fur is found in conditions of marked prostration, and serious illness, such as uraemia, general peritonitis, and severe pneumonia, and may then be associated with the collection of sordes on the teeth, gums and lips.

In most cases, a dry tongue is an indication of dehydration and calls for the administration of fluids. A very dry tongue is always a grave sign, but, if it shows evidence of becoming moister, there is usually an associated improvement in the condition of the patient.

After a heavy coating of fur has disappeared, the tongue remains red and raw and, if the organ is still dry, painful cracks may develop on its surface.

It has already been seen that the tongue is sometimes affected by thrush; the characteristic 'strawberry' appearances seen in scarlet fever are described on p. 51. (See also pernicious anaemia, in which the tongue is clean, smooth and almost devoid of papillae, p. 178.)

The tongue is frequently the site of injury and ulceration **Injury** may be caused by biting, especially in epilepsy. It is for this reason that if possible a gag is placed between the teeth of a patient in a fit.

Ulceration of the tongue may be of four types:

1. Simple, associated with dyspepsia, stomatitis and with broken teeth.
2. Tuberculous, a complication of tuberculosis of the lungs.
3. Syphilitic.
4. Malignant; cancer of the tongue which usually presents as a chronic ulcer with hard, raised margins.

Diseases of the Salivary Glands

The saliva is secreted by three pairs of salivary glands, the parotid, submandibular and sublingual. Its function is to perform the first stage of carbohydrate digestion by the action of the enzyme ptyalin, which converts starch into sugar. It also acts as a lubricant for the swallowed food and keeps the mouth moist. One to two pints (0·5–1 litre) are normally secreted daily, excessive secretion being called salivation. Inflammation of the parotid gland occurring in **mumps** has already been described (p. 72).

Infection sometimes spreads up the duct of the gland in severe or neglected cases of stomatitis and in gravely ill patients and may result in the formation of an abscess (**suppurative parotitis,** p. 199), which may need incision. This may be avoided in some cases by the use of penicillin or other antibiotic.

Occasionally **salivary calculi** form in the ducts producing painless swelling of the glands after meals. These concretions can be seen by x-ray and may be removed by operation.

Difficulty in Swallowing (Dysphagia)

The act of swallowing has two consecutive stages:

1. The passage of food from the mouth, through the pillars of the fauces into the pharynx. This is a voluntary act in which the tongue, palatal and pharyngeal muscles take part.
2. The involuntary peristaltic contractions of the oesophageal muscles which carry the food to the cardia.

It follows, therefore, that difficult or painful swallowing may have a number of causes, e.g.:

  (i) Stomatitis and glossitis: painful movements of the jaw such as occur in parotitis and mumps.
 (ii) Tonsillitis, quinsy and pharyngitis.
(iii) Paralysis of muscles of the pharynx or palate such as may occur in poliomyelitis (bulbar paralysis), diphtheria and other diseases of the nervous system.
 (iv) Conditions affecting the oesophagus.
  (v) Hiatus hernia.
 (vi) Achalasia, in which the lower oesophageal sphincter fails to relax.
(vii) Hysterical patients sometimes complain of dysphagia (p. 406).

Disease of the oesophagus

Affections of the oesophagus, causing **dysphagia** and obstruction to the passage of food, may be considered in the following way (see also p. 4):

1. Obstruction to the Lumen of the oesophagus. A foreign body, for example a swallowed tooth-plate, coin, or bone, may become fixed in the oesophagus. This impaction is liable to occur at two positions (*a*) behind the cricoid cartilage, (*b*) at the cardia, where the oesophagus enters the stomach.

2. Obstruction due to Disease of the Wall. A stricture of the oesophagus may be caused by (*a*) the contraction of scar tissue following injury to the wall as a result of swallowed corrosive poisons, (*b*) cancer of the oesophagus, the commonest sites of which are also at the level of the cricoid cartilage and at the junction of the oesophagus with the stomach (the cardia).

3. Obstruction due to Pressure on the oesophagus from outside. Tumours in the mediastinum or growing from the lung, retrosternal goitre and aneurysm of the aorta may press on the oesophagus and thereby cause dysphagia.

4. Interference with the neuromuscular mechanism. A rare condition in which the muscle at the lower end of the oesophagus fails to relax and to allow the contained food to pass into the stomach, produces similar symptoms. This is known as **achalasia of the cardia** or **cardiospasm.** Treatment is by instrumental dilatation but in some cases operation (Heller's myotomy) is necessary.

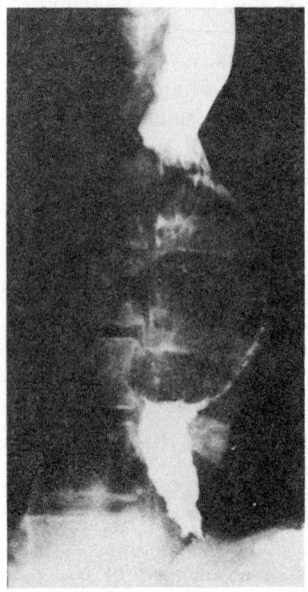

Fig. 43 Carcinoma of the oesophagus (barium swallow)

Symptoms of oesophageal obstruction. The patient is conscious of the food being held up. If the condition is of long duration, gradual starvation occurs, owing to the fact that insufficient food reaches the stomach. There is progressive emaciation and acetone may appear in the urine as a result of the semi-starvation produced.

The passage of solid food is more difficult than semi-solids or liquids and, for this reason, the diet should consist mainly of milk foods, including Benger's, arrowroot, etc., beaten-up eggs, thickened soups, custard, fruit juice and sugar, given frequently and in small quantities at a time.

Diagnosis and treatment. The diagnosis is made on the

statement of the patient that he is unable to swallow properly, and may be aided by giving a barium meal the progress of which is watched by x-rays. The level and character of the obstruction can then be determined. In other cases, the obstruction can be seen by passing an illuminated tubular instrument known as the oesophago-scope. This investigation, known as **oesophagoscopy**, may be performed in many instances without the use of general anaesthesia.

The treatment depends on the cause of the obstruction. Foreign bodies are removed with the aid of the oesophagoscope and strictures may be dilated with bougies under direct vision by the use of this instrument.

Carcinoma of the oesophagus may be treated by means of deep x-ray therapy. In some instances a growth may be removed by operation. In other cases, a tube is inserted into the oesophagus to prevent its closure by growth.

In severe cases of oesophageal obstruction, which cannot be dealt with by these means, it is necessary to make an artificial opening into the stomach (gastrostomy), and to feed the patient with liquid or semi-solid food by this route.

Diseases of the stomach

Food, after leaving the oesophagus, passes into the stomach where further stages in the process of digestion go on.

Ptyalin, contained in swallowed saliva, continues to act for some time and converts starch into sugar. Pepsin, secreted by the stomach, transforms protein into peptone in the presence of hydro-chloric acid. The food is mixed thoroughly with the gastric juice and passed on, in small quantities at a time, through the pylorus into the duodenum. The process of mixing is carried out by rhythmic wave-like contractions of the muscular tissue of the stomach wall (peristalsis).

Methods of gastric examination

In addition to investigating the symptoms presented by the patient, the following aids to diagnosis may be employed:

1. X-ray.
2. Pentagastrin test.
3. Examination of the stools for altered blood.
4. Gastroscopy.
5. Gastric camera.
6. Telemetering devices, e.g. a pH capsule.

1. X-ray (Barium meal). The patient swallows half to one pint of a mixture containing barium sulphate, which is opaque to x-rays and which shows clearly the outline of the stomach and duodenum. In this way, the shape, size and position of the organ, together with the character of the peristaltic waves, may be seen.

The rate at which the barium leaves the stomach can be observed, and any irregularities of its surface caused by ulceration or by new growths may be visible.

It is important that the stomach be empty before this examination is made and it is the duty of the nurse to see that the patient has no food or drink for at least four hours prior to a barium meal.

2. The pentagastrin test. This investigation is carried out in order to ascertain the presence and amount or absence of hydrochloric acid in the gastric juice. An excess of acid is spoken of as hyperchlorhydria, a diminished amount as hypochlorhydria. If no hydrochloric acid is found the condition is called achlorhydria or achylia (which also implies the absence of pepsin and intrinsic factor).

All three states may be found in normal individuals, but hyperchlorhydria is common in duodenal ulcer; hypochlorhydria in chronic gastritis and cancer of the stomach; and achlorhydria in cancer of the stomach, pernicious anaemia and simple achlorhydric (hypochromic) anaemia (p. 181).

Hyperchlorhydria may be found in duodenal ulcer.

Hypochlorhydria ,, ,, ,, ,, $\begin{cases} \text{chronic gastritis.} \\ \text{cancer of the stomach.} \end{cases}$

Achlorhydria ,, ,, ,, ,, $\begin{cases} \text{cancer of the stomach.} \\ \text{pernicious anaemia.} \\ \text{simple hypochromic} \\ \quad \text{anaemia.} \end{cases}$

The test is carried out in the morning before food has been taken. The patient is instructed to swallow a Ryle's tube. A good deal of patience may be required in order to persuade a nervous individual to swallow the tube. He should be told to place it within the lips, to take deep breaths through the nose and then swallow. Any tendency to retching must be counteracted by deep breathing, and saliva should be ejected into a receiver and not swallowed. When the tube is in the stomach, as confirmed by x-ray, the resting juice is collected by continuous aspiration with a suction pump for one hour. Pentagastrin is then given subcutaneously, in a dose of 6 micrograms per kg of body weight, and gastric juice is collected for another hour. Throughout the collection, the patient lies on his left side. The hydrochloric acid output, before and after stimulation by pentagastrin is calculated from measurement of the collected volumes of juice and the results of titration against a standard solution of alkali.

The amount and character of the resting juice is important. A large quantity indicates obstruction at the pylorus, for a stomach emptying at a normal rate will not contain anything taken the night before. If, in addition, it is foul-smelling and contains altered blood it is suggestive of cancer.

The 'Diagnex' test. The presence of hydrochloric acid in the stomach can also be determined by this test on the urine. 'Diagnex' contains a blue dye which is only absorbed from the bowel and excreted in the urine if it has been acted on by hydrochloric acid in the stomach. The urine is collected and tested two hours after the 'Diagnex' has been taken. This test is much easier to carry out than the test meal, and in some cases gives all the information required.

3. Occult blood in the faeces. When bleeding occurs in the upper part of the alimentary tract, the blood is passed on to the intestine and is subjected to the actions of the digestive juices and bacteria; by the time it is expelled from the body in the faeces, it is no longer recognizable as such to the naked eye. If the bleeding has been severe the stools are dark in colour and tarry in consistency **(melaena)**. The altered blood from slight bleeding can, however, be detected by chemical tests and is referred to as hidden or occult blood.

Care must also be taken that blood resulting from epistaxis or injuries about the mouth has not been swallowed. Occult blood is frequently detected in the stools in gastric and duodenal ulcer and in cancer of the stomach also in some patients who are taking aspirin.

Fresh, red blood in the stools suggests bleeding from the colon or rectum in conditions such as ulcerative colitis, carcinoma and haemorrhoids.

4. Gastroscopy. The gastroscope is an instrument consisting of an upper rigid metal portion and a lower flexible part into which are fixed a series of lenses. The instrument is illuminated by an electric battery and is passed down the oesophagus into the stomach. A fiberscope allows a particularly good view of the gastric antrum.

No food should be given to the patient for 8 hours before the examination. One hour beforehand he is given a hypodermic injection of morphine with atropine or scopolamine. A local anaesthetic (decicain 2%, with adrenaline) is painted on the back of the tongue and pharynx, which is also sprayed with the same solution to include the upper part of the larynx. The patient then lies on his left side with his head supported by an assistant, and the gastroscope, lubricated with K-Y jelly, is passed.

In this way the interior of the stomach can be seen. It is often possible to demonstrate the presence of an ulcer and to decide whether or not it is malignant.

5. *The Gastric Camera* allows good colour photographs to be taken of the interior of the stomach.

6. *Telemetering devices* permit a continuous assessment of changes (of pH, for example) in the patient's stomach. They are only used in special cases and in research.

Symptoms of gastric disturbances

The main symptoms of gastric disorders are: loss of appetite (anorexia), flatulence, hiccough, pain, nausea and vomiting.

Anorexia. Loss of appetite is common in chronic gastritis and cancer of the stomach. It is also seen in toxaemic conditions such as the acute fevers and tuberculosis, and in heart failure. It is a matter of great importance to the nurse. In those cases in which organic disease is present a suitable, light and appetizing diet must be given and the patient encouraged to take as much as he can digest. Frequent small feeds are usually taken more readily than large meals. It is sometimes possible to increase the appetite by giving small doses of insulin.

Not infrequently, however, anorexia occurs in the absence of organic disease in anxiety states and hysteria. In such cases tact and firmness are essential and they may be helped by psychological treatment.

Anorexia nervosa is a rare but more serious psychological condition often precipitated by some emotional crisis, in which food is refused and the patient becomes progressively emaciated. It may be looked upon as a weight phobia in which the patient avoids or vomits all 'fattening' foods. Unconsciously the patient fears not only the normal adolescent weight changes which will fill out her figure into womanhood but is afraid of the psychosocial implications of puberty. It is more common in adolescent females (only 5% of patients are boys) and may be accompanied by amenorrhoea, hirsuties, severe constipation, hypotension, slow pulse and a poor peripheral circulation. The basal metabolic rate is low and the serum cholesterol level tends to be elevated. Disorders of electrolyte and fluid balance may occur. Severe oedema is sometimes seen.

Several months of inpatient care may be needed under the close supervision of a psychiatrist. Phenothiazine drugs (e.g. chlorpromazine) may be helpful. Electroconvulsive therapy (ECT) is applied in some cases. Patients must be retrained to eat meals containing adequate carbohydrate.

Death may occur from suicide or, less often, from malnutrition.

Gastric Flatulence. Gastric flatulence, or the accumulation of gas in the stomach, is a common condition and is nearly always due to swallowed air. The patient feels some discomfort in the upper abdomen which he thinks is due to wind and which he imagines he can displace by bringing it up. The attempts at eructation only result in swallowing more air, so that the stomach becomes more and more distended. After a number of attempts have been made the stomach becomes do distended that the gas is at last expelled noisily and the patient obtains relief. The condition may be associated with organic disease of the stomach, such as gastric ulcer or cancer, or with disease of the gall-bladder, but more often it is due to nervous dyspepsia, a condition frequent in neurotic and hysterical individuals. It is important to recognize this state of affairs and to explain to the patient the mechanism of the introduction of gas into the stomach. This is usually effective in the case of an intelligent patient who is willing to co-operate. Temporary relief can be obtained by sipping hot water or by taking a little oil of peppermint on a lump of sugar. Air swallowing is also known as **aerophagy.**

Hiccough. Hiccough is due to a spasm of the diaphragm occurring at irregular intervals and may have a number of causes. It is essentially a reflex action with a nerve centre in the 3rd, 4th and 5th segments of the cervical portion of the spinal cord. Two varieties may be considered. The first when the attack is mild and of short duration, the second in which it is persistent.

(*a*) *Hiccough of short duration.* This is a very common condition and is usually associated with distension or overloading of the stomach. In these cases, simple measures such as pressure on the eyeballs, holding the breath, the trick of drinking water from the distant side of a glass which causes drawing in of the abdominal muscles; drawing the thighs up to the abdomen or pressure on the epigastrium, are usually effective. If not, a carminative such as peppermint or ginger may be given. Rebeathing into a bag for a short time, thereby increasing the carbon dioxide in the blood, is helpful.

(*b*) *Persistent hiccough.* This is often very troublesome and may go on for many hours or days. The common causes of prolonged attacks are acute abdominal conditions such as peritonitis in which it is a serious sign, intestinal obstruction, uraemia and encephalitis. Sometimes firm traction on the tongue for several minutes will cut short an attack. In other cases chlorpromazine and inhalation of amyl nitrite may be required. Barbiturates, morphine or inhalation of chloroform are also effective in some cases.

Pain. Pain due to gastric disease is felt either in the epigastrium or behind the sternum. It is usually related to the intake of food, coming on soon after meals, and is described as being of a gnawing or burning character. The occurrence of epigastric pain at definite intervals of time, which the patient can foretell with considerable accuracy, is a common feature of organic disease of the stomach or duodenum.

Nausea. Nausea, or the sensation of feeling sick frequently precedes vomiting and is relieved when emesis has taken place.

Vomiting

Vomiting or emesis is a very common symptom and may be due to a number of causes. The process of vomiting may be divided into three stages.

1. Salivation, nausea and sweating.
2. Deep inspiration with contraction of the diaphragm and abdominal muscles.
3. Ejection of the vomitus while the breath is held.

The mechanism by which it occurs can be explained if it is re-remembered that a special vomiting centre is present in the nervous system (the medulla). The sensory or afferent nerves pass from the stomach and other abdominal viscera to the vomiting centre and the

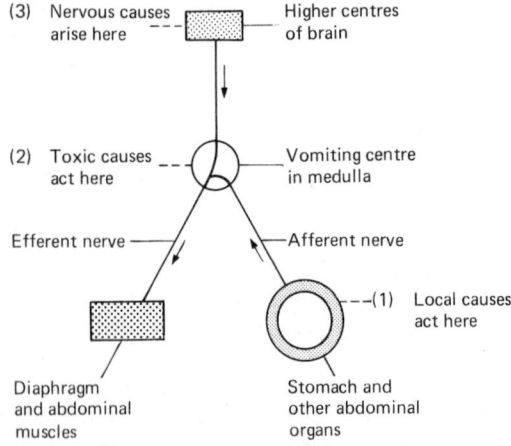

Fig. 44 Diagram illustrating the mechanism of vomiting.

efferent or motor nerves pass from the medulla to the diaphragm, abdominal and stomach muscles. The stimuli which cause vomiting may arise (*a*) in the stomach or abdominal organs and pass, via the afferent nerves, to the medulla. (*b*) The centre itself may be affected by toxic processes or (*c*) may receive stimuli from the higher centres in the brain. In other words, the causes may act locally or centrally, the local causes producing vomiting by the process of reflex action. Some of the common causes may be classified thus:

A. LOCAL AND REFLEX CAUSES
　　1.　Irritation of the pharynx (e.g. tickling the back of the throat).
　　2.　Alimentary conditions.
　　　　(*a*) Gastritis, gastric ulcer, pyloric stenosis, cancer of the stomach.
　　　　(*b*) Peritonitis, intestinal obstruction, appendicitis.
　　　　(*c*) Constipation and gall-bladder disease
　　　　(*d*) Painful stimuli (e.g. biliary or renal colic).
　　　　(*e*) The action of drugs (emetics) on the stomach, including a number of poisons.

B. TOXIC CAUSES (acting directly on the vomiting centre).
　　1.　The onset of any acute infection.
　　2.　Nephritis and uraemia.
　　3.　Pregnancy.
　　4.　Emetic drugs acting directly on the centre (e.g. apomorphine). After anaesthetics.

C. NERVOUS CAUSES (due to stimuli from higher centres).
　　1.　Psychological stimuli (e.g. revolting smells or sights).
　　2.　Meningitis, cerebral tumour, migraine, concussion.
　　3.　Sea- or motion-sickness, due to impulses from the labyrinth.

Special characters of vomiting. Early morning vomiting is characteristic of pregnancy and of gastritis, especially when due to alcohol. Vomiting after food is most likely to occur in gastric and other abdominal conditions. When there is no relation to food the cause is usually of nervous or toxic origin.

It is a matter of great importance for the nurse to observe the character and quantity of the vomited material. The vomitus may consist of:

(*a*) Food, which is usually partly digested. In some cases, material taken the previous day or many hours before can be detected, an observation which indicates obstruction to the outlet of stomach contents at the pylorus.

(*b*) Fluid, which may appear either watery or bile-stained.

(*c*) Blood. This may occur either in the form of bright red blood after recent haemorrhage; or as dark brown material, usually described as having the appearance of 'coffee grounds,' which is due to the blood having been in the stomach sufficiently long for the gastric juice to cause its partial digestion. The vomiting of fresh or altered blood is called **haematemesis** (p. 221).

(d) 'Faecal' fluid. Dark brown fluid with a foul, faeculent odour is often vomited in the later stages of intestinal obstruction.

The term projectile vomiting is used when the stomach contents are ejected with great force. It is liable to occur in pyloric stenosis (especially the congenital type in infants, p. 226) and in cases of cerebral disease, e.g. cerebral tumour.

In cases of gastroenteritis, vomiting is associated with diarrhoea.

Treatment. Vomitus should be collected in a suitable receiver, measured and retained for inspection. This is particularly important in cases of suspected poisoning. If possible, the patient should lean forward and the head should be supported. All traces of vomit must be removed as soon as possible, the night clothes or bed linen being changed if necessary. The actual treatment of vomiting must in every case depend on its cause. 'Avomine', chlorpromazine ('Largactil'), perphenazine ('Fentazin') or metoclopramide ('Maxolon') are effective in some cases. A little brandy in water is sometimes useful, or a mixture containing kaolin or bismuth may be given. If much fluid has been lost intravenous salines with glucose are given. After prolonged or severe vomiting, acetone may appear in the urine.

Great care must be taken to see that an unconscious patient does not inhale vomit into the trachea and lungs. This may lead to sudden death from asphyxia or, if the patient survives, to pneumonia. An unconscious patient who is vomiting should not be left unattended. The head must be turned to one side and all vomited material removed from the mouth and pharynx without delay using a suction apparatus.

Dyspepsia

Dyspepsia or indigestion is a common condition, having three main symptoms:

(a) *flatulence* and eructation of gas, with the associated feelings of epigastric discomfort and distension;

(b) *heart-burn,* or the sensation of substernal and precordial pain, which is due to spasm of the oesophagus and to the regurgitation of the acid contents of the stomach into its lower end;

(c) *water-brash* or pyrosis which is the regurgitation of watery fluid into the mouth, consisting mainly of swallowed saliva.

The common *causes* of dyspepsia may be classified thus:

1. General causes.
    (a) Imperfect mastication due to bad or deficient teeth.
    (b) Hurried or irregular meals.
    (c) Constipation.
    (d) Anxiety states.
    (e) Air-swallowing (aerophagy) and flatulence.
2. Errors of diet.
    (a) Indigestible food, new bread, unripe fruit.
    (b) Excess of alcohol, tobacco or condiments.
    (c) Overdrawn tea.
3. Organic diseases.
    (a) Gastritis, gastric ulcer or cancer, hiatus hernia, duodenal ulcer.
    (b) Diseases of the liver or gallbladder.
    (c) Chronic heart disease.

The **treatment** of simple dyspepsia is similar to that of chronic gastritis but organic causes must be excluded.

Gastritis

Inflammation of the mucous membrane of the stomach may be acute or chronic. The common causes of **acute gastritis** include some drugs (e.g. aspirin), unripe fruit, decomposed tinned meat, shellfish, excess of alcohol and corrosive poisons, such as strong acids or alkalis. The main symptoms are epigastric pain and tenderness, vomiting and constipation which may be followed later by diarrhoea.

If vomiting is very severe, intravenous salines may be necessary. Anti-emetic drugs, belladonna and kaolin or an antacid may be given. A diet consisting of small frequent feeds of soda-water or diluted milk is taken at first and gradually increased as the symptoms abate.

Chronic gastritis may follow recurrent attacks of acute gastritis or may be due to any of the causes of dyspepsia. The symptoms are mainly dyspeptic, consisting of anorexia, flatulence, nausea and occasional vomiting especially in the early morning. The tongue is furred and constipation is often present.

The **treatment** consists in attention to the teeth, supplying dentures if necessary, and insisting on proper mastication and regular meals. The food should be light and easily digested. Alcohol is prohibited, tea must be weak and freshly made and all condiments and tough meat should be avoided. The bowels are kept regular by saline aperients, and a bitter or alkaline mixture (e.g. Mistura Gentianae Alkalina, BPC) may be given before meals, in order to increase the appetite and to stimulate the secretion of gastric juice. The patient should take regular exercise, with rest before and after meals.

In chronic gastritis and dyspepsia, the following are suitable articles of diet:—Mutton, chicken, fish, eggs, milk, farinaceous food, toast, asparagus, spinach and cauliflower.

The following should be avoided:—Fried foods, pork, game, shell-fish, twice-cooked meat, new bread, pastry, cabbage, carrots and turnips.

Atrophic gastritis, in which the gastric mucosa is abnormally thin and acid secretion is diminished or absent, is found in a number of conditions, e.g. pernicious anaemia, hypopituitarism and Addison's disease. Localized patches of atrophic gastritis occur in cases of gastric ulcer and gastric carcinoma. An erosion may form in the atrophic mucosa and may bleed.

Peptic ulcer

This is a common condition and includes:
1. Gastric ulcer.
2. Duodenal ulcer.
3. Anastomotic ulcer, e.g. at the site of a gastro-enterostomy.

The actual cause of these conditions is not fully explained but certain facts are known.

1. The common factor in all ulcers in the upper part of the alimentary tract is the presence of gastric juice which has digestive properties. Similar ulcers may be found in the lower end of the oesophagus, the stomach, duodenum and at the junction of a gastro-enterostomy after this operation has been performed. Hence the term **'peptic ulcer'** is often used to cover all these conditions.

2. Two types of gastric juice may be considered: (*a*) the resting or fasting juice, (*b*) the secretion produced by the intake of food. Clearly the latter can have little effect in the production of an ulcer because it is immediately 'buffered' or neutralized by the food. On the other hand the fasting juice may be excessive in amount and high in acid in cases of peptic ulcer.

3. Even this is not a full explanation because a high acid fasting juice does not necessarily produce an ulcer. It follows, therefore, that in ulcer

cases the gastric mucous membrane is less resistant to injury than that of the normal stomach and presumably has lost some of its natural protective immunity to the action of gastric juice.

4. Gastric secretion is influenced by the involuntary (autonomic) nervous system, the impulses from which reach the stomach in the vagus nerve. Emotional disturbances can influence not only gastric secretion

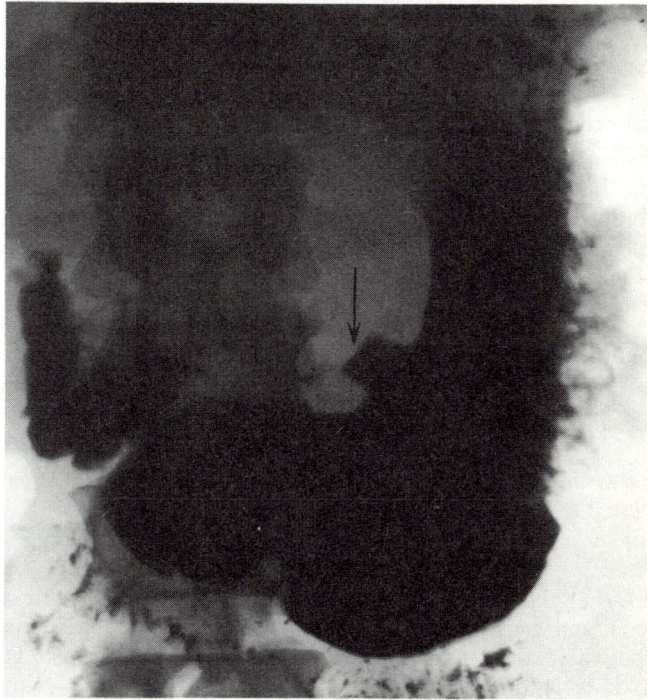

Fig. 45 X-ray of stomach (barium meal) showing deep ulcer crater on lesser curvature.

but also the movements of the stomach and the capillaries in its mucous membrane through the vagus nerve. In the same way that an emotion can cause blushing, which is increased capillary dilatation in the skin, so can it produce 'blushing' of the mucous membrane of the stomach. This phenomenon can be observed through the gastroscope.

5. It is therefore possible to consider a peptic ulcer as being produced by the action of gastric juice on the mucosa of a stomach or duodenum which has lost the natural power of resisting this action. This result is provoked by stimuli reaching the stomach through the vagus nerve which

may be of emotional origin and which produce excessive gastric secretion and movement and abnormal capillary dilatation.

6. It is also known that various hormones play their part in the secretion of gastric and other intestinal juices, and in some cases they influence the production or treatment of a gastric ulcer.

The importance of this theoretical conception has its bearing on the modern treatment of ulcer which lays less emphasis on the details of dietetic treatment and more on the factors just mentioned.

It should be noted that peptic ulcers are rare in children. Duodenal ulcer is more common in patients belonging to blood group O.

Gastric ulcer

Ulceration of the stomach is common and may be either acute or chronic. The process of ulceration consists of erosion of the mucous membrane of the stomach which may involve a blood vessel or which may penetrate the muscular coat and reach the peritoneal covering of the organ. If the ulcer is on the posterior aspect of the stomach it may become adherent to the pancreas.

Symptoms. *1. Pain.* The most important symptom is epigastric pain, often described as 'burning' in character, occurring at regular intervals (usually one quarter to one hour) after food has been taken. Attacks may last for several weeks and then subside, only to recur later.

2. Tenderness. This is present in the epigastrium and may be associated with some rigidity of the abdominal muscles.

3. Vomiting. This sometimes occurs after food and may relieve pain.

4. Other features. The tongue is clean, there is frequently some anaemia, and constipation is common. As a rule, the appetite is not lost, but the patient may be afraid to eat on account of the pain which food will bring on.

Complications and Results. *1. Healing.* With medical treatment the majority of early ulcers heal. (*a*) A small ulcer will heal without leaving any signs. (*b*) If the ulcer is large and is situated close to the pylorus, the contraction of scar tissue associated with healing may so narrow the pylorus that there is an obstruction to the passage of food into the duodenum, a condition known as pyloric stenosis. (*c*) The same process of contraction of scar tissue in an ulcer situated in the middle of the stomach may result in a narrowing of the body of the organ, so that it becomes divided into two halves, communicating with each other by a narrow opening. This condition is called 'hourglass' stomach.

2. Perforation. It has been pointed out that an ulcer may penetrate the walls of the stomach and reach the peritoneum, in the same way that a typhoid ulcer involves the bowel (p. 42). A perforation may occur which permits the stomach contents to enter the general peritoneal cavity and, unless treated at once, will result in peritonitis. The main symptom of this acute surgical emergency is the sudden onset of severe and continuous epigastric pain, in a patient who gives a history of previous indigestion. The pulse rate rises and the muscles of the abdominal wall become rigid. The treatment is immediate operation to close the perforation. If the operation is performed within a few hours the prognosis is good, but delay over 6 or 8 hours renders the condition less favourable.

3. Haemorrhage. As in typhoid ulceration, a blood vessel may become eroded. Bleeding from an ulcer, if severe, results in haematemesis (p. 221) and melaena. In other cases, it causes the presence of occult blood in the stools.

4. Cancer. In a few instances, a chronic ulcer of the stomach may be followed by cancer at the site of the ulcer.

Diagnosis. The diagnosis of the condition is made by considering the history of abdominal pain related to food, the appearance of occult blood in the stools and, in many instances, the demonstration of the ulcer as an irregularity of the surface of the stomach as seen by x-rays after a barium meal, or by gastroscopy.

Duodenal ulcer

This is the most common type of peptic ulcer. The main points of difference between the symptoms of gastric and duodenal ulcer are that in the latter the onset of pain is generally delayed until 3 or 4 hours after food has been taken (hunger pain) and that the pain is relieved by taking more food. This pain may wake the patient during the night. Vomiting and haematemesis are less common, but perforation, melaena and the presence of occult blood in the stools occur as in gastric ulcer. The condition is more common in men and shows a tendency to recur at intervals after apparent recovery An acid secretion test often shows hyperchlorhydria and a barium meal may demonstrate an ulcer or a deformity of the duodenal cap.

Treatment of gastric and duodenal ulcer

The treatment of these conditions may be either medical or surgical, the line of action adopted being determined by the circumstances in each individual case. The main indications for **surgical treatment** may be summarized thus:

1. Perforation.
2. Pyloric stenosis.
3. Recurrent haemorrhage.
4. Failure of medical treatment to produce lasting results.
5. Social and economic factors which interfere with prolonged medical treatment.
6. A suspicion of malignancy.

In other words, the majority of uncomplicated ulcers should be given a trial with medical treatment before operative measures are undertaken.

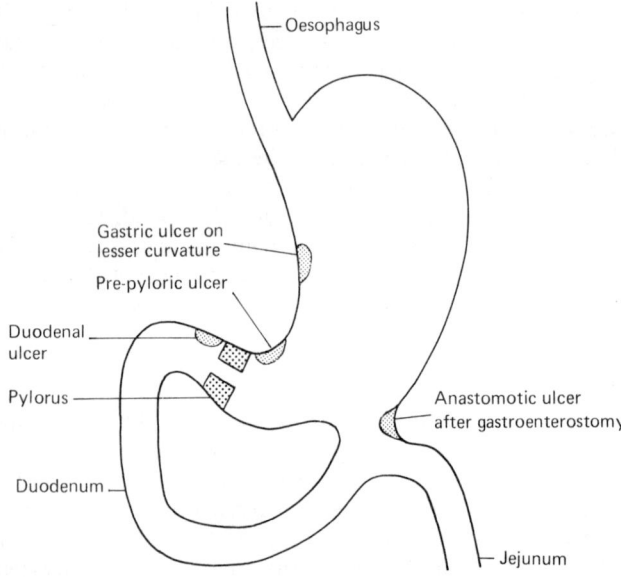

Fig. 46 The common sites of peptic ulcer.

The nurse in the course of her training and experience will probably meet with methods of **medical treatment** which differ from one another in a number of ways. It is her duty to carry out in detail the instructions given in each case.

Physical and mental rest with freedom from emotional strain are essential. It will frequently be observed that the pain of an ulcer will disappear after a few days' rest in bed without any other special treatment. A tranquillizer may be administered to help to allay anxiety. Belladonna diminishes the action of the vagus nerve and not only reduces gastric secretion but also lessens the movements of the stomach. 'Probanthine' and similar drugs may be used instead of belladonna.

The objects of the medical treatment of peptic ulcer are to:

(a) give symptomatic relief
(b) promote healing of the ulcer
(c) prevent recurrence.

These objectives may be achieved by:

1. Adequate physical rest.
2. Removal of anxiety.
3. Control of hyperacidity.
4. Diminution of gastric peristalsis.
5. Cessation of smoking.
6. Avoidance of aspirin in any form.
7. Suitable dietetic measures.

Physical and mental rest with freedom from emotional strain are essential. The use of various drugs is also important:

1. To neutralize acid as far as possible by the administration of antacids (alkalis), e.g. magnesium trisilicate, aluminium hydroxide or special compressed tablets of these or similar substances which are allowed to dissolve slowly between the cheek and lower jaw, at the rate of two or three an hour, such as 'Nulacin', 'Gelusil', 'Prodexin'.

2. To give a general sedative such as phenobarbitone or sodium amytal or a tranquillizer such as diazepam.

3. To give a drug which diminishes the secretion of acid and reduces peristalsis and muscular spasm, e.g. atropine or belladonna, propantheline ('Probanthine'), 'Merbentyl', 'Wyovin'. The latter anticholinergic drugs are not necessarily more helpful than belladonna.

4. It has been shown that gastric ulcers heal more rapidly when carbenoxolone ('Biogastrone') is administered 3 times a day *after* meals for 6 weeks.

'Duogastrone' capsules are used for duodenal ulcer; they are specially made so as to deliver carbenoxolone directly into the duodenum and they must be taken 15 to 30 minutes *before* meals. Carbenoxolone is a derivative of liquorice. Patients may remain ambulant and even working during treatment with carbenoxolone and less attention to diet is necessary. These drugs may cause electrolyte disturbance with potassium loss. Caved-S is an alternative liquorice preparation which contains antacids and frangula bark (an antispasmodic) in addition to liquorice.

Diet. Formerly very strict and dull dietetic measures were imposed, essentially based on the 'Sippy method'. However, the main points of dietetic measures persist:

(a) The diet should produce the least possible mechanical stimulation of the stomach and irritation of the ulcer.

(b) It must produce the minimum amount of gastric secretion.

(c) Adequate nourishment including a sufficiency of vitamins, especially vitamin C, must be supplied in order to improve the general condition and, thereby, promote healing.

(d) Feeds should be small so that the stomach is not overloaded, and at first should be given at intervals of two hours when the patient is awake.

The following indicates the sort of diet which might be used in acute cases:

STAGE I (May be necessary for a few days, when acute symptoms are present.)

(a) Bed rest except for visits to lavatory.

(b) Two-hourly feeds of milk 150 ml (5 oz) with Horlick's, Benger's, Ovaltine, arrowroot, custard, junket to which sugar, cream, chocolate, etc. may be added to taste. Strained orange or tomato juice two or three times daily.

(c) In most cases at the three main meal-times rusks, thin bread and butter with honey or a lightly boiled egg may be taken.

(d) Thick soup or purée may replace one or more of the milk feeds.

STAGE II Two-hourly feeds continue.

On waking:	Milk or weak milky tea.
Breakfast:	Milk, milky tea or milk flavoured with coffee. Cereal with milk and sugar and cream to taste.
	One egg, lightly boiled, poached or scrambled, or steamed fish.
	Bread and butter.
Mid-morning:	Milk drink.
Lunch:	Thick soup or purée.
	Steamed fish, chicken, rabbit, minced beef or mutton.
	Mashed or creamed potatoes.
	Sieved vegetables.
	Milk pudding or cream cheese with plain biscuit and butter.
Tea:	Milk or milky tea.
	Bread and butter with jam, honey or Marmite.
	Sponge cake.
Supper:	As lunch.
Bed time:	Milk drink.

General measures and post-ulcer regime. In all cases the teeth should, if necessary, receive attention. The patient must eat slowly and masticate food properly. Hunger should be avoided at all times and if the patient wakes during the night a milk drink or biscuits followed by a dose of antacid should be taken. Smoking should be avoided or at most only allowed in strict moderation after meals.

Foods to be avoided (see also chronic gastritis p. 214) include:

1. Obviously hard and indigestible foods.
2. Highly spiced foods and irritating condiments such as mustard and pepper.
3. Fried and greasy foods.
4. Fruit skins and pips.
5. Coarse vegetables.
6. Alcohol, strong tea and coffee.

In fact, this is largely a matter of common sense. Immediately any symptoms return the patient may find a Stage I or II diet comforting for a few days until they subside.

Continuous drip therapy. It is possible to neutralize the hydrochloric acid in the gastric juice continuously by giving milk by a drip feed directly into the stomach. A Ryle's tube, made non-irritant by smearing with 2% cocaine ointment, is passed through the nostril and fixed in position to the cheek by strapping. It is changed, cleaned and boiled every other day. If the nasal method is not tolerated the tube may be passed through the mouth. From a height of 2 feet (61 cm) a continuous drip of milk, which may be citrated, is given from a suitable container such as a transfusion bottle at the rate of 40 drops a minute. This will provide 5 pints (2·8 l) of milk in 24 hours. Glucose and 10% casein hydrolysate may be added in the proportion of 1 pint to 5 pints (0·5–2·8 l) of milk. 'Aludrox' may be added to the drip ($\frac{1}{2}$ fl oz to each pint of milk; 15 ml to 0·5 l). This method may be used for short periods in selected cases.

Haematemesis

Haematemesis or the vomiting of blood is an important and common condition which may be due to a number of causes:

1. Local **disease of the stomach,** especially gastric ulcer. Other lesions include acute gastritis, particularly if due to corrosive poisons, hiatus hernia, carcinoma of the stomach and some cases of duodenal ulcer when the blood flows back through the pylorus into the stomach.
2. **Swallowed blood,** e.g. after epistaxis, haemoptysis, fractured

base of the skull when the roof of the nasopharynx is injured, or operations about the nose and throat, such as tonsillectomy.

3. Congestion of blood in the portal vein (**portal hypertension**) due to cirrhosis of the liver. In this condition the veins at the lower end of the oesophagus, where the portal veins anastomose with those of the general circulation, become dilated and varicose. They may rupture and the escaping blood is subsequently vomited (page 253).

4. Certain **blood diseases,** such as purpura and leukaemia.

5. **Aspirin,** especially if taken on an empty stomach, may cause haematemesis in some individuals.

By far the most important cause is haemorrhage from a peptic ulcer. This may be slight, or profuse and even repeated so that the patient becomes very collapsed and anaemic. The skin becomes cold and sweating, the pulse rate increases and the blood pressure falls. Unless successfully treated without delay, death may occur.

It has already been pointed out that the vomited blood may be bright red if the loss is very recent, or dark brown, like 'coffee grounds', if it has been in the stomach sufficiently long to be acted on by the gastric juice.

It is usually acid in reaction to litmus. Some blood always passes into the duodenum and is expelled in the faeces. In severe cases, when the amount is large, actual **melaena** occurs; in others, occult blood is found in the stools (p. 207).

Haematemesis must not be confused with haemoptysis. The latter consists of the coughing up of bright red frothy blood from the lungs which is alkaline in reaction and usually followed by bloodstained sputum. It is not always as easy as it might seem to differentiate the two conditions. So often, all the patient will say is that he 'brought up blood'. Unless the condition is actually observed, a careful history is necessary.

The treatment of haematemesis. The essential point in the medical treatment of haematemesis due to peptic ulcer is to keep the patient absolutely quiet at rest in bed, and for this purpose morphine 15 mg (gr $\frac{1}{4}$) may be injected to allay restlessness. It may be repeated at intervals of 4 to 6 hours. The disadvantage of giving morphine is that it may cause vomiting. The foot of the bed is raised on blocks in order to combat shock and cerebral anoxia.

In all cases, blood grouping is carried out and preparations are made for blood transfusion which is often required. Dextran may be given intravenously until blood is available.

In the most severe cases, in addition to blood grouping, the following points require notice:

1. Careful attention must be given to the toilet of the mouth at frequent intervals.
2. An hourly pulse chart should be kept.
3. The blood pressure should be recorded at regular intervals according to the severity of the case.
4. A blood count or haemoglobin estimation should be carried out at intervals of 12 to 24 hours at first.
5. The blood urea should be estimated.
6. The bowels should be left alone for 4 or 5 days if necessary, after which an enema may be given.

Diet. In the most severe cases it may be decided that nothing should be given by mouth for 1 or 2 days. In such instances the patient may use chewing-gum to help to keep his mouth moist. The practice of giving ice to suck, except in very small quantities, is generally considered undesirable. The patient is then given 120 ml (4 fl oz) of half-strength normal saline every 4 hours for 12 hours. This is taken in small quantities at a time and is later followed by citrated milk 30 ml (1 fl oz) every 2 hours, increasing gradually up to 150 ml (5 fl oz).

In the majority of cases, however, feeding can commence within a few hours of the patient having settled down in hospital.

Surgical treatment of haematemesis. Many cases of haemorrhage from peptic ulcer recover satisfactorily with medical treatment, but there are some in which the bleeding continues in spite of the measures adopted and are likely to prove fatal. This is particularly liable to occur in older patients whose arteries are hard and in those who have very chronic ulcers which have bled before. It is important therefore that a surgeon should have the opportunity of seeing the patient before his state becomes desperate. If it is decided that surgery is necessary, blood transfusion is continued and an operation (e.g. partial gastrectomy) performed.

Postoperative complications include:—

(*a*) haemorrhage,
(*b*) anastomotic ulcer when gastro-enterostomy has been performed,
(*c*) 'dumping syndrome' in which the patient feels faint, sweats and is sometimes very distended after a meal. This may only be relieved by vomiting,
(*d*) anaemia,
(*e*) loss of weight.

Cancer of the stomach

This is a common variety of cancer, which occurs more frequently in men than in women and is usually seen between the ages of 40 and 60 years. It may commence at the pylorus (60%), on the lesser curvature or at the cardia, and in some cases may possibly develop at the site of a chronic gastric ulcer.

Symptoms. In a few instances there is a long history of chronic dyspepsia, suggesting that a simple ulcer has been present. In the majority, there is a rapid onset of weight loss, anaemia or gastric symptoms in an individual who has previously had a good digestion.

The main symptoms are:

1. Loss of appetite, often with a special repugnance for meat.
2. Flatulence.
3. A varying degree of epigastric pain or discomfort.
4. Nausea and vomiting.

In addition, there is loss of weight and general strength. Anaemia either of the hyperchromic or hypochromic type may develop and a tumour is frequently palpable in the abdomen in the later stages.

A deformity of the stomach is often seen by x-rays. The test meal shows hypo- or achlorhydria and occult blood is generally present in the faeces. Gastroscopy may be helpful in diagnosis.

Complications. The commonest complication for which surgical treatment may be required is pyloric stenosis, the growth obstructing the flow of food into the duodenum with consequent dilatation of the stomach (p. 225).

Severe haematemesis is rare, although vomited material may contain small quantities of blood or 'coffee grounds'.

Obstructive jaundice may develop later as a result of secondary deposits in the liver.

Prognosis and treatment. Unless the growth can be removed completely by surgical means, the average duration of life, after the first appearance of symptoms, is 3 months to 1 year. In some cases if there are no secondary deposits in the liver or other organs, excision of the portion of the stomach containing the cancer is successful.

When the growth causes pyloric obstruction with dilatation of the stomach, temporary relief may be given by joining the stomach to the jejunum, thereby allowing food to enter the small intestine directly, without having to pass through the pylorus. This operation is called gastro-jejunostomy.

In all cases, the mouth must be kept clean and the patient made

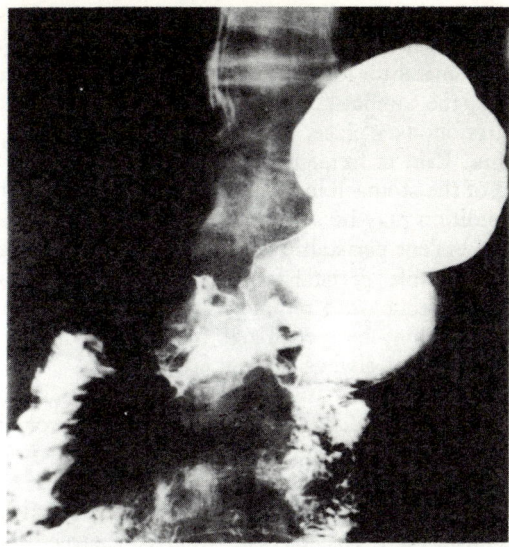

Fig. 47 Cancer of the stomach (barium meal).

as comfortable as possible. Passing a stomach tube and washing out the organ shortly before a meal is due often relieves vomiting. Analgesics, including morphine or pethidine, may be required in the later stages for the alleviation of pain.

A light nutritious diet is generally necessary and should be given in small frequent feeds, but the patient may be allowed to eat and drink what he likes provided it does not increase the severity of symptoms.

Pyloric stenosis and gastric dilatation

Contraction of scar tissue, resulting from the healing of a gastric or duodenal ulcer situated in the neighbourhood of the pylorus, or the presence of a cancerous new growth, may so narrow the canal that difficulty is experienced in passing the stomach contents into the duodenum. The stomach endeavours to overcome this obstruction and the mechanical principles involved in this process are the same as those employed when the heart is working at a disadvantage and endeavouring to force its contained blood through a valve narrowed by disease (see p. 110).

If the obstruction is slight, hypertrophy of the muscle of the stomach enables peristaltic contractions of greater strength to overcome the mechanical disadvantage present. If the degree of obstruction increases, the stomach is unable to empty completely and progressive dilatation takes place.

Symptoms. Pain is frequently marked and is due to the violent contractions of the stomach in its endeavour to overcome the obstruction. The condition may be so marked that the outline of the dilated organ and the violent peristaltic waves may be seen on the surface of the abdomen (visible peristalsis). Vomiting of large quantities of material usually occurs and remnants of food taken many hours or even days before may be recognized. Wasting is usually rapid and constipation is almost always present.

An excessive amount of resting juice, e.g. up to 300 ml (10 fl oz) is obtained in a test meal. The fluid is often dark in colour, offensive and may contain food remnants.

Treatment. Some relief may be obtained by passing a stomach tube and washing out the stomach, the patient being given small and frequent liquid feeds. If possible, either partial gastrectomy or gastrojejunostomy are performed.

Congenital hypertrophic pyloric stenosis

This is a condition affecting infants, particularly breast-fed males between 4 and 13 weeks after birth. The symptoms consist of vomiting, constipation and progressive emaciation. Often a small tumour can be felt in the abdomen, and visible peristalsis may be observed after feeds. Copious stomach contents are usually ejected violently and may travel for some distance. This characteristic is referred to as 'projectile vomiting'.

The lesion consists of hypertrophy of the muscle fibres at the pylorus which fails to relax properly as each peristaltic wave reaches it. As in pyloric stenosis from other causes, there is associated dilatation of the stomach which may be confirmed by x-ray. Similar symptoms are produced if the pyloric muscle is affected by simple spasm, a condition which may be relieved by twice daily gastric lavage.

Treatment may be:
1. Surgical. (The treatment of choice.)
2. Medical.

When marked hypertrophy is present an operation is generally

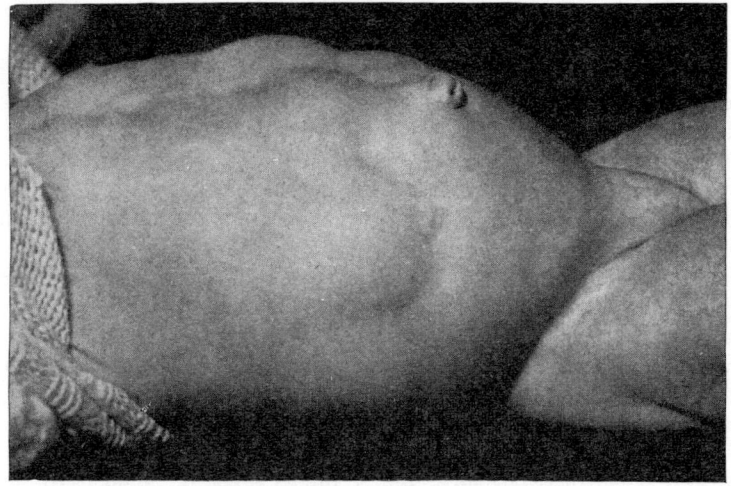

Fig. 48 Waves of gastric peristalsis going from left to right in a case of pyloric stenosis.

performed, an incision being made through the muscle of the pylorus down to the mucous membrane (Rammstedt's operation).

The postoperative care and feeding is most important. Gastro-enteritis is a dangerous complication and must be avoided by:

1. Scrupulous cleanliness in the preparation of feeds.
2. Isolation from other children with upper respiratory infections and cases of gastro-enteritis.

Postoperative feeding commences a few hours after operation on the following lines:

(a) Glucose saline, 1 teaspoonful (5 ml) hourly for 4 hours, followed by 2 teaspoonfuls (10 ml) hourly for 4 hours.

(b) Milk feeds, preferably breast milk, 15 ml ($\frac{1}{2}$ oz) every $1\frac{1}{2}$ to 2 hours for 24 hours, followed by 60 ml (2 oz) every 3 hours for 24 hours, and 75 ml (3 oz) three-hourly for a further 24 hours. The child's usual diet can then be resumed.

Some cases are successfully treated by medical measures. In addition to gastric lavage, an antispasmodic drug similar to atropine, known as **'Eumydrin'** (atropine methonitrate 0·6%), is given in a dose of 1 to 3 drops, half an hour before each feed for several weeks.

The treatment of dehydration which is often present is of great importance. Saline is given intravenously (usually by a scalp vein drip), or subcutaneously with 'Hyalase'. Ketosis may also occur.

Acute dilatation of the stomach

This is a very serious condition which may come on some hours or even days after abdominal operations, injuries to the spine and, less frequently, during the course of other acute illnesses.

The organ rapidly becomes very dilated as a result of loss of tone in its muscular walls. The patient becomes collapsed and vomits large quantities of fluid which is often dark in colour. The abdomen is distended.

Treatment. Prompt measures are essential. The patient must be placed on his face or slightly turned on his left side, with a pillow under the pelvis and the foot of the bed raised. The stomach is washed out with normal saline at intervals or a Ryle's tube may be swallowed and the stomach contents aspirated repeatedly or by continuous suction. Injections of carbachol or pituitary extract may be ordered. Intravenous fluids are given to relieve dehydration and to restore electrolyte balance and a binder may be applied to the abdomen.

Diaphragmatic or Hiatus Hernia

Sometimes a portion of the upper end of the stomach protrudes through the diaphragm into the thorax at the site of the usual oesophageal opening. This can give rise to dyspepsia, and sometimes haematemesis or melaena followed by anaemia. Symptoms are especially likely to occur if the patient lies down after meals. A simple diet of the peptic ulcer type, together with antacids, weight reduction and the advice to sleep in a semi-upright position and to avoid stooping may be all that is required. In other cases the opening in the diaphragm may be repaired surgically.

The condition is demonstrated by a barium meal.

Diseases of the intestine

After leaving the stomach and duodenum the food continues its passage through the intestinal tract. The process of digestion by the action of enzymes secreted by the pancreas and glands of the intestine goes on. Absorption of fluid and broken-down foodstuffs takes place. Finally, the residue is subjected to the action of bacteria in the colon and leaves the body through the rectum and anus by the act of defaecation.

In addition to vomiting, the main **symptoms** of intestinal disorders are:

I. Alteration in character of the faeces.
II. Abdominal colic.
III. Distension with gas (tympanites or meteorism).
IV. Diarrhoea.
V. Constipation.

I Alteration in Character of the Faeces

1. Quantity. Faeces consist of unabsorbed food residue and water together with large numbers of dead and living bacteria. In an adult the average daily amount passed is 200 g (5–6 oz); in an infant of one year about 100 g (3 oz).

The type of food taken modifies the bulk of the faeces. If it is easily digested, e.g. milk, the faecal residue is small, whereas vegetables, fruit and coarse wholemeal bread are not fully broken down and leave much unabsorbed material. Advantage is taken of this fact in the dietetic treatment of constipation by prescribing food which will leave a large residue. This residue or 'roughage' acts as a stimulus to the peristaltic movements of the bowel.

2. Colour. The normal dark-brown colour of faeces is due to the altered bile pigments which they contain. If the passage of intestinal contents is hurried, as in diarrhoea, the alteration in the pigments is less marked, so that the faeces are lighter in colour and, in the case of infants, actually green.

In certain varieties of jaundice, especially when the bile ducts are obstructed and bile is unable to reach the bowel, the faeces are devoid of pigment and may be described as clay or putty coloured.

In melaena, the stools are tarry in consistency and black in colour. Black stools also occur as a result of eating liquorice or taking certain medicines, including iron, bismuth and charcoal.

3. Consistency. Normal faeces are semi-solid in consistency and are sufficiently soft to be moulded into a cylindrical form by their passage through the anal canal.

In diarrhoea, the stools are abnormally liquid, while in constipation they tend to form hard lumps, described as scybala.

In pancreatic disease or when bile is absent the stools are bulky and pale. In addition, they are frothy and oily in character, because the digestion and absorption of fats is defective in the absence of bile salts and the pancreatic enzyme, lipase. Such stools may be difficult to wash from a bed-pan or to flush down a lavatory pan.

The 'pea soup' stools of typhoid fever are described on p. 43.

4. Odour. The odour of faeces is characteristic. Very offensive stools may be associated with diarrhoea and excessive putrefaction of proteins. In pancreatic disease the presence of rancid fat is responsible for their offensive nature.

5. Abnormal contents. Excess of mucus is seen in constipation, in diseases of the colon, and frequently in children after the administration of aperients.

Fresh blood, bright red in colour, can be seen in the motions when its source of origin is low down in the alimentary canal, and may be due to ulcerative colitis, cancer of the colon and rectum, or haemorrhoids.

Pus is present if an abscess bursts into the lower bowel and may also be found in colitis and cancer.

Intestinal parasites, including round-worms, thread-worms and portions of tape-worms may be seen in the faeces (p. 245).

Other abnormalities are discovered by chemical or microscopic examination, including occult blood (p. 207), the ova of intestinal parasites, amoebae and abnormal bacteria, such as typhoid and dysentery bacilli.

The nurse must observe and report any abnormality noticed in the stools, including foreign bodies such as coins or pins which may have been swallowed and passed through the alimentary tract, and it is her duty to keep an accurate record of the number passed.

II Abdominal colic

Intestinal colic is a form of generalized abdominal pain caused by spasmodic contraction of the colon or other parts of the bowel. It is often very severe in type and may be accompanied by nausea, vomiting or sweating.

Its characteristics are sudden onset with equally rapid cessation and a tendency to recur at short intervals. Abdominal tenderness may be present but is seldom marked; in fact, firm pressure on the abdomen frequently gives relief. The patient is usually restless, a point of contrast with cases of gastric perforation, or peritonitis in which the patient is still and anxious.

The most common cause of intestinal colic is eating indigestible and irritating foodstuffs, such as unripe fruit, shell-fish, pork or ices and may be associated with either diarrhoea or constipation. It occurs, also, after taking the more violent purgatives.

It is seen in serious conditions such as intestinal obstruction from any cause, lead poisoning and in connection with certain nervous disorders.

The treatment will depend on the cause of the condition. In the absence of any serious lesion, gentle massage, or application of heat to the abdomen may be tried. An aperient or an enema may be ordered, provided it is certain that no serious lesion is present.

The condition is common in infants and is characterized by attacks of screaming in which the abdomen becomes hard and the baby draws up the legs. It is generally due to flatulence, excessive, irregular or too rapid feeding, but may be associated also with serious conditions such as intussusception. In the simple variety, relief is obtained by the passage of flatus. To encourage this the child may be picked up and placed face downwards on one hand or held by the left arm with the belly pressed firmly against the nurse's chest while the other hand gently strokes or pats the back. A simple carminative, such as Dill Water, is often useful and applications of warmth to the abdomen or a small warm water enema (40·5 °C, 105 °F) are of value.

III Distension with gas (tympanites, meteorism)

Distension of the intestines with gas or flatus is called tympanites. The gas may be formed in two ways:

1. Excessive fermentation of carbohydrates.
2. Increased putrefaction of proteins.

It is due to a number of causes, the most serious of which are acute abdominal states such as intestinal obstruction and peritonitis requiring treatment by operative means. The condition itself frequently follows abdominal operations and is also seen in typhoid fever (p. 43). Simple causes include chronic dyspepsia and indigestion caused by unsuitable foods and it may be associated with intestinal colic.

The accompanying internal rumblings, due to movements of flatus in the intestines, are called borborygmi.

The abdomen gives a resonant tympanitic note on percussion and the distension may cause respiratory and cardiac embarrassment.

In simple cases relief is obtained by heat and massage to the abdomen. The passage of a rectal tube or enemata (simple or turpentine) are useful. Injections of pituitary extract or carbachol may be ordered.

IV Diarrhoea

The term literally means 'a running through' and is applied to the frequent passage of unformed motions of loose consistency. It may occur in acute attacks or assume a chronic and persistent form. There are many causes of this symptom, although the important factor present in most cases is excessive peristaltic movement of the intestinal tract leading to undue speed in the progress of its content.

(1) GENERAL CAUSES

1. Dietetic, including unsuitable food, alcoholic excess, unripe fruit.
2. Chemical irritants, including aperients and poisons such as mercury and arsenic. Oral antibiotics.
3. General infections including the onset of acute fevers.
4. Toxaemia such as uraemia or thyrotoxicosis.

(2) LOCAL DISORDERS OF THE ALIMENTARY TRACT

1. Gastric disturbances. Gastro-enteritis. Virus infection.
2. Inflammation of the small intestine (enteritis), and large intestine (colitis). Ulcerative colitis.
3. Specific intestinal infections such as typhoid fever, dysentery, cholera and food poisoning.
4. Cancer of the colon or rectum.
5. Disorders of pancreatic secretion and intestinal absorption (steatorrhoea, e.g. coeliac disease and sprue).

(3) NERVOUS CAUSES, especially as a result of emotion or fear.

Diarrhoea is frequently associated with colic and may be accompanied by vomiting as in gastro-enteritis. Apart from the symptoms due to the actual cause of the condition, marked prostration and collapse may follow severe diarrhoea as the result of loss of fluid from the body and electrolyte disturbances.

The details of **treatment** vary in individual cases, but may be summarized in the following way:

1. Treat the primary cause, e.g. sulphonamides or antibiotics in infections of the bowels.
2. Replace fluid loss in the following ways (a) fluids by mouth, (b) intravenous or subcutaneous (with 'Hyalase') salines in severe cases.
3. Rest in bed especially if there is pyrexia or marked weakness.
4. Keep the body warm by hot blankets and bottles. Apply heat to abdomen for the relief of pain.
5. Check the irritation and excessive movements of the bowels by mixtures such as Chalk and Opium Mixture (BNF), or

kaolin mixtures. 'Lomotil' (diphenoxylate) is another useful drug.

6. In severe cases no solid food should be given for at least 24 hours. Plenty of water may be taken, also arrowroot, gruel and milk. Later, milk puddings and bread and butter may be added. A little whisky or brandy is often useful if collapse and exhaustion are marked. Pulped apple diet is sometimes given. Anti-emetic drugs may be needed for associated vomiting.

In cases of diarrhoea the nurse must keep an adequate record of the number of stools passed and inspect them for the presence of abnormalities. She should be able to give an accurate description of their appearance and, if necessary, save specimens for subsequent examination. Rectal swabs may be taken for bacteriological examination.

In infectious cases, the stools and bed linen must be disinfected and the rules suggested for preventing the spread of infection in typhoid fever (p. 47) carried out.

If the patient is unable to visit the lavatory, a bedpan should be provided at once.

In severe cases the anus must be cleaned with wool or soft material moistened with soap and water if necessary and carefully dried and powdered because the frequent passage of stools renders the part sore and tender. The local application of barrier cream or silicone spray may be useful.

Food Poisoning. This may be due to eating 'foods', such as certain toadstools, which are themselves poisonous or to eating foods contaminated with chemicals, bacteria or viruses. Bacterial food poisoning may be either of the 'toxin type' or the 'infection type'. The 'toxin type' is due to toxins produced by the organism, e.g. the *Staphylococcus pyogenes*, from the septic finger of a food-handler. The toxin is not destroyed by cooking and causes symptoms within 6 hours of the contaminated food being eaten.

In the 'infection type' of food poisoning, symptoms are delayed for 12–48 hours after the offending meal because the organism (e.g. *Salmonella typhimurium*) has to multiply before it can cause toxaemia.

The patient's vomitus, faeces and suspected food, if any remains, should be sent to the laboratory. The District Community Physician (M.O.H.) must be notified of suspected cases of food poisoning.

Treatment includes bed rest and fluid replacement. If oral fluids, including normal or half-normal saline cannot be retained, or if water-deficiency is severe, the intravenous administration of dextrose-saline will be necessary. Food should be withheld until nausea and vomiting have subsided. Re-feeding should then commence with light, easily-digested, low-residue foods.

Drugs used in cases of food poisoning include anti-diarrhoeal preparations (see above) and antibiotics such as neomycin, colomycin and ampicillin.

Staphylococcal entero-colitis. Although antibiotics may be used in the treatment of some cases of diarrhoea due to infection, the use of oral antibiotics for other purposes may so alter the bacteriological content of the bowel that resistant staphylococci may grow. The development of acute staphylococcal enteritis is a very serious condition both in children and adults. The treatment includes prompt replacement of fluids and electrolytes, and the administration of erythromycin, cloaxcillin or neomycin to which staphylococci are sensitive. Steroids may be useful.

Diarrhoea in infants

The condition is commonest up to the age of 12 months and affects mainly bottle-fed infants of the poorer classes.

There are two main types:
1. Simple diarrhoea (dietetic).
2. Acute infective gastro-enteritis.

1. Simple diarrhoea. This type is not infrequently associated with the onset of an acute fever or dentition. It may also be due to minor errors of diet such as excess of carbohydrate or fat in artificially fed infants. The motions vary in number between two and ten daily and may be light brown or, more commonly, green in colour. They are loose rather than watery, sour and offensive in odour, and contain undigested food. Moderate pyrexia may be present, the child is fretful and suffers from colic and flatulence.

In mild cases, adjustment of the diet after a preliminary period of twelve hours in which milk is replaced by glucose saline or similar solution, may be sufficient. In severe cases treatment similar to that described under infective gastro-enteritis is required.

2. Acute infective gastro-enteritis. This is a serious condition which is liable to occur in epidemic form in any locality and any age may be affected. Outbreaks also occur in institutions, residential and day nurseries and hospital wards. The incidence and mortality have fortunately fallen very considerably since the early years of this century. The older the child, the better is the outlook.

It is most likely to appear during the hot summer months, but cases may be seen at any time.

The actual causes are not clear, but various organisms, including special types of *Esch. coli*, have been found in the stools and it is generally agreed that it is of bacterial or virus origin. In some outbreaks dysentery bacilli (e.g. Sonne type) may be found, and it is therefore wise to take rectal swabs for bacteriological examination in all cases, although in many it is not possible to identify the organism. In others, it may be associated with otitis media or a focus of infection elsewhere. Infected milk, dirty bottles, teats, and comforters are factors in its incidence, while flies, dust, overcrowding and general lack of cleanliness play an important part in its spread. Some cases are associated with upper respiratory infection and it is possible that droplet infection may play some part in its spread.

The infection is very prone to spread in a hospital ward and, once a case has occurred, the strictest isolation is essential.

The following account refers mainly to the condition as it affects infants, but the same general principles apply to adults.

The cardinal symptoms are diarrhoea with green stools and vomiting: these are associated with pyrexia (39·5–40·5 °C, 103–105 °F), tachycardia, abdominal colic and evidence of loss of fluid from the body. Infants withstand the loss of fluid badly; there is rapid emaciation and loss of weight, the skin becomes inelastic, the eyes sunken, the fontanelle depressed and the face pinched. These are the characteristic features of dehydration. The extremities feel cold, although the rectal temperature may be high.

In addition to the purely gastro-intestinal symptoms there is evidence of marked toxaemia, affecting especially the nervous system. Convulsions may occur. There may be restlessness, drowsiness or coma. Irregular, rapid and deep breathing, known as 'air hunger', is often seen in severe cases.

It must be clearly understood that the severity of the malady varies in individual cases and in different epidemics. Some are relatively mild, while in others the process is so acute that death may ensue in a few hours. In any outbreak, however, the mortality tends to be high. Soreness of the buttocks, stomatitis, otitis media and bronchopneumonia are the most frequent complications.

Treatment
1. Prophylaxis.
2. Treatment of the acute stages.
3. Return to a normal diet.

1. PROPHYLAXIS. This is of great importance in preventing outbreaks and in limiting the spread of the malady.

(*a*) Weaning should be avoided as far as possible in very hot weather and when an epidemic is known to exist.

(*b*) Boiling or pasteurization of all milk, which is carefully protected from flies and dust. Whenever possible milk should be kept in a refrigerator or ice chest. A separate 'milk kitchen' is always desirable on children's wards.

(*c*) Utmost cleanliness of bottles and teats which are boiled after use and kept in 'Milton'.

(*d*) *Isolation.* When cases are nursed in hospital strict bed-isolation must be observed, preferably in a separate ward or cubicle. Transfer to a special infectious unit may be desirable. Soiled napkins must be removed at once and placed in a special container. If possible, it should be arranged that the nurse changing the infants should take no part in feeding them or other children. Masks and gowns should be worn and the hands carefully washed in running water before and after attending to the infant.

2. TREATMENT OF THE ACUTE STAGES

(*a*) General measures.

(*b*) Restoration of fluid loss.

(*c*) Diet.

(*d*) Administration of drugs.

(*e*) Treatment of special symptoms.

(*a*) *General measures.* Good and careful nursing are of very great importance. The infant must be kept warm in bed in a well-ventilated room or in the fresh air. Napkins must be changed directly they become wet or soiled and removed at once from the room. There is a tendency for the buttocks to become sore and excoriated, but this can be avoided by careful attention. The surrounding skin must be washed with warm water, dried and powdered after each motion, care being taken that folds of skin are not overlooked. If the buttocks become red, a square of linen or lint smeared with soft paraffin, Lassar's paste or zinc and castor oil may be applied before the napkin is put on. A silicone, water-repellent cream, e.g. 'Siopel', is also useful.

(*b*) *Restoration of fluid loss.* Loss of body fluid is always a serious matter in young children, and one of the most important and urgent parts of the treatment in these cases is to remedy this deficiency. Intravenous, subcutaneous (with 'Hyalase') and intra-peritoneal fluids are employed in all severe cases, and the nurse is often required to prepare for their administration.

For intravenous injection one fifth normal saline with 5% glucose may be used. The amount at first required is about 90 ml (3 oz) per pound of body weight in 24 hours, given at the rate of about 10 drops per minute (30 ml per hour).

Small transfusions of blood or plasma are sometimes used.

(c) *Diet.* All milk and other food is withheld for 12 to 36 hours, and is replaced by fluids such as plain water, glucose-saline, one fifth normal saline or an electrolyte solution in amounts of 15 to 30 ml ($\frac{1}{2}$ to 1 fl oz) every hour. In other cases the oral administration of a dilute solution containing sodium chloride and lactate and potassium chloride in doses of 50 ml every half to one hour may correct water deficiency (dehydration) and electrolyte loss within 12 hours. The total daily intake of fluid both oral and intravenous should be carefully recorded.

(d) *Drugs.* Sulphonamide drugs are sometimes used. Oral antibiotics such as ampicillin, neomycin, streptomycin, or tetracycline, may also be tried in some cases. A combination of streptomycin with sulphonamides ('Streptotriad') is of value.

(e) *Treatment of special symptoms, etc.* Collapse may be treated by hydrocortisone intravenously, which may 'buy time' for the infant until water and electrolyte deficiency has been corrected and antibiotics have had time to act.

Diluted brandy often improves the general condition.

3. RETURN TO NORMAL DIET. This often presents difficulties and must be a gradual process, determined by the progress of the child. As soon as food seems to be tolerated a weak milk mixture is given in small amounts every 2 to 3 hours. Milk must be well diluted and skimmed in order to reduce the fat content, or one of the half-cream dried or acid milks (Lacidac) may be tried. Later, a little sugar is added in the form of dextrimaltose; finally dried milk or ordinary milk mixtures may be employed. Ascorbic acid or, for older children, orange juice and cod-liver oil may be added to the diet.

V Constipation

Constipation may be defined as delay in evacuation of the faeces.

There are two types:

1. Intestinal stasis or delay in the progress of intestinal contents.
2. Dyschezia or delay in emptying the rectum.

1. Intestinal stasis. In this type, the delay is in the colon, the contents of which are not moved on at their normal rate. This may occur for a number of reasons, the main one being inefficient contraction of the muscular tissue in the wall of the gut.

In order that peristalsis may take place it is necessary for the bowel to contain an adequate amount of unabsorbed food material or 'roughage' which acts as a stimulus. Inefficient contraction also occurs in the absence of intestinal juices and if the bowel contents are deficient in fluid.

It is for this reason that constipation is liable to occur in acute febrile diseases when all three factors are present. The secretion of intestinal juice is diminished, and on account of this a light non-stimulating diet is taken because a full diet, leaving adequate roughage, could not be digested; while the body fluids are diminished as a result of increased loss by sweating.

In individuals who are otherwise healthy, the same process may occur if the diet is unsuitable, or if they do not take sufficient fluids by mouth. The habitual use of aperients may, in fact, contribute to the development of chronic constipation.

Actual mechanical obstruction to the progress of the intestinal contents, as a result of adhesions between loops of bowel or due to a new growth, etc., may also produce constipation, which, if complete, constitutes **intestinal obstruction** which is a surgical problem.

2. Dyschezia or delay in emptying the rectum. When faeces reach the rectum they produce distension of the cavity and stretching of its walls. This causes impulses to pass to the spinal cord and eventually reach the brain where they arouse the conscious sensation of the desire to defaecate. If this call is neglected, the rectum accommodates itself to its contents by relaxation of the muscle in its walls, the impulses cease to travel to the spinal cord and the desire to defaecate passes off. The arrival of more faecal material in the rectum causes further distension and more impulses pass to produce the desire to defaecate. If opportunity is still not taken to answer these calls of nature, the over-stretched rectum becomes insensitive. It fails to send further impulses, and remains over-distended with hard dry faecal material.

If this habit is allowed to continue the rectum remains permanently over-stretched and does not regain its normal tone, so that subsequently a large quantity of faecal material must accumulate before any nervous impulse reaches consciousness.

This is the most common variety of constipation and is due almost entirely to habitual failure to respond to the conscious desire to defaecate when it arrives.

Failure to obey the call to defaecate may be due to conditions such as piles when the act is painful and the patient deliberately postpones it. In the majority of cases, however, failure to make a habit of emptying the rectum at a regular time each day, social inconveniences or shyness are responsible.

The voluntary act of defaecation consists of raising the pressure within the abdomen and thereby causing compression of the rectum at the same time as the sphincter muscle of the anus is relaxed.

The breath is held and the diaphragm is fixed. The muscles of the abdominal wall and pelvic floor then contract.

The power of defaecation may to some extent be impaired if the muscles of the abdominal wall and pelvic floor are weakened, e.g. after operation or child-birth and in old age.

The main causes of constipation may be summarized in the following way:

1. Delay in passage of the intestinal contents:
    (a) due to unsuitable diet and lack of fluids,
    (b) due to general diseases, febrile conditions,
    (c) due to local causes, mechanical obstruction, cancer, etc.
2. Delay in emptying the rectum:
    (a) faulty habits,
    (b) local causes, piles, etc.,
    (c) weakness of the abdominal muscles.

Symptoms. The actual symptoms produced by constipation are variable. Many individuals only have their bowels opened 2 or 3 times a week and remain in perfect health. Others worry so much about slight irregularity that their mind is not at rest unless a daily action occurs. There is no doubt that a daily action at a regular hour should be aimed at in every case, but if an individual is able to re-main healthy and free from symptoms with fewer motions it is better that he should do so than take large and frequent doses of aperients in order to ensure daily evacuation.

The symptoms which may be associated with constipation include general lassitude, headache, abdominal discomfort, furred tongue and loss of appetite. Chronic constipation may lead to impaction of faeces, and overflow faecal incontinence (spurious diarrhoea).

Treatment

A distinction must be made between the acute type of constipation due to febrile diseases and the chronic type associated with improper diet and faulty habits.

In the first variety the use of aperients is both justifiable and necessary in many cases. On the other hand, the use of purgatives in some patients who are acutely ill is dangerous. It must be re-membered that a copious watery motion means loss of fluid from the body and, if several such motions are passed, this fluid loss may be a serious matter, for in many acutely ill cases attempts which are being made to induce the patient to take an adequate amount of liquid by mouth will be wasted if large amounts are being lost by the bowel at the same time.

Aperients are drugs and, therefore, should be ordered by the doctor, rather than be left to the nurse to administer at will, for there is no doubt that there is still much lack of discretion in their use.

As a general rule, enemata are preferable in acute and severe illness, and there need be no cause for anxiety if the rectum is not emptied for two or three days (except, of course, in cases of actual intestinal obstruction). Glycerin or 'Dulcolax' (bisacodyl) suppositories are often useful.

In the second variety, the repeated use of drugs only results in irritation of the bowel and gradual impairment of its peristaltic activity so that the constipation becomes more marked and aperients of increasing dosage and strength are required.

Many aperients are available, the more common ones being Epsom salts, senna and cascara (see also p. 506).

The treatment of chronic constipation is based on general hygienic grounds. Adequate exercise must be taken; the diet should form a large residue in order to act as a stimulant to the peristaltic action of the colon and, therefore, contains green vegetables, fruit such as prunes and apples, wholemeal bread and porridge. Additional faecal bulk may be obtained by the use of bran or methyl cellulose granules. Water is taken before meals, and half to one pint should be drunk on rising in the morning.

The bowels can be educated to act at a regular time each day and the habit of visiting the lavatory should be made at an hour convenient to the routine life of the individual which in most cases is in the morning. This is important because taking food into the empty stomach causes stimulation of the movements of the colon by the process of reflex action (**gastro-colic reflex**) and the colonic contents are moved on into the rectum, so that in most individuals the rectum is full and ready to be emptied after breakfast.

In addition to taking a suitable diet, the attempt to re-form regular habits may in the first place require some assistance. Liquid paraffin or lactulose ('Dulphalac') are of value when the faeces are hard and dry. Small warm water enemata in the morning may help to start a regular rhythm of bowel action, or a suppository may be used.

Cases in which the abdominal musculature is weak will be helped by abdominal exercises.

Intractable cases may, however, require regular doses of mild aperients such as milk of magnesia, lactulose, salts, senna or cascara.

Occasionally, in elderly patients, hard masses (**scybala**) accumulate in the rectum and their removal by a gloved finger is necessary, an unpleasant procedure for all concerned.

Inflammation of the intestines. Various portions of the intestines may become inflamed. If the small intestine is affected the condition is called **enteritis.** This is frequently associated with acute gastritis and may be due to food poisoning or the action of various irritants on the bowel. The main symptoms are abdominal pain and diarrhoea. The varieties of gastro-enteritis peculiar to infants have already been described. Regional ileitis (Crohn's disease) is a chronic inflammatory disease of the small bowel. Its cause is unknown and its treatment is unsatisfactory.

Ulcerative colitis

This is a disease in which ulcers develop in the mucous membrane of the colon. In appearance the ulcers resemble those seen in dysentery, but there is no connection between the two conditions other than a similarity in some of the symptoms.

The disease may be acute, chronic or relapsing in type. In the latter variety, intervals of some months or even years may intervene between relapses.

Causes. There are two age peaks for the onset of this disease, people in their 4th and 5th or in their 7th decades being most often affected but it may occur in children. It is more common in women than in men. The actual cause of the condition is unknown. Although emotional upsets precipitate relapses they are not the underlying cause. It is possible that hypersensitivity to an allergen, e.g. milk proteins, cheese, etc., may provoke antibodies in some individuals which in some way affect the colon. Such patients may improve when milk products are excluded from the diet. There is some evidence that ulcerative colitis may belong to the group of 'auto-immune' diseases. Many patients with the disease have, in their blood, antibodies to human colon (colon antibodies). It is possible that these are formed, in the first place, as antibodies to certain bacteria in the colon and that they subsequently act as auto-antibodies.

Symptoms. These consist of diarrhoea with the passage of frequent stools containing blood, pus and mucus. In acute cases there is pyrexia, tachycardia and wasting and the patient may go downhill rapidly. The number of motions may be increased to as many as 10 or even more daily and may sometimes consist almost entirely of blood and mucus. The patient complains of colicky pains and the abdomen may be tender. Because of the blood loss some degree of anaemia is usually present and may be severe. Water deficiency and disturbance of the electrolyte balance occurs in acute cases. Complications also include arthritis, iritis, erythema nodosum, liver disease, and perforation of the bowel with peritonitis which may prove fatal. Some chronic cases may later develop cancer.

The diagnosis may be confirmed by sigmoidoscopy, when bleeding points and ulcers can be seen in the oedematous mucous membrane of the colon and upper part of the rectum. Bacteriological examination of the stools does not reveal any abnormal organisms.

Treatment

1. *General.* Rest in bed during the acute stages.

2. *Diet.* The general nutrition must be maintained by a high calorie, high protein, low residue diet supplemented by vitamins. As already mentioned, milk products may have to be excluded if a trial suggests that these are in any way causal.

3. *Anaemia.* This is treated by blood transfusions repeated sufficiently often to maintain a normal haemoglobin level. When this has been attained and the acute symptoms have subsided, iron may be given by injection.

4. *Dehydration.* In the acute stages intravenous fluids are required to correct dehydration and electrolyte loss, especially potassium.

5. *Steroids.* Oral prednisolone (20–60 mg daily) or intravenous hydrocortisone are often used during acute attacks. In addition, a rectal drip containing hydrocortisone or a prednisolone enema may be employed; a short course of tetracycline may be given at the same time.

6. *Sulphonamide.* A special sulphonamide, sulphasalazine ('Salazopyrin'), which appears to have an effect on connective tissue, may be given with advantage between attacks and in the more chronic cases. The average dose initially is 1 to 2 g every 6 hours. Smaller doses are used in maintenance.

7. *Psychotherapy* may be helpful in some cases but is not curative. Sedative drugs such as phenobarbitone or tranquillizers such as diazepam may be of value.

8. *Surgery.* This may be necessary in very acute cases if medical treatment fails or if complications such as stricture resulting from healing of ulcers or the development of polypi which may become

malignant occur. The operations include (*a*) total proctocolectomy and a permanent ileostomy, and (*b*) subtotal excision of the large bowel with preservation of the rectum and ileorectal anastomosis. This is feasible only if the rectum appears relatively healthy. After incomplete removal of diseased bowel there remains the risk of cancer developing in the rectal stump.

Starch and opium enemas are sometimes given to check diarrhoea in acute cases. They are most useful at night in order to give the patient some undisturbed sleep.

Spastic colon. This chronic condition, formerly known as **mucous colitis,** may be regarded as a variety of chronic constipation associated with pain in the left iliac fossa and the passage of shreds of mucus in the stools which are hard and dry. A low residue diet, methyl cellulose, liquid paraffin and drugs such as propantheline, mebeverine and tranquillizers are the main principles of treatment.

Cancer of the colon (carcinoma coli). This is a fairly common form of cancer; the main symptom being increasing constipation which may alternate with diarrhoea. Blood, mucus and pus may appear in the stools and a tumour is often felt in the abdomen. The lesion may be demonstrated by giving a barium enema and examining the patient by x-rays; and, if close to the rectum, may be seen on sigmoidoscopy. It is a common cause of intestinal obstruction and the treatment is surgical.

Hirschsprung's disease (megacolon). This is a rare and usually congenital condition which occurs in infants in which the colon becomes enormously dilated, probably due to a disorder of the neuromuscular mechanism with failure of the sphincter, situated at the junction of the pelvic colon and rectum, to relax as peristaltic waves fail to reach it normally. This is similar to what occurs in achalasia of the cardia (p. 204). Constipation is present and the enlarged colon may be demonstrated by means of a barium enema. Operative measures are usually necessary.

Diverticulosis. Small sac-like diverticula commonly protrude from the mucous membrane of the colon, particularly the sigmoid and, in themselves cause no symptoms and do not call for any special treatment. An increase in the fibre content of the diet may be beneficial, however, and may be taken as bran.

Diverticulitis. This means that inflammation, acute or chronic develops in the sac usually because the neck of the sac has become obstructed. Pain, local tenderness and fever, diarrhoea or constipation and local abscess formation with peritonitis may occur. Urinary symptoms develop if the inflammation impinges on the bladder.

Treatment includes dietetic restriction, adequate fluids and electrolytes, antibiotics, analgesics and sometimes surgery.

Coeliac disease (idiopathic steatorrhoea) is a chronic condition which mainly affects children and consists of the inability to absorb fat and other nutrients from the intestine due to sensitivity to the wheat-protein, gluten. The stools, containing excess of fat, are pale, bulky and offensive. There is general under-nourishment, stunting of growth, abdominal distension, chronic diarrhoea and rickety changes may occur in the bones. The treatment consists of excluding ordinary wheat flour containing the protein gluten which most of these patients are unable to tolerate and a gluten-free diet is the most important factor in treatment. Relapses may occur if adults return to a normal diet. Special gluten-free flour is available. It may also be necessary to diminish the fat content of the diet to the amount which the individual can digest and absorb. Bananas are a useful addition to the diet. Calcium is given in large doses and iron or vitamin B_{12} administered according to the type of anaemia which may be present. Vitamins A, B and D are also essential. Folic acid may also be given (p. 180).

Idiopathic steatorrhoea (adult coeliac disease or non-tropical **sprue**) may sometimes occur in adults and may be associated with a macrocytic type of anaemia, resembling pernicious anaemia. Tropical sprue is a cause of malabsorption and anaemia in the tropics. It usually responds to folic acid. Tetracycline may also be helpful.

Rectal examination

Examination of the rectum is an important procedure in all cases of abdominal disease. A view of the interior of the cavity may be obtained by the use of the **proctoscope**. Digital examination is made with the gloved finger smeared with soft paraffin or similar lubricant to facilitate introduction. It is possible to demonstrate the presence of inflammation of the rectum (proctitis)—or haemorrhoids (piles). In addition, an ulcer or cancerous growth may be felt in the rectum, or the presence of a tumour in a neighbouring organ may be discovered. In young girls it is possible to investigate the size and state of the uterus in this way.

Investigation of intestinal disorders

The methods which may be employed to investigate diseases of the intestine may be summarized thus:

  1. History and physical examination of the abdomen.

2. Examination of the faeces (bacteriological, microscopic and chemical).
3. Following through by x-rays a barium meal given by mouth or a barium enema.
4. Sigmoidoscopy.
5. Rectal examination and proctoscopy.
6. Biopsy; for the jejunum (e.g. in coeliac disease) a special capsule (the Crosby capsule) containing a little guillotine is swallowed and is triggered off by the doctor when it reaches its destination.

Intestinal parasites

The intestinal canal may be the home of various parasites, the common ones being worms, of which four important varieties are found:

(a) Thread-worms   (c) Tape-worms.
(b) Round-worms   (d) Hook-worms.

The eggs or ova of the parasites usually enter the human being (the host) in contaminated food or water. They reach the intestine where they mature into the fully grown worm.

They are usually recognized by the presence of the worm or the ova in the faeces.

Certain drugs, known as anthelmintics, are used in order to kill the worms when they are present in the intestine.

Thread-worms (oxyuris vermicularis). These are the commonest and least harmful of the worms and are usually found in children. They appear in the faeces as small white threads 0·5 to 1·3 cm ($\frac{1}{4}$ to $\frac{1}{2}$ inch) in length, and may be seen wriggling about in recently passed motions. They inhabit the large intestine and when they reach the rectum may cause general irritability and itching of the anus which is worse at night. Vulvo-vaginitis may occur in female children. The ova gain entrance to the body in the food or by direct infection from one child to another, as a result of contamination of the clothes or the fingers.

Treatment. The usual treatment is to give one of the salts of piperazine either in the form of a tablet or elixir for a week, the dose being adjusted to the age of the patient. Proprietary preparations include 'Antepar' and 'Entocyl'. 'Pripsen', which also contains a laxative, is taken as a single dose. This is repeated after 2 weeks in order to cover the possibility of reinfestation. Viprynium ('Vanquin'), used in the same way, is another drug effective against thread-worms.

A bland ointment may be applied to the anus for the relief of itching. The child should be prevented from re-infecting itself by cutting the nails short, tying the nightdress below the feet at night so that the fingers cannot reach the anus, or by splinting the arms.

Night clothes and bed linen should be boiled after treatment. All members of a family, including adults, should be investigated and treated at the same time.

Round-worms (Ascaris lumbricoides). This worm is 15 to 25 cm (6 to 10 inches) long and resembles the ordinary earth worm in general appearance but is yellowish-white in colour. As a rule, not more than one or two parasites are present in each host, and both adults and children may be affected.

The symptoms are very variable, but abdominal pain, itching of the nose and, occasionally, convulsions in children may occur. Sometimes these worms wander into the bile ducts and produce jaundice or into the stomach from which they are subsequently vomited. In the early (larval) stage the lungs may be affected.

The main drug used in **treatment** is piperazine taken in a single dose.

Tape-worms. The two varieties encountered in this country are called **Taenia solium** (the pork tape-worm) and **Taenia saginata** (the cattle tape-worm). They are called tape-worms on account of their flat appearance which resembles a piece of tape, 3–5 metres (10 to 15 feet) in length. Each worm consists of a head or scolex having either small hooklets or suckers by which it attaches itself to the intestinal mucous membrane, and a large number of oblong or square segments. Those near the head are small, but they become increasingly large at the opposite extremity where they measure 1·3 cm ($\frac{3}{4}$ inch) in length by 0·5 cm ($\frac{1}{4}$ inch) in breadth. The lowest segments when fully developed drop off and appear in the faeces.

Tape-worms differ from the other intestinal parasites in not being directly transmitted from man to man. They require what is called an intermediate host. That is, ova after leaving the human host are consumed by animals such as pigs or cattle (the intermediate hosts) in which they undergo a further stage in development. A human being may subsequently become infected by eating the diseased meat if it is insufficiently cooked. The parasites form small cysts in the infected flesh which on account of its appearance is referred to as 'measly'.

The symptoms are indefinite and usually consist of abdominal pain and general depression; the diagnosis being made on the appearance of segments in the faeces.

A fresh-water fish tape-worm is also found in Northern Europe. This may interfere with the absorption of Vitamin B_{12} causing an anaemia similar to pernicious anaemia.

Treatment. 1. PROPHYLAXIS. (*a*) the routine inspection of meat by Public Health Authorities has done much to reduce the incidence of tape-worms. (*b*) if meat is properly cooked the parasites are destroyed. (*c*) The stools of affected persons must be disposed of carefully after disinfection.

2. TREATMENT.

(*a*) A salicylamide compound **niclosamide**, ('Yomesan') 2 g, kills and partly dissolves tape-worms. Four tablets well chewed followed by two more an hour later are taken without previous starvation or dieting. A laxative is given 2 hours later.

(*b*) Dichlorophen ('Anthipen') (70 mg per kilo body weight) may be used for *taenia saginata* without preliminary fasting or subsequent purgation.

(*c*) **Mepacrine** (1 g) is best given by a duodenal tube.

The motions passed are collected in warm water and a search is made for the head of the worm. If this is not found the treatment is repeated in ten days, for if the head is not detached and expelled, the tape-worm will form again, and segments will reappear in the motions in about 3 months.

(*d*) **Male fern** (*Filix Mas*).

The following routine is carried out. In order that the anthelmintic drug may come into full contact with the worm, the stomach and intestines should be as empty as possible. The patient is, therefore, starved for two days, fluids only, e.g. milk, soup, being given, and saline aperients are administered. On the third morning capsules containing 4–6 ml (60 or 90 minims) of liquid extract of male fern (Extractum filicis) are given either as a single dose or 3 doses at intervals of half an hour. Two hours later a full dose of Epsom Salts (magnesium sulphate) 8 g (120 grains) is taken. On no account must castor oil be used, as poisonous symptoms may be caused by its action on male fern.

Hookworm (ankylostomiasis). Although hook-worm infection is not common in Europeans, the ova are sometimes found in the stools of coloured people arriving in this country.

The worm enters the skin, e.g. of persons walking barefoot, and finds its way via the bloodstream and the lungs to the intestines. Anaemia, dyspepsia and pneumonia may occur.

'Alcopar' (bephenium), 5 g as a single dose or tetrachlorethylene (3 ml) may be used in treatment.

DISEASES OF THE LIVER

Functions of the Liver. The liver plays an active part in various metabolic processes and in the formation of bile. The latter has two important constituents, bile pigments and bile salts. The pigments, called bilirubin and biliverdin, are formed from haemoglobin derived from worn-out and broken-down red cells. The salts are necessary for the proper digestion and absorption of fat from the intestine.

Bile is produced in the liver cells from constituents in the bloodstream and secreted into the bile capillaries which unite to form larger ducts. It leaves the liver by the hepatic ducts and is stored and concentrated in the gallbladder. When required for digestive purposes, it leaves the gallbladder by the cystic duct and flows along the common duct to reach the duodenum.

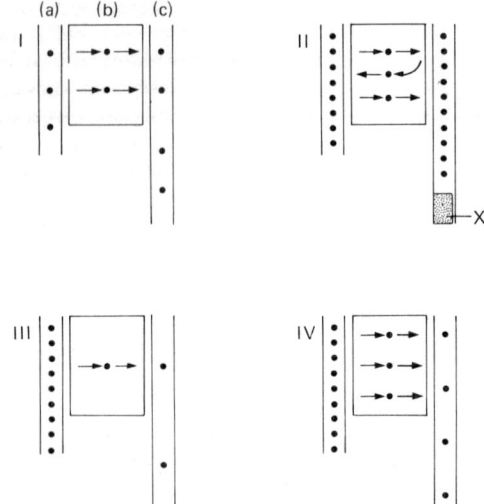

Fig. 49 Diagram illustrating the types of jaundice. (*a*) Bloodstream. (*b*) Liver cell. (*c*) Bile duct.

I. Represents normal amount of bile in blood, passing through liver cell and into bile duct.

II. Obstruction (X) of bile duct results in accumulation of bile in the duct behind the obstruction. The excess of bile is reabsorbed through the liver cells into the bloodstream.

III. In toxic jaundice the liver cell is damaged and the bile from the bloodstream is unable to pass through.

IV. Haemolytic jaundice, in which there is more bile in the bloodstream than the liver can deal with.

Jaundice (icterus)

By jaundice is meant the accumulation of bile pigments in the blood, which manifests itself by yellow coloration of the skin and mucous membranes. The excess of pigment is excreted in the urine, which becomes dark brown in colour.

It is a symptom rather than a disease and may be due to a variety of causes. There are three main types:

   I. Obstructive.

  II. Toxic and infective (Hepatic jaundice).

 III. Haemolytic.

I Obstructive jaundice. Complete obstruction of the ducts prevents bile from reaching the duodenum. It, therefore, accumulates in the liver and is subsequently reabsorbed into the bloodstream, with the production of jaundice. The lack of bile salts in the intestine leads to inefficient digestion and absorption of fats, so that the stools are bulky and contain excess of fat. In addition, in the absence of bile pigments the faeces are pale or clay-coloured.

Obstruction may be caused in the following ways:

1. Obstruction in the lumen of the ducts (gallstones).
2. Obstruction due to disease of the wall of the bile ducts, e.g. Inflammation (cholangitis), cancer of the bile ducts.
3. Pressure on the ducts from outside, e.g. tumours of the liver, stomach, pancreas or neighbouring lymph glands.
4. Chlorpromazine and methyltestosterone may produce bile stasis in the fine canals in the liver. The former drug also damages the liver cells.

II Toxic of hepatic jaundice. This variety differs from the last in the fact that the ducts are not obstructed, but bile pigment accumulates in the blood because the liver cells are damaged and therefore unable to secrete it properly.

The toxins concerned may be derived from a virus, bacteria or may be of chemical origin. Jaundice of this type occurs in infective hepatitis, septicaemia and occasionally, in typhoid fever and pneumonia. It is seen also in toxic conditions associated with pregnancy. Poisoning with arsenic, benzene, chloroform and phosphorus produces similar damage to the liver cells.

III Haemolytic jaundice. This is a third type of jaundice which is sometimes seen. It results from an excessive destruction of the red cells so that there is an accumulation of bile pigments in the blood because the liver cells are unable to excrete more than a certain amount at a time. However, in the absence of any obstruction to the bile ducts, the stools are not clay-coloured.

Because of the excessive destruction of red cells the condition is usually associated with haemolytic anaemia (p. 182).

The commonest **varieties of jaundice** seen are:

(*a*) Infective hepatitis (catarrhal jaundice) which is associated with damage to the liver cells and catarrhal inflammation of the bile ducts and may occur in epidemics.

(b) Jaundice due to gallstones.

(*c*) Jaundice due to cancer of the liver or pancreas.

(*d*) Other rarer causes include Weil's disease, the jaundice of the new-born associated with a positive Rhesus factor and jaundice following incompatible blood transfusion.

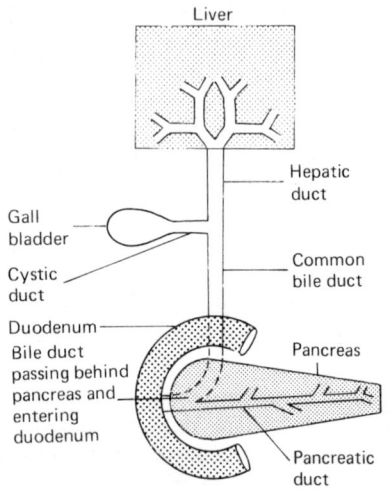

Fig. 50 Diagram illustrating the biliary apparatus.

Symptoms of Jaundice. In addition to the appearance of bile in the urine and the yellow discoloration of the skin which, in severe and long-standing cases, may assume a greenish-brown hue, the patient frequently complains of itching, general depression and irritability of temper. Nausea and dyspepsia are common and the pulse tends to be slow.

Viral hepatitis

There are two types of viral hepatitis, namely Infective hepatitis (due to Virus A) and Serum hepatitis (due to Virus B). Clinically the two diseases are very similar but the incubation period of the first is 2 to 6 weeks, whereas that of the second is 2 to 6 months.

Infective hepatitis (Catarrhal jaundice). It may be transmitted by faecal contamination of food or water, and possibly by droplet infection in the early stages. There is some catarrh of the bile ducts together with a variable amount of toxic damage to the liver cells. It tends to affect children and young adults and sometimes occurs in epidemics which are most common in autumn and winter. The severity of attacks varies.

The **symptoms** include anorexia, vomiting and epigastric pain as well as those of jaundice, with yellow staining of the skin and mucous membranes. There is usually some enlargement of the liver which may be tender. The stools are pale and bile is present in the urine. Most cases recover in a few weeks without special treatment but a few may slowly progress to cirrhosis of the liver, or develop acute yellow atrophy.

Rest, not necessarily strict, is advisable during the acute stages and a subsequent period of convalescence may be necessary. During the first few days of the illness the patient is often nauseated and, in particular, cannot tolerate fats. These should, therefore, be avoided during this period but a prolonged fat-free diet is unnecessary.

A short course of steroids lasting not more than 21 days may be helpful in those cases in which jaundice is prolonged.

Severe itching may be relieved by antihistamine drugs.

Immuno-globulin given before and during the incubation period may help to attenuate the disease and is useful in limiting epidemics in schools and institutions and in pregnant women who are liable to severe attacks.

In view of the fact that the virus is present in the faeces for some days before the jaundice appears and for 2 to 4 weeks after, great care must be taken in the disposal of excreta and in the washing of hands. Disposable instruments and supplies should preferably be used for patients with infective hepatitis. Instruments which are to be re-used should be cleaned and then sterilized by autoclaving for thirty minutes at 15 p.s.i. Re-usable articles in the hospital room should be autoclaved or cleaned with soap and water and soaked for 24 hours in a solution of 0·5% iodine in 70% ethanol or isopropanol. Books, magazines and newspapers should be incinerated.

Because of the damage to the liver cells the patient should be advised to take no alcohol for at least 6 months.

Serum hepatitis is a form of virus hepatitis which may be conveyed by blood transfusion or the use of unsterile needles and syringes. It has assumed particular importance because of outbreaks in haemodialysis units. These have endangered the lives of staff working in the units; paradoxically the threat to patients is small. Attempts are made to ensure that donated blood does not contain the virus. The presence of **hepatitis associated antigen** (HAA) is regarded as a sign of infected blood and ideally all donated blood is now screened for this antigen.

Treatment. The treatment of jaundice depends on its cause and type, obstructive jaundice usually being a surgical problem. In general because of the lack of bile in the intestine the amount of fat in the diet should be reduced. No cream is allowed, butter is permitted in small quantities only, and milk should be skimmed. A high protein diet is often necessary. Itching is relieved by antihistamine drugs. If the biliary obstruction is incomplete, cholestyramine will relieve itching by increasing bile salt excretion.

Weil's disease (leptospirosis) is caused by leptospira excreted in the urine of rats and is therefore most often seen in sewer workers. The main symptoms are jaundice, pyrexia, haematuria and purpura. Full doses of penicillin or tetracycline are used in treatment.

Acholuric jaundice. (Congenital haemolytic anaemia.) This is a disease which tends to occur in families. It is characterized by mild jaundice without the appearance of bile in the urine. The spleen is enlarged and the red cells are abnormally fragile. The usual treatment is splenectomy.

Cirrhosis of the liver

This is a disease seen less frequently now than in the past. It affects mostly males between the ages of 40 and 50 years. An excess of fibrous tissue, replacing many of the normal cells, is present in the liver which becomes hard and has an irregular, 'hob-nail' surface. Alcohol, malnutrition and possibly some unknown toxins play a part in its aetiology. Rarely cases appear to follow infective hepatitis. The first symptoms are mainly dyspeptic, and the liver and sometimes the spleen are found to be enlarged. Later, haematemesis and ascites may occur on account of the associated congestion in the portal vein.

Treatment. The treatment in the early stages consists of leading a regular life and avoiding alcohol. A high-protein diet supplemented by vitamins, in particular vitamin B, is given. If this is strictly carried out, the progress of the disease may be checked. Some patients benefit from corticosteroid therapy. Thiazides (e.g. chlorothiazide, bendrofluazide), frusemide ('Lasix'), ethacrynic acid ('Edecrin' and spironolactone ('Aldactone-A') may be used in an attempt to control the ascites. Very vigorous diuretic therapy may cause grave electrolyte problems. In order to keep the doses of diuretics as low as possible, dietary sodium is restricted to 22 mEq daily. It may be necessary to remove ascites by paracentesis of the abdomen, a procedure which should preferably not be repeated because valuable protein is lost in the ascitic fluid.

Patients with advanced liver failure may not tolerate more than 40 g of protein daily. Faecal bacteria breakdown excess protein in the colon to ammonia, which is absorbed into the portal circulation. A normal liver removes this ammonia but a failing one cannot and it affects the brain, causing mental symptoms (encephalopathy). **Lactulose** ('Duphalac') is a drug which acidifies the faeces and results in decreased absorption of ammonia from the colon.

It should be particularly remembered that sedative drugs, especially morphine and paraldehyde, are potentially dangerous in patients with impaired liver function, as their detoxication is slower than normal.

Surgical measures to relieve portal hypertension are sometimes tried, e.g. joining the portal vein to the inferior vena cava (portocaval anastomosis).

Portal congestion or hypertension. Congestion of the portal vein and the areas from which it drains blood is an important condition and may be due to a number of causes.

Tributaries pass to the portal vein from the contents of the peritoneal cavity, including the lower end of the oesophagus, the stomach, the intestines and the spleen. The portal vein reaches the liver where it divides into venules and capillaries and the blood is eventually collected up in the hepatic veins which enter the inferior vena cava. It has been seen in connection with heart failure that congestion or 'back pressure' in the inferior vena cava affects also the hepatic veins, causing enlargement of the liver and congestion in the portal vein and the areas drained by it. The same effect is produced in the spleen and abdominal viscera if there is obstruction to the flow of blood through the liver, as in cirrhosis, or if the portal vein is pressed on by a tumour before it enters the liver.

It is clear that the organs pouring their blood into the portal circulation will become congested if their venous return is impaired. Rupture of engorged veins at the lower end of the oesophagus and upper part of the stomach, which become varicose, accounts for the occurrence of haematemesis in cirrhosis of the liver. Distension

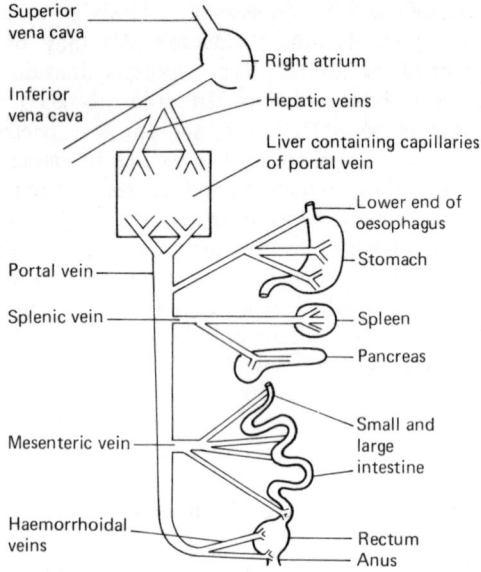

Fig. 51 Diagram illustrating the portal circulation.

and varicosity of the veins of the rectum producing haemorrhoids is also common. The accumulation of fluid in the peritoneal cavity (ascites) in heart failure and in cirrhosis of the liver is also explained by this congestion in the portal circulation. Ascites is really the outpouring of oedema fluid in the peritoneal cavity and is produced in the same way as oedema of a limb by the exudation of fluid from the capillaries and veins when the venous return to the heart is impeded, or as a result of inflammation.

Cancer of the liver

The occurrence of primary cancer in the liver is very rare, but secondary deposits of malignant growth arising in organs such as the stomach, colon, rectum, breast, lung, etc., are common.

The general condition of the patient is poor, the liver is enlarged and irregular, and obstructive jaundice and ascites are common. Once secondary deposits of any size are present in the liver, the duration of life is short.

Other conditions. Generalized inflammation of the liver substance is called hepatitis. **Acute yellow atrophy** (acute hepatic necrosis) of the liver is a severe and often fatal condition which may occur in toxaemia of pregnancy and poisoning from certain chemical substances, such as phosphorus and carbon tetrachloride. Very rarely, drugs such as sulphonamides and paracetamol in excessive dosages may be responsible. Abscesses may occur in its substance as a result of amoebic dysentery, or as part of a general pyaemia.

Hepatic coma. Liver failure and disturbance of consciousness may complicate various liver diseases such as acute yellow atrophy, acute hepatitis and late cirrhosis especially after taking certain drugs such as barbiturates or potent diuretics. In cirrhosis the immediate cause may be sudden haemorrhage, excessive alcoholic intake, severe general infection or rapid tapping of ascites. Drowsiness and abnormal behaviour may progress to deep coma and even death. One of the most striking features, especially in cirrhosis, is that the level of consciousness may vary markedly from day to day and even from hour to hour. The mental disturbance seems to be due to a breakdown product from the action of enzymes or bacteria on proteins in the intestine and the aim of treatment is to remove protein and destroy the bacteria. Protein is strictly excluded from the diet, and a broad spectrum antibiotic and regular enemas are given. Calories are supplied in the form of glucose by mouth or by intravenous infusion and electrolyte balance is maintained. In cases of acute liver failure (for example those due to viral hepatitis or paracetamol overdosage) the liver is often able to regenerate sufficiently for the patient to recover if the patient can be tided over the few critical days. Efforts are being made to perfect an 'artificial liver'; a recently developed haemoperfusion system perfuses the blood through charcoal and ion-exchange resins to remove toxins normally dealt with by a healthy liver.

Van den Bergh's test is an investigation of the amount and type of bile pigment present in the blood.

Other tests of liver function which are carried out on a specimen of blood include:

1. Colloidal gold (positive in cases of infective hepatitis, cirrhosis and Weil's disease, but usually negative in obstructive jaundice).
2. Thymol turbidity (raised in hepatitis, negative in obstructive jaundice).
3. Serum alkaline phosphatase (raised in obstructive jaundice).
4. Estimation of the serum proteins.
5. Estimation of the serum transaminase.

In special cases liver puncture (biopsy) is carried out and the material obtained examined microscopically.

DISEASES OF THE GALLBLADDER AND BILE DUCTS

Cholecystitis

Inflammation of the gallbladder may be acute or chronic. The main symptoms are epigastric pain, with tenderness over the gallbladder at the tip of the 9th rib, nausea, vomiting and flatulence.

In acute cases the temperature is raised. If suppuration is present, rigors occur and operation may be necessary, unless the condition subsides with antibiotic therapy, e.g. ampicillin.

Gallstones (cholelithiasis)

Most gallstones (biliary calculi) are composed predominantly of **cholesterol,** which is admixed with calcium salts and which clusters around a bile pigment centre. In some cases the abnormality is apparently in the liver cells, which produce bile supersaturated with cholesterol. The cholesterol precipitates out of solution in the gall-bladder and the crystals adhere together to form gallstones. In other cases, inflammation of the gallbladder may be responsible for stone formation. One big stone or a large number of smaller ones are formed.

While the stones remain in the gallbladder they may cause no symptoms or only those of dyspepsia due to associated cholecystitis. A gallstone may, however, pass down the cystic duct and reach the common bile duct. The passage of a stone down the ducts causes attacks of excruciating pain in the epigastrium and in the back in the neighbourhood of the right shoulder. It is associated with vomiting and sweating and is referred to as gallstone or **biliary colic.**

If the stone is a small one it will pass down the bile duct into the duodenum, but as multiple stones are usually present further attacks of biliary colic may occur when others escape from the gallbladder.

If a large calculus is present it may fail to pass into the duodenum and the bile duct will become obstructed with the subsequent development of jaundice.

Treatment. Many cases of cholecystitis and gallstones require operative treatment. If medicinal measures are employed the patient

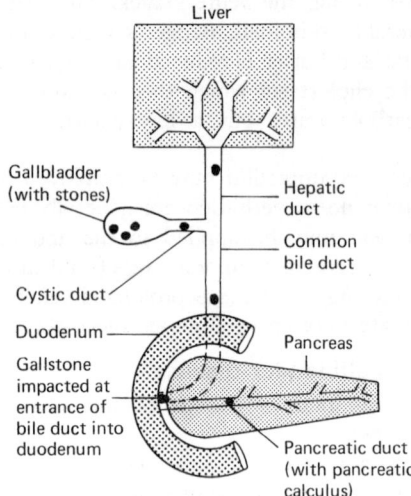

Fig. 52 Diagram showing the positions in which gallstones may be found.

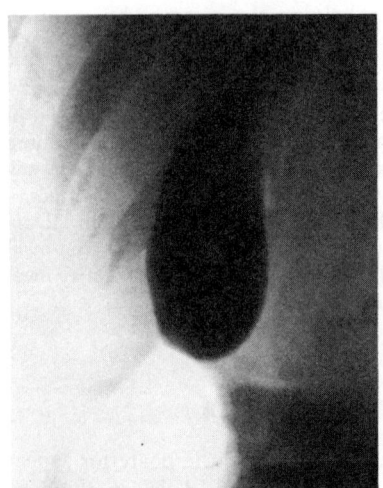

Fig. 53 Normal cholecystogram, showing shadow of gallbladder containing dye.

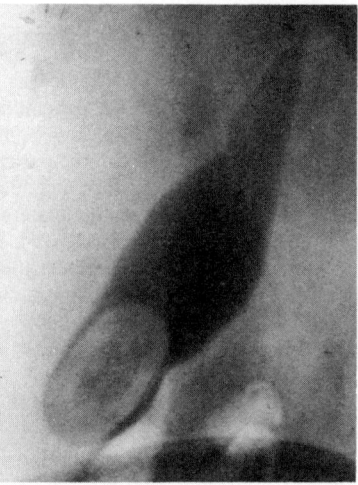

Fig. 54 Cholecystogram showing gallstone.

must rest in bed during the acute stages. The diet will consist of broth, milk preferably skimmed, Benger's food and later boiled fish. The amount of fat and butter is reduced and eggs are given sparingly on account of the cholesterol which they contain, i.e. low fat, high protein, high carbohydrate, but a low calorie diet if obesity is present.

Antibiotics such as ampicillin may be employed for acute cases. Morphine and atropine or pethidine are generally required for gallstone colic and heat may be applied to the abdomen. Sublingual glyceryl trinitrate may give temporary relief and intramuscular propantheline bromide may give more prolonged relief of biliary colic. Magnesium sulphate is often used as an aperient.

Investigation of gallbladder disease

1. *X-ray*. A radiogram of the gallbladder area may show the presence of gallstones.

2. *Cholecystography*. Certain substances, conveniently referred to as 'Gallbladder dyes', which are opaque to x-rays, are excreted by the liver in the bile. In normal cases they are concentrated and stored for a short time in the gallbladder. Advantage is taken of this fact to obtain x-ray pictures of the outline of the gallbladder.

Various methods of administration are employed, but the following account may be of assistance in helping the nurse who is often responsible for administering the dye.

One of the preparations such as iopanoic acid ('Telepaque') is generally used. On the day before the examination is carried out the amount of fat in the diet is reduced to a minimum. The patient has a light supper containing no fat at 7 p.m. At 10 p.m. the patient swallows 6 'Telepaque' tablets. X-ray pictures are taken the following day, approximately 14, 18 and 19 hours after the drug has been administered (i.e. 12 noon, 4 p.m. and 5 p.m.). During this period no food is allowed, but water may be drunk. The first meal of the day is given 1 hour before the last x-ray. This consists of a fatty meal and may include bread and butter, and bacon with a cup of tea.

DISEASES OF THE PANCREAS

The pancreas is a glandular organ lying across the posterior aspect of the abdomen behind the peritoneum. The head lies in the concavity formed by the duodenum, and the body extends across the vertebral column to the left, so that the tail reaches the neighbourhood of the spleen.

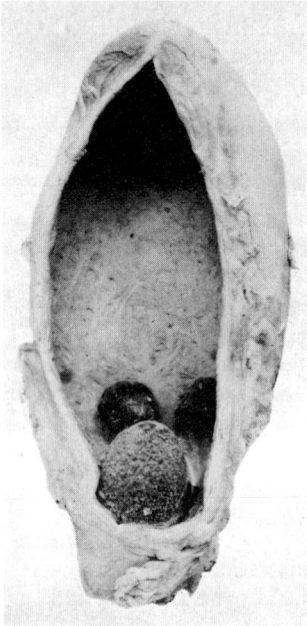

Fig. 55 Enlarged gallbladder with gallstones.

The duct of the gland joins the lower end of the common bile duct and pours its secretions into the duodenum. Specialized groups of cells, called the Islets of Langerhans, secrete insulin directly into the bloodstream and disorder of their function results in **diabetes** (p. 439).

Obstruction to the flow of the external secretion (pancreatic juice) which contains the fat-splitting enzyme, lipase, is followed by inefficient digestion and absorption of fat so that the stools become bulky, oily and frothy in character (p. 229). This may occur if the duct is obstructed by pancreatic calculi, or if the lower end of the bile duct is obstructed by a gallstone below the level of the entrance of the pancreatic duct (see Fig. 52, p. 257). Inflammation of the pancreas (pancreatitis) may produce similar symptoms. Cancer of the head of the pancreas is common and gives rise to jaundice owing to pressure on the bile duct.

DISEASES OF THE PERITONEUM

Peritonitis

Inflammation of the peritoneum may be acute or chronic. Acute peritonitis generally follows surgical conditions such as appendicitis, perforation of a gastric or typhoid ulcer, or any condition in which the cavity becomes contaminated by the contents of the bowel.

Secondary deposits of cancer are frequently seen in the peritoneum and may cause ascites.

Chronic peritonitis may be caused by the tubercle bacillus.

Tuberculous peritonitis is of two types. The first is associated with outpouring of fluid into the peritoneal cavity and the development of ascites. In the second the inflammatory process results in dense adhesions between various loops of bowel.

The symptoms consist of enlargement of the abdomen, increasing weakness and loss of weight. There is usually some pyrexia and abdominal pain. The condition mainly affects children and adolescents but is not now common. The treatment consists of rest in bed, and the administration of streptomycin, para-amino-salicylic acid (PAS) and isoniazid over a long period.

Ascites

The accumulation of fluid in the peritoneal cavity has been frequently mentioned, and it has been explained that the condition is of the nature of oedema of the cavity. It may be an entirely local condition or part of a generalized oedema of the body.

The common causes are:
1. Obstruction to the portal vein (portal hypertension).
    (*a*) Cirrhosis of the liver.
    (*b*) Cancer of the liver or neighbouring parts.
2. Congestion in the portal vein.
    (*a*) Chronic heart failure.
    (*b*) Constrictive pericarditis.
3. Chronic inflammation of the peritoneum.
    (*a*) Secondary cancer of the peritoneum.
    (*b*) Tuberculous peritonitis.
4. Part of generalized oedema.
    e.g. Nephrotic syndrome.

The treatment will to some extent depend on the cause of the condition, e.g. when due to heart failure it may respond to a salt-

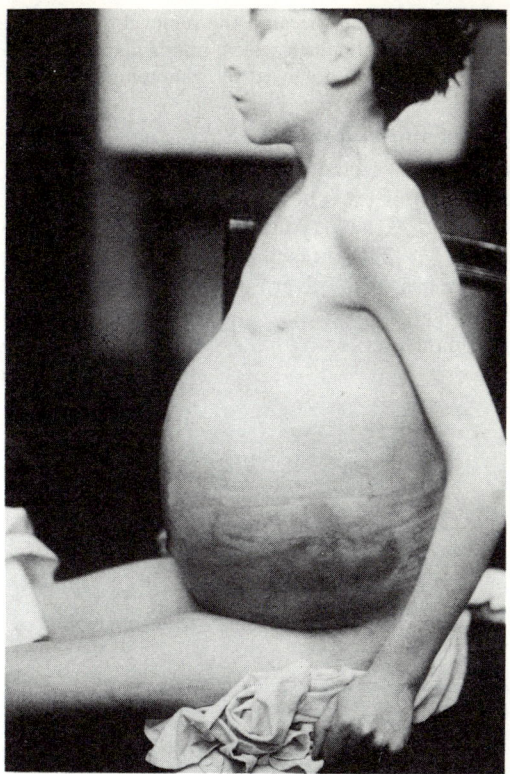

Fig. 56 Ascites (severe).

free diet, restricted fluid intake and diuretics. It may be necessary, however, to remove the excess of fluid from the peritoneal cavity. This operation is referred to as paracentesis of the abdomen.

Paracentesis abdominis. The following accessories are required. Sterile towels and swabs, iodine, a trocar and cannula, and a syringe, needle and procaine or similar local anaesthetic.

The patient is placed in Fowler's position if possible. The trocar and cannula is inserted either in the iliac fossa or in the mid-line of the abdomen between the umbilicus and the pubes. For this reason it is essential that the patient be catheterized before the operation is performed, because a distended bladder may be injured if the tapping is performed in the mid-line. An abdominal binder or many-tailed bandage is placed in position before the operation commences, and it is the duty of the nurse to see that this is kept tight while the fluid is escaping and for 24 hours afterwards. This is necessary because the removal of fluid causes a lowering of pressure inside the abdomen which, unless maintained by the external pressure of a binder, may be followed by symptoms of collapse.

Enlargement of the abdomen

The common causes of enlargement of the abdomen are:
1. Accumulation of fat (obesity).
2.   ,,   ,, gas (tympanites)⎱ For causes, see
3.   ,,   ,, fluid (ascites) ⎰   pp. 231, 260.
4. Large tumours of the liver, spleen or kidney.
5. Ovarian cysts.
6. The pregnant uterus.

6 Diseases of the Respiratory System

The respiratory system may be conveniently described as consisting of the upper and lower air passages.

1. The upper air passages include:
   (a) The nose and accessory air sinuses (i.e. the maxillary antrum, the frontal, sphenoidal and ethmoidal sinuses).
   (b) The nasopharynx, pharynx and the tonsils.
   (c) The larynx and trachea.
2. The lower air passages, situated within the cavity of the thorax:
   (a) The bronchi.
   (b) The bronchioles.
   (c) The alveoli or air cells in the lung.

1. Diseases of the upper air passages

Acute coryza (the common cold)

Acute catarrhal rhinitis or inflammation of the nasal mucous membrane occurs in the common 'cold in the head' and is sometimes referred to as **coryza.** This condition is due to a virus often followed by bacteria. It is highly infectious, the organisms being conveyed mainly by droplet infection.

The symptoms are dryness in the nose and nasopharynx followed by sneezing, nasal obstruction and watery discharge which later becomes muco-purulent. A varying degree of malaise and, sometimes, pyrexia is present.

The complications which may ensue are:

(a) Spread of infection to the nasal sinuses, especially the maxillary antrum, which may become filled with pus (sinusitis).

(b) Downward spread of the inflammation causing laryngitis, tracheitis or bronchitis. The general term '**upper respiratory infection**' is often used.

There are, in fact, a number of acute febrile catarrhal illnesses ranging in severity from the common cold and pharyngitis to influenza and pneumonia due to infection with different types of virus. One attack produces very little subsequent immunity and children are more susceptible than adults.

The treatment of colds is frequently neglected, but they can be made more tolerable by putting the patient to bed and inducing sweating by the use of blankets, hot drinks and drugs such as aspirin.

Inhalations of oil of eucalyptus, benzoin or menthol and decongestant sprays or nasal drops, e.g. 'Otrivine', help to relieve the nasal obstruction.

Chronic nasal catarrh also occurs and is associated with thickening of the mucous membrane over the turbinate bones.

Infection of the nasal mucous membrane by the diphtheria bacillus (nasal diphtheria) has already been described (p. 56).

Adenoids

Adenoids consist of hypertrophied lymphoid tissue situated in the nasopharynx which becomes enlarged as a result of chronic infection in the same way as the tonsils.

The condition is common in children and is associated with frequent colds, nasal obstruction, mouth-breathing and snoring. The swollen tissue may cover the openings of the Eustachian tubes and, by preventing air from entering the middle ear, cause deafness. If infection spreads up the tubes, otitis media may develop.

The treatment consists of improving the general health by abundant fresh air and good nourishment. If this fails to effect a cure the adenoids are removed by operation.

Nasal obstruction. Patients frequently complain of inability to breathe through one or both nostrils. This may be due to rhinitis, adenoids, deflection of the nasal septum to one or other side, foreign bodies in the nose or new growths.

Epistaxis

Bleeding from the nose is a common symptom and may be due to local or general causes.

LOCAL CAUSES

   (*a*) Injury to the nose.

   (*b*) Fracture of the base of the skull.

   (*c*) Ulceration of the nasal mucous membrane.

GENERAL CAUSES

(a) High blood pressure.

(b) Venous congestion associated with heart disease (commonly mitral stenosis).

(c) Blood diseases, such as leukaemia and purpura.

(d) Menstruation (very occasionally).

(e) Typhoid fever.

Treatment. The patient should sit erect and the clothing round the neck loosened. A cold compress or ice-bag may be applied to the nose. If the bleeding occurs from a point on the septum near the anterior nares, as it often does, pinching the nose for 5 minutes may be sufficient to stop haemorrhage. If these methods fail, the affected side must be plugged gently with ribbon gauze which is sometimes soaked in adrenaline solution or hydrogen peroxide. The plugging should be removed in 12 to 24 hours since it is liable to become septic. If it is necessary to retain the plug in position for a longer period, it should be moistened frequently with hydrogen peroxide which checks bacterial growth. Cauterization of the bleeding point may be possible. Very severe cases may require injections of morphine and blood transfusion may be necessary.

Hay fever (see p. 16).

Acute Tonsillitis

Acute inflammation of the tonsils is a common and often painful condition, which should not be neglected on account of the serious complications which sometimes occur, e.g. acute rheumatism and nephritis.

The causal organism is usually a streptococcus. The following varieties are described:

1. Superficial, in which the tonsil is involved in general inflammation of the pharynx.

2. Follicular, a very common form, in which the crypts of the tonsil become filled with pus and can be seen as small yellowish spots scattered over the surface of the red and swollen organ.

3. Suppurative, when the infection spreads into the surrounding tissues producing a peritonsillar abscess or **quinsy**. As a rule, this very painful condition only affects one tonsil and the swelling may extend into the soft palate. The pain is sometimes referred to the ear.

4. Special types of tonsillitis due to diphtheria, syphilis or associated with infectious diseases such as scarlet fever are described with those maladies.

Symptoms. Acute tonsillitis is abrupt in onset. The patient complains of soreness of the throat and painful swallowing (dysphagia). The temperature is usually high, up to 40 °C (104 °F), and is associated with malaise, headache and pains in the limbs. The tonsils are found to be red and swollen and, in the follicular variety, the characteristic patchy exudate from the crypts can be seen. The cervical glands are enlarged and tender.

It is of the utmost importance that cases of acute tonsillitis should be distinguished from the rare cases of diphtheria in order that anti-toxin may be administered early in the latter condition. If there is any doubt about the diagnosis, a throat swab is taken and, in some cases, antitoxin is given before the result is obtained.

Treatment. The patient should usually be kept in bed until the fever has subsided and isolation should be maintained as far as possible since the condition tends to be infectious. It is well known how quickly sore throat will spread round a hospital ward or affect several members of one family.

Frequent hot gargles (glycothymoline or phenol) are comforting. A kaolin poultice may be applied to the neck in order to relieve the pain of cervical adenitis. Aspirin may be given for pain and headache and may also be used as a gargle. An aperient may be desirable in some cases. Penicillin or one of the other antibiotics are often used. The prompt treatment with adequate doses of penicillin in infections of the upper respiratory tract due to haemolytic streptococci is important in the prevention of rheumatic fever and nephritis. Antiseptic lozenges such as 'Tyrozets', or 'Dequadin', are sometimes given.

A **quinsy**, if its progress is not checked by antibiotics, requires opening with a scalpel and sinus forceps. Evacuation of the pus is followed by immediate relief. Owing to the risk of inhaling septic material, endotracheal intubation is necessary if a general anaesthetic is required.

The patient should be encouraged to drink as much fluid as possible, but if swallowing is very painful, semi-solids are taken more easily than liquids. The diet should include eggs and milk, custard, jellies and thick soups. Ice-cream is usually appreciated.

Tonsillectomy. There should always be a clear indication such as quinsy or recurrent acute attacks of tonsillitis before tonsillectomy is considered. Among conditions not favourably influenced by operation are acute rheumatism, nephritis, asthma and anaemia.

The tonsils form part of a ring of lymphoid tissue which is situated in the upper air passages and consists of these organs together with the lymphoid tissue in the nasopharynx which is sometimes referred to as the pharyngeal tonsil and when hypertrophied constitutes adenoids.

This lymphoid tissue is the first line of defence of the body against infection entering either by the respiratory or digestive tracts. The second line of defence consists of the cervical glands which drain it.

Vincent's Angina. This is an uncommon condition in which the mouth, gums or tonsils may be affected and which is due to the combined action of a spirochaete and a bacillus. A membrane resembling diphtheria may be seen on one or both tonsils which, on separating, leaves a slowly healing ulcer. The diagnosis is confirmed by bacteriological examination. Most cases respond to penicillin.

Acute pharyngitis

The symptoms consist of pyrexia, difficulty in swallowing and dryness of the throat which appears red and inflamed. The treatment is similar to that employed in acute tonsillitis. Chronic pharyngitis is a fairly common condition but rarely calls for any special nursing treatment.

Acute epiglottitis (*Haemophilus* epiglottitis)

This is a serious condition which affects young children. The epiglottis may swell so much as to obstruct the airway and cause cardiac arrest or death. Treatment includes chloramphenicol, hydrocortisone and tracheostomy. Attendants dealing with the patient's airway should protect themselves from *haemophilus* pneumonia and other *haemophilus* infections by wearing masks.

Laryngitis

This condition may be either acute or chronic and frequently follows a downward spread of catarrhal inflammation from the nasopharynx or tonsils. It is seen in measles and influenza and may also be due to excessive strain on the voice and to the inhalation of irritating vapours.

Special varieties caused by tuberculosis, syphilis or new growth also occur. Therefore, hoarseness persisting for more than three weeks should be specially investigated.

The characteristic symptom is hoarseness or loss of voice

(aphonia) which is associated with a dry cough and, sometimes, pain on swallowing.

Treatment. In acute cases the patient should remain indoors and, if necessary, be confined to bed. Rest of the voice is essential. In the most severe cases absolute silence is required. In others, the patient should speak in a whisper, without using the vocal cords. Inhalations of friar's balsam (Tinct. benzoin. co.) or laryngeal sprays are generally employed.

Very severe inflammation, syphilis and new growths may cause obstruction to breathing sufficiently marked to necessitate tracheostomy.

Laryngeal diphtheria has already been described (p. 56).

Sometimes loss of voice with inability to speak other than in a whisper may be due to hysteria.

Laryngismus stridulus. This is an uncommon condition which is seen in children about the age of 1 year who are subject to rickets. The characteristic features are recurrent spasms in which the respiration ceases for some seconds while the child struggles for breath and becomes cyanosed. Each spasm of breath-holding is followed by a long crowing inspiration as the spasm relaxes. These symptoms may be mistaken for laryngeal diphtheria but are rarely fatal.

Treatment during a spasm consists of the administration of intravenous calcium gluconate. A small dose of chloral is sometimes given. The associated rickets also requires treatment.

Stridor is a term used to describe a harsh, high-pitched crowing noise as air passes in and out of a partially obstructed larynx or trachea. It may be caused by such conditions as:

(*a*) Obstruction in the lumen, e.g. a foreign body.

(*b*) Disease of the walls, e.g. inflammation, tumour, etc.

(*c*) Pressure from without, e.g. tumours of the thyroid, aortic aneurysm, malignant new growths and glands.

(*d*) Paralysis of the vocal cords due to injury to the laryngeal nerves, e.g. post thyroidectomy.

(*e*) Laryngismus stridulus, tetany and temporary spasm of the vocal cords.

Tracheitis

Acute inflammation of the trachea which may occur by itself or in association with other upper respiratory infections. It is characterised by cough and soreness behind the upper part of the sternum. Soothing inhalations and linctus are usually all that are needed in treatment.

2. Diseases of the Lower Air Passages

Examination of the lungs

Physical examination. The nurse frequently observes the physician when he is making an examination of the chest. The routine of inspection, palpation, percussion and auscultation is carried out, and the following observations are made:

1. Inspection. The shape, the movement and expansion on respiration, the rate and type of breathing.

2. Palpitation. Confirmation of the observations made by inspection. The vibrations caused by the voice are transmitted to the hand placed on the chest wall when the patient says 'ninety nine', etc.

3. Percussion. The chest normally gives a resonant sound, but if fluid be present in the pleural cavity or if the lung is solid and airless the percussion note is dull.

4. Auscultation. The sound produced by air entering and leaving the bronchioles and alveoli on respiration can be heard and may be altered by disease processes. In addition, bubbling sound (râles) or highly pitched musical squeaks (rhonchi) may be detected.

Radiography. Further investigation may be carried out by means of radiography. In addition to an ordinary x-ray picture, 'Dionosil', which is opaque to x-rays, is used in certain cases (e.g. bronchiectasis, lung abscess and cancer of the lung). This may be injected (*a*) with a special syringe and needle above the cricoid cartilage after the skin and superficial tissues have been anaesthetized or (*b*) through a nasal catheter so that the liquid falls directly into the larynx. The walls of the bronchi are clearly outlined on the x-ray plate by this means. This is called a **bronchogram.**

A tomogram consists of a series of x-ray pictures of a localized portion of the lung each one of which is specially focused to an increasing depth. This may help to determine the nature of a shadow shown on a routine film.

Bronchoscopy. The state of the bronchi may also be investigated by the passage of the bronchoscope, an illuminated, flattened, tubular instrument resembling the oesophagoscope, which is passed through the larynx and trachea. Foreign bodies in the air passages may be removed through it and conditions such as new growths may be visible from which a portion may be removed for microscopic examination (biopsy).

Spirometer test, see lung function tests p. 275.

Examination of sputum. Bacteriological examination of the sputum is of value in the diagnosis of pulmonary disease. E.g.

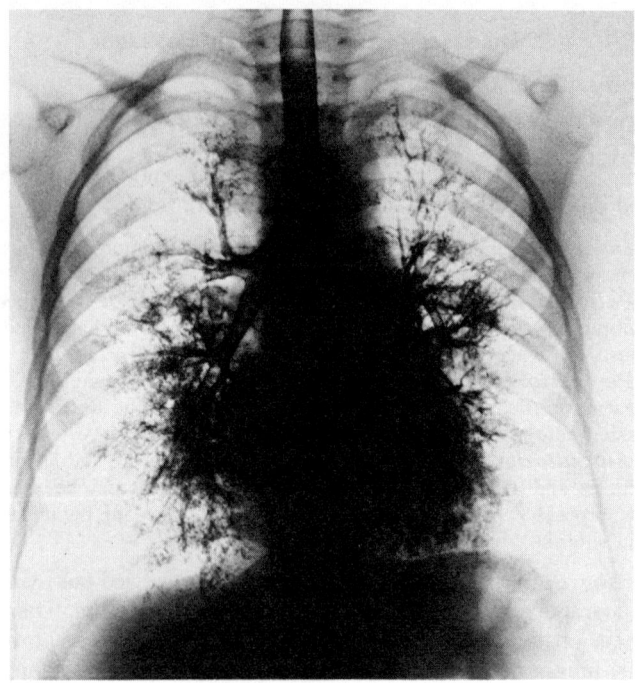

Fig. 57 Normal bronchogram.

(a) Tubercle bacilli in pulmonary tuberculosis. (b) Sensitivity to anti-biotics of organisms present in pneumonia and bronchitis. (c) Microscopic examination for the presence of cancer cells. (d) Microscopic examination for the presence of eosinophils in asthmatic bronchitis; thick green sputum is not always due to purulent infection.

Breathing. The normal rhythmic movements of respiration are automatic and under the control of the respiratory centre situated in the medulla, but can be consciously modified by the individual. Each breath consists of inspiration and expiration and occurs in the adult regularly at the rate of 18 to 20 respirations per minute.

The pulse rate is normally about four times the respiration rate and the correlation of these figures is referred to as the **pulse-respiration ratio.**

In febrile states the respiration rate is often quickened, the increase, however, being in proportion to the acceleration of the pulse. When the rapidity of the respirations exceeds this proportion the existence of some respiratory disorders may be inferred. For example, in pneumonia the rate of breathing becomes so increased that the ratio approximates 3 : 1, or 2 : 1, while in some cases of poisoning when the respiratory centre is depressed (e.g. morphine) the opposite state of affairs exists and the respirations are so slow that the ratio becomes altered to 6 : 1, i.e.:

	Pulse Rate	Respiration Rate	Ratio
Normal	72	18	4 : 1
In pneumonia	120	40–60	3 : 1, 2 : 1
In morphine poisoning	72	12	6 : 1

The respiration rate should be counted while the patient is quiet and, if possible, without attracting his attention to what is being done since, in a nervous patient, the rate may alter if he knows what is happening. The count may be performed by watching the movements of the chest or by placing the hand lightly upon it while the fingers are still on the radial pulse.

Dyspnoea. Difficulty in breathing is called dyspnoea and is generally accompanied by an increase in the rate and depth of respiration. This normally occurs after exercise. It is also seen in heart disease, in diseases of the respiratory system, especially bronchitis, pneumonia and asthma, and in cases where there is obstruction to the entry of air into the lungs, such as the presence of a foreign body in the larynx or in laryngeal diphtheria.

When the condition is so severe that the patient is forced to remain in the sitting posture it is called **orthopnoea** (e.g. in heart failure).

Other abnormalities in breathing. Deep sighing respirations occurring without increase in the general rate are sometimes seen in cases of diabetic coma, and after severe haemorrhage, both external and internal. This state is known as **'air hunger'.**

Stertorous breathing consists of noisy, snoring inspirations and is heard during anaesthesia, in cerebral haemorrhage and other conditions which may render the patient unconscious.

Cheyne-Stokes breathing is a peculiar type of respiratory rhythm usually seen in serious conditions such as heart failure or cerebral disease, when the patient is comatose and death is imminent, although occasionally recovery takes place. It is characterized by periods in which successive respirations gradually get deeper and more rapid until a maximum is reached and then shallower until breathing ceases. After a period lasting some seconds shallow respiration again commences and becomes increasingly deeper only to fade away into another period (**apnoea**) in which the respiratory movements are absent. The condition sometimes responds to intravenous injections of aminophylline.

Cough. A cough consists of a forcible, noisy expiration preceded and followed by a prolonged inspiration. It may be a voluntary act or may occur as a result of reflex action caused by irritation of any part of the respiratory mucous membrane.

The nurse should observe the character of a cough, its frequency and duration, its effect upon the patient and the factors which influence its occurrence.

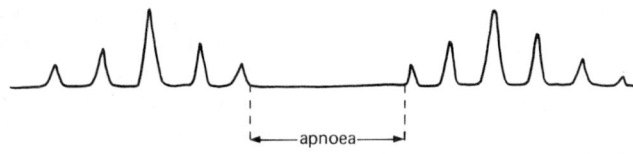

Fig. 58 Diagram illustrating the respiratory movements in Cheyne-Stokes breathing.

Three common types of cough may be described:

(*a*) The dry or tight cough. (*b*) The moist or loose cough. (*c*) The spasmodic cough.

(*a*) The dry cough without expectoration occurs in affections of the throat, laryngitis and the early stages of pneumonia. It is often the first symptom of pulmonary tuberculosis while, in some cases, it may be entirely of nervous origin.

(*b*) The moist cough with expectoration is seen in bronchitis, in the more advanced states of pulmonary tuberculosis and in the later stages of pneumonia and in bronchiectasis.

(*c*) The characteristic example of the spasmodic type is whooping-cough. Spasms of coughing associated with hoarseness of the voice also occur in laryngeal diphtheria (croupy cough).

The brassy cough of aortic aneurysm is referred to on p. 155.

Sputum. Sputum consists of the material coughed up from the respiratory passages and lungs (although mucus or muco-pus may trickle into the pharynx from nasal catarrh or sinusitis), and it is the duty of the nurse to provide a suitable carton into which a patient may expectorate if necessary. Sputum should be preserved for inspection as a matter of routine. The following points about its character are to be observed:

1. Quantity. 2. Consistency. 3. Colour. 4. Odour.

1. QUANTITY. The quantity expectorated is very variable but, if it appears to be excessive, the daily amount should be measured. It is especially liable to be copious in conditions such as bronchiectasis, lung abscess and advanced pulmonary tuberculosis.

2. CONSISTENCY. Sputum may be either mucoid or purulent in quality. The first type is clear and often very tenacious but, in conditions such as oedema of the lungs, it is watery and frothy. All degrees of purulent sputum may be seen from what is referred to as muco-purulent to almost pure pus. In the later stages of pulmonary tuberculosis it may form flat, round masses rather like small coins in the bottom of the sputum cup, and is then referred to as being 'nummular' in character.

3. COLOUR. Mucoid sputum is colourless; purulent sputum is yellow or greenish. The sputum in pneumonia often has a rusty colour. Blood may be coughed up alone or the sputum may be stained red by streaks of blood, for example, in pulmonary tuberculosis, mitral stenosis and pulmonary infarction.

4. ODOUR. As a rule, sputum is odourless, but in cases of bronchiectasis and abscess of the lung it has a very foul smell.

Sputum is frequently required for bacteriological examination in pulmonary tuberculosis when it is often possible to demonstrate the presence of the tubercle bacillus. As a rule, an early morning specimen should be reserved. In other cases, such as bronchitis and pneumonia, the bacteriology of the sputum may be required in order to test the sensitivity of the organisms to the various antibiotics. Great care must be taken that the receptable is properly marked with the patient's name and the date.

Sputum may be highly infectious and therefore, unless required for examination, must always be received either into a special destructible carton or into a quantity of antiseptic solution, such as phenol (carbolic) or lysol (1 in 40 to 1 in 80) which, in addition to destroying some of the organisms present, prevents expectoration from sticking to the side of the mug and becoming dry.

Hypoxia is a general term indicating under-oxygenation of the tissues and may be due to many causes, e.g. respiratory depression and diseases of the lung, circulatory disorders and anaemia.

Lung Function Tests

The function of the lungs is to enrich the blood with oxygen and to clear it of excess carbon dioxide, which is a waste product. The effectiveness of the process can be gauged by the partial pressures of these gases in blood samples from an artery. Normal values at rest are as follows:

Partial pressure of oxygen in arterial blood
$$(Pao_2) = 80 - 110 \text{ mm Hg}$$
Partial pressure of carbon dioxide in arterial blood
$$(Paco_2) = 36 - 44 \text{ mm Hg}$$

Sometimes the degree of **saturation** of arterial blood with oxygen (Sao_2) is measured and the normal range is 93–98%. It is reduced not only in certain lung diseases but also when there is shunting of blood from the right side of the heart to the left side, as in Fallot's tetralogy (see p. 137).

Instead of measuring $Paco_2$ directly, the partial pressure of carbon dioxide is often measured in alveolar air which has been breathed into a collecting bag. The result $(Paco_2)$ is practically identical to the Pco_2 of mixed venous blood which, at rest, is 6 mm Hg higher than the $Paco_2$.

Respiratory failure is characterized by carbon dioxide retention, indicated by a high $Paco_2$, and hypoxaemia, indicated by a low Pao_2.

Proper gaseous exchange depends on the processes of **ventilation** (the mass movement of air in and out of the lungs) and **gas transfer** (movement of gases between the air in the alveoli and the blood in the lung capillaries). For ventilation to be fully effective there must be proper **distribution** of the air throughout the air spaces and proper **perfusion** of blood throughout the capillary system. That is, there must be a balance between ventilation and perfusion. Ventilation of unperfused segments of lung (e.g. where blood supply is impaired by pulmonary emboli) is ineffective and, conversely, so is perfusion of unventilated lung tissue (e.g. in the consolidated lobe of lobar pneumonia). Ventilation and perfusion are considered together by expressing them as a ratio, V/Q.

Ventilation

It may be helpful to know some of the terms used and their abbreviations. Examples of normal values are quoted, but it should be remembered that age, sex and physique influence the measurements.

Compliance. With changes in pressure in the pleural cavity there are changes in lung volume. A lung which is not very compliant, perhaps because it is stiffened by oedema fluid, will expand less for a given pressure than would a normal lung. Normal compliance = 0·1 to 0·2 l per cm H_2O pressure.

The **Total Lung Capacity** (TLC) is the volume of gas in the lungs at the end of a full inspiration. Normal = 6 l (litres).

The **Vital Capacity** (VC) is the maximum volume of gas which can be expelled from the lungs after a full inspiration. Normal = 4·8 l. This measurement varies widely among individuals and its main use is in the periodic assessment of any one patient, when it will indicate improvement or deterioration.

The **Residual Volume** (RV) is the volume of air left in the lungs after a vital capacity measurement. Normal = 1·2 l.

The TLC and the RV are increased in emphysema and the ratio RV/TLC, which is normally 1/5, is also increased.

The **Functional Residual Capacity** (FRC) is the volume of air left in the lungs at the end of a normal quiet expression. Normal = 3 l. This is increased in emphysema.

The **Tidal Volume** (TV) is the volume of air inspired with each breath during normal quiet ventilation. It is normally about 500 ml.

The **Maximal Voluntary Ventilation** (MVV) or **Maximal Breathing Capacity** (MBC) is the maximal volume of air that can be breathed in and out in 1 minute. The normal is more than 150 l/min for men and more than 100 l/min for women aged 20 years. Any condition which impairs the mechanics of breathing will decrease the MVV. Poliomyelitis does so by weakening the respiratory muscles and emphysema does so by causing diffuse obstruction of the airways.

The **Forced Expired Volume** is usually measured over the course of one second and is then abbreviated to FEV_1. The FEV_1 is the volume of air expired in one second, after a full inspiration, when the patient is expiring air as fast as possible. It is usually expressed as a percentage of the vital capacity and it is normally above 75%.

The **Peak Expiratory Flow** (PEF) or **Peak Flow Rate** (PFR) is the rate of maximum flow of expired air. This is measured with a Wright Peak Flow Meter which is easy to use at the bedside.

FEV_1, expressed as a percentage of the VC, is reduced only in diseases causing airways obstruction, such as bronchial asthma and emphysema. In the former, the obstruction is relieved by the inhalation of a bronchodilator such as isoprenaline; in the latter it is irreversible. The PFR is reduced by all conditions which impair ventilation, be they obstructive or non-obstructive. An example of a non-obstructive condition is a pleural effusion, which ranks as a

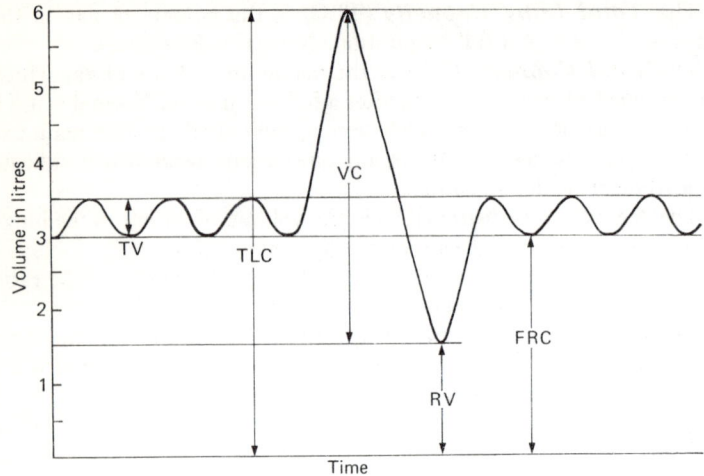

Fig. 59 Normal lung volumes.

restrictive condition because it prevents proper expansion of the lung.

In summary, ventilation may be reduced by **obstruction** of airways or by **restriction** of the chest or lung movements. **Air-trapping** contributes to the ventilatory defect in obstructive lung diseases; air may get into cystic spaces but be unable to get out easily.

Gas Transfer

The exchange of oxygen and carbon dioxide between the air in the alveoli and the blood in the lung capillaries depends upon:

1. The balanced distribution of ventilation and perfusion (V/Q).
2. Diffusion.
3. Chemical reactions in the red blood cells.

Gases are exchanged by diffusion through the air, the alveolar fluid, the alveolar membrane, the capillary membrane, the plasma and the red cell membrane.

From the diagram it can be seen that the alveolar-capillary membrane is formed from the adjoining walls of the alveolus and the capillary.

The **diffusing capacity** or, more correctly, the **transfer factor**, is the rate of transfer of gas through a membrane in relation to a constant pressure difference across it. It is often measured using a small quantity of carbon monoxide (CO) as the test gas and the total diffusing capacity is abbreviated to DLco. The normal DLco at rest is 15–25 ml/min/mmHg.

Some diseases, e.g. pulmonary oedema, idiopathic fibrosis and sarcoidosis, thicken the alveolar-capillary membrane and might therefore be expected to interfere with diffusion. Such interference has been referred to as 'alveolar-capillary block'. It is doubtful, however, whether exchange of gases is ever, in practice, seriously impaired by such a mechanism; inequalities of ventilation and blood flow are far more important in reducing gas transfer.

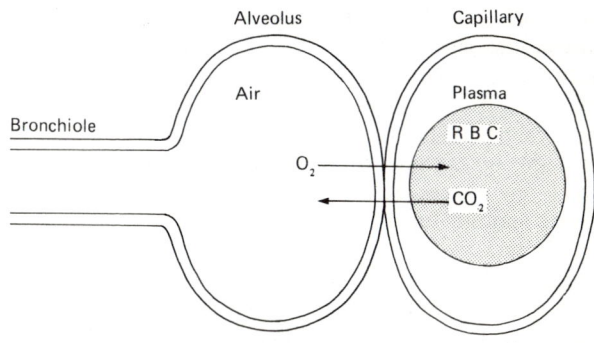

Fig. 60 Gas transfer.

Common Symptoms of Respiratory Diseases

The main symptoms which indicate pulmonary disease are:
  (*a*) Cough, with or without expectoration.
  (*b*) Dyspnoea and alterations of respiratory rate.
  (*c*) Cyanosis (p. 124), and hypoxia.
  (*d*) Pain in the chest.
  (*e*) Haemoptysis.
Pain in the chest in affections of the lungs is almost always due to inflammatory involvement of the pleura and is described under pleurisy (p. 291).

Haemoptysis

Haemoptysis means coughing up of blood. In true haemoptysis the blood comes from the larynx, trachea, bronchi or lungs. False haemoptysis may occur when the bleeding comes from the mouth, nose or pharynx. In other words, while present in diseases affecting the lungs, it may also be due to other conditions which result in bleeding into the respiratory tract.

The common causes are:

I PULMOTARY DISEASE

 e.g. Pulmonary tuberculosis.
   Cancer of the lung.
   Innocent tumours.
   Injury to the chest.
   Pulmonary embolism.
   Bronchiectasis and lung abscess.

II VENOUS CONGESTION OF THE LUNGS

 e.g. Mitral stenosis.

III OTHER LESS COMMON CAUSES include rupture of an aortic aneurysm into a bronchus, and certain blood diseases, e.g. leukaemia.

Haemoptysis may be very copious, as much as a pint of blood being brought up at one time; on other occasions, it may only amount to a few ounces. It is generally followed by the appearance of bloodstained sputum for a few days. A very large haemoptysis may prove rapidly fatal.

Coughing of blood from the respiratory tract (haemoptysis), although it may be swallowed and subsequently vomited, must not be confused with vomiting of blood from the alimentary tract haematemesis, p. 221). The main points of difference are indicated in the following table:

Haemoptysis	Haematemesis
1. The blood is coughed up.	The blood is vomited.
2. Blood is bright red and frothy.	Blood is not frothy and often dark.
3. Blood may be mixed with sputum.	Blood may be mixed with food particles.
4. Blood is alkaline in reaction.	Blood is acid in reaction if mixed with gastric juice.
5. Is frequently preceded by a tickling sensation in the throat.	May be accompanied by nausea and fullness in the epigastrium.
6. Is followed by bloodstained sputum.	No sputum. Often melaena.
7. Often a history of cough.	Often a history of abdominal pain.

Investigation of a case of haemoptysis calls for a full examination of the patient, x-rays, examination of the sputum, and often broncho-scopy. Sometimes no obvious cause is found.

The treatment of haemoptysis

Slight forms of haemoptysis do not require urgent treatment, but the more severe ones must receive immediate attention. All cases of haemoptysis require careful investigation in order to ascertain the primary cause of this symptom.

The condition is very alarming both to the patient and to his relatives and every effort must be made to reassure them. In this connection, it is well to remember that haemoptysis in early pulmonary tuberculosis and in mitral stenosis is rarely fatal.

In severe haemoptysis the patient is placed in bed and kept absolutely quiet. Morphine (15 mg, gr $\frac{1}{6}$ to $\frac{1}{4}$) is generally injected and has the effect of allaying restlessness and checking the cough, thereby affording an opportunity for blood to clot in the eroded vessel.

The posture of the patient is important. If it is known from which lung the haemorrhage has come (as in pulmonary tuberculosis involving one lung), the patient should lie on the affected side. In other cases he should be placed with the shoulders slightly raised, and the head low. By these means it is possible to limit the spread of blood into the other bronchial tubes. Sometimes it is necessary for him to be propped up with pillows.

Absolute rest must be insisted on. The patient is fed and everything is done for him. The diet at first consists of cold liquids given in quantities of 100 ml (3 or 4 fl oz) every four hours. Ice may be given to suck during the intervals. The diet is gradually increased and the patient is allowed to do more for himself in the course of several days or weeks.

In addition to morphine, a linctus may be given to diminish the cough, but care is needed not to depress the cough reflex lest an aspiration pneumonia should develop.

Blood transfusion may be required if the loss of blood is severe.

Diseases of the lungs

The lungs are covered by pleura and consist of bronchi, bronchioles, and alveoli or air cells, the latter being surrounded by blood vessels and connective tissue.

There is a tendency for inflammatory processes affecting the upper air passages to spread to the lower ones and, it may be stated as a general rule, that the farther the spread the more serious does the condition become.

Thus, bronchitis may occur and, if the inflammation descends to the bronchioles and air cells, the condition is referred to as broncho-pneumonia. Inflammation of the alveoli also occurs in lobar pneumonia, and pleurisy (inflammation of the pleura) is common. Sometimes in these conditions permanent damage is done to the mucous membrane, or the inflammatory process may involve the connective tissue in the lung substance. When the latter occurs, an excess of fibrous tissue is formed which tends to contract like scar tissue and a condition referred to as fibrosis of the lung results. It is for these reasons that recurrent attacks of respiratory infections are liable to take place and that chronic chest troubles are so frequent.

It has been seen that the lungs may become congested with blood in cardiac failure (pp. 119, 124). In addition, they may be the site of tuberculosis and cancer.

Bronchitis

Bronchitis is defined as inflammation of the mucous membrane of the bronchial tubes and may be acute or chronic in type. When the smallest tubes (bronchioles) are involved the condition is sometimes referred to as bronchiolitis and is similar to broncho-pneumonia (p. 289).

Acute bronchitis

Cause. The condition is of bacterial origin (with the exception of those cases caused by the inhalation of irritating vapours). It occurs most frequently in winter and foggy weather and is especially common in old people and children.

The common predisposing causes are:
1. Downward spread of an upper respiratory infection, e.g. nasal catarrh, laryngitis, etc.
2. Inhalations of irritant vapours, tobacco smoke and air pollution.
3. Association with measles, whooping-cough, influenza, etc., as a symptom or complication.
4. Exposure to wet, cold and fog, especially in the elderly and subjects of chronic bronchitis and emphysema.

Pathology. The invading organisms, often streptococci, *Haemophilus influenzae* or pneumococci, cause inflammation of the bronchial mucous membrane which becomes red, swollen and congested with blood. This accounts for the tightness in the chest and the dry cough which are present in the early stages. Later, the glands in the bronchial mucous membrane are stimulated by the process of inflammation to secrete an excess of mucus, which is coughed up as sputum. The mucous secretion is at first frothy, but after a short time becomes purulent.

Symptoms. The onset is fairly rapid. Pyrexia, accompanied by soreness in the chest and a dry cough, which later becomes loose, is usually present. Some dyspnoea often occurs and, in severe cases, may be associated with cyanosis. Breathing is 'wheezy' and rhonchi can be heard with a stethoscope all over the lungs. The acute inflammation subsides in the course of one or two weeks, but in old people and children the condition may spread to the bronchioles and cause broncho-pneumonia. In the elderly, the strain on the heart caused by bronchitis may be serious and may lead to heart failure.

Treatment. The patient should be kept in bed in a warm room. In the early stages when the chest is tight and a dry cough is present, relief may be obtained by inhalations of friar's balsam (Tinct. Benzoin. Co.) or by increasing the moisture in the atmosphere by means of a steam kettle. Various expectorant cough mixtures are given which assist the bronchial mucous membrane to secrete mucus and, thereby, loosen the cough. The drugs which may be used in cough mixtures include ipecacuanha, ammonium carbonate and tincture of squills. Broncho-spasm and wheezing may be relieved by antispasmodic drugs such as 'Choledyl' and aminophylline suppositories. Ampicillin or co-trimoxazole ('Septrin', 'Bactrim') may be given.

If the cough is very troublesome, a linctus containing opium (Linctus Scillae Opiatus), methadone ('Physeptone'), pholcodine or codeine may be used at night. Cyanosis or associated heart failure will require oxygen, or the administration of special drugs.

A fluid diet may be given to the more severe cases in the early stages. Hot drinks of lemon sweetened with sugar or honey are very comforting and should be given frequently. As the patient improves a full diet is gradually introduced.

Acute laryngo-tracheo-bronchitis

This condition, though rare, is dangerous and occurs especially in young children. It is usually due to a cold virus preparing the way for secondary infection by streptococci or other organisms. The mucous membrane of the respiratory tract becomes acutely inflamed and oedematous and pneumonia may develop. Dyspnoea, cyanosis with signs of respiratory obstruction, pyrexia and toxaemia are the main symptoms. The important points of treatment, which is urgent, are a humid atmosphere (steam kettle or oxygen-tent), antibiotics and, if necessary, tracheostomy.

Chronic bronchitis

Chronic bronchitis may follow repeated acute attacks but is usually a distinct and separate disease entity. It is especially liable to occur in older people with emphysema and those whose hearts are affected by myocardial degeneration. The condition generally manifests itself in the colder months and affected individuals are liable to a 'winter cough' each year.

Town fogs, air pollution and heavy smoking are all contributory causes.

Symptoms. The main symptoms are cough, with a variable amount of sputum, shortness of breath especially on exertion, and wheeziness of the chest. There is no pyrexia unless an acute attack supervenes.

The condition should not be neglected because of the frequent presence of myocardial degeneration. In these circumstances, the associated respiratory disorder causes an increased strain to fall upon the heart which often results in cardiac failure (Cor pulmonale). When this occurs or an acute attack is superimposed upon the chronic chest trouble, the patient may become seriously ill. Cyanosis is marked and some oedema of the extremities may be present. Some of these cases prove fatal.

Treatment. The main point is to avoid or ward off acute episodes. Susceptible persons should avoid chills and fog and must give up smoking. If possible, residence in a warm climate during the winter is advisable and in any case warm clothing is necessary. Regular doses of tetracycline or other suitable drug, including co-trimoxazole ('Septrin') during the winter months, are sometimes given with a view to diminishing the severity of acute attacks, especially those with purulent sputum.

'Bisolvon', 8 mg tds by mouth, may help to reduce the viscidity and volume of mucoid sputum. Steam inhalations may also help if the sputum is thick.

Various cough mixtures and antispasmodic drugs are given as in acute bronchitis and complications are treated as they arise.

Bronchial asthma

This condition may be defined as recurrent attacks of dyspnoea associated with spasm of the bronchial muscles. It must not be confused with the attacks of dyspnoea which occur in cardiac and renal disease and which are sometimes referred to as cardiac and renal asthma respectively.

The smaller bronchi contain a certain amount of muscular tissue in their walls which, when it contracts, causes narrowing of the lumen of the tubes (bronchospasm). This takes place in bronchial asthma, and may also be associated with some swelling of the bronchial mucous membrane and the accumulation of tenaceous secretion in bronchioles. The narrowing of the bronchi causes difficulty in breathing air in and out, particularly out, of the alveoli. In order to obtain sufficient ventilation of the lungs in the presence of this increased resistance to the air-flow, the respiratory movements are forced and, in addition to the muscles normally used in respiration, others are brought into action (the so-called accessory muscles). The accessory muscles used in inspiration are stronger than those employed for expiration, with the result that the individual experiences more difficulty in emptying the lungs than in filling them. The characteristic feature of breathing in asthma, therefore, is difficult and prolonged expiration without much increase in the respiration rate.

Asthma may be of **extrinsic** (allergic) or **intrinsic** type. People with extrinsic asthma have positive reactions to skin tests with allergens. Asthma starting after the age of 40 years is usually of the intrinsic type.

The actual cause of the malady varies in different cases, and in many cannot be determined although many sufferers appear to have an inherited allergic constitution. In some cases oversensitiveness to foreign proteins, such as those contained in the dandruff of various animals (cats, dogs, horses, etc.), feathers, pollen, house dust, and certain foodstuffs, is responsible, so that the affected individual develops an attack when he comes in contact with even minute quantities of these substances. For example, if an individual is sensitive to cow's milk, goat's milk should be substituted. Asthma of this nature is said to be of the **allergic** type (see p. 15). The principal culprit in house dust is the house dust mite (*Dermatophagoides pteronyssinus*), measuring about 0·3 mm long and 0·2 mm wide, which is a normal inhabitant of human skin and is shed as the superficial epidermal cells are shed. The mite feeds on human dandruff and is found in dust from mattresses and armchairs. The seams of mattresses may harbour many of the mites and a patient's asthma may be worse at night when he is inhaling them. Most patients with extrinsic asthma have positive skin reactions to extracts of the house dust mite. The mite flourishes in damp low-lying districts and is not found at high altitudes.

Emotional stress and suggestion sometimes determine the onset of an attack in a susceptible person; for example, an asthmatic aware that he is sensitive to the perfume of a certain flower may develop an attack if he sees an artificial one.

Infection may precipitate an attack of asthma. Many cases of asthma are associated with bronchitis. In a few instances, associated disease of the nose (polypi, deflected septum, sinusitis, etc.) may be present.

Asthma may be seen at any age and is not uncommon in children, especially those who have been subject to eczema and other chronic skin conditions.

Asthma commencing: (a) in infancy is often due to food allergy, (b) between the ages of 10 and 30 to inhalants, e.g. dust, (c) after 45 to respiratory tract infections.

Symptoms. The attack comes on rapidly. Increased respiratory movements are present and expiratory dyspnoea is marked. The patient bends forward and throws the head back in order to bring into action the accessory muscles of respiration. There is usually some cough which is dry at first but becomes looser as the paroxysm passes off. The passage of air in and out of the contracted bronchi is accompanied by musical wheezing sounds (rhonchi) which can be heard by an observer.

The patient may appear very ill and sometimes cyanosed during a paroxym and is exhausted after it has subsided. Attacks may last for a few minutes or may be prolonged for many hours ('**Status asthmaticus**') and may prove fatal.

Treatment. The management of asthma has undergone changes in recent years coinciding with the introduction of both hand-operated nebulizers and pressurized metered-dose aerosols, both of which, however, contain varying doses of bronchodilator drugs such as adrenaline and isoprenaline with or without atropine methonitrate. Steroids are also used in selected cases.

Treatment must, therefore, be considered:

(a) Self-administered by the patient.

(b) Treatment of a severe attack and status asthmaticus, usually in hospital.

(c) Management between attacks.

(a) There is no doubt that the prompt use of an appropriate nebulizer or pressurized aerosol atomizer will cut short many attacks, e.g. Salbutamol ('Ventolin') which may also be taken in tablet form.

The puffs should be made during inspiration. In other instances sublingual isoprenaline (10 mg) is effective. Nevertheless the patient must be fully advised in their use, especially in the case of a pressurized aerosol, according to the maker's instructions. (For example not more than every quarter-of-an-hour for weaker solutions or two-hourly for the stronger ones containing atropine.) It must be remembered that isoprenaline is a powerful cardiac stimulant and may predispose to cardiac arrhythmias which may prove serious.

(b) If the attack is severe or status asthmaticus has developed the patient is usually admitted to hospital and therapy is urgent. Hydrocortisone, 100 mg, is given intravenously and over the next 24 hours a further 200 mg is given by intravenous drip. For less severe attacks, a 10-day course of prednisolone, starting with 50 mg daily, in divided doses, and reducing, may suffice. Subcutaneous adrenaline (1 ml of 1/1000 solution) or intravenous aminophylline, 500 mg, given very slowly (5 to 10 minutes) are employed. Oxygen is usually necessary and intravenous electrolyte fluids may be required if the patient is dehydrated. Any infection is treated with antibiotics.

Morphine and similar respiratory depressants are dangerous and contra-indicated. Sedatives should also be avoided during attacks.

(c) Between attacks the general health requires attention. Every effort is made to find an allergic cause for the condition and for this purpose a personal and family history of allergic conditions is sought. Skin testing to various allergens is often necessary and if this should prove positive special desensitizing injections may be indicated. An offending allergen should be avoided if possible. The asthmatic's mattress should be cleaned with a vacuum-cleaner once a week and his bedroom should be kept free of dust.

Drugs which help to diminish the liability to bronchospasm may be taken regularly, e.g. ephedrine (15 to 60 mg, $\frac{1}{4}$ to 1 gr), choline theophyllinate ('Choledyl'), salbutamol ('Ventolin') tablets or aminophylline suppositories at night. Proprietary preparations, e.g. 'Felsol' and 'Franol,' are helpful to some patients. Disodium cromoglycate ('Intal'), which is extremely helpful in some cases, is not a bronchodilator. It inhibits the release of spasm-inducing agents and blocks the asthmatic response.

A small maintenance dose of prednisolone is sometimes required but the aim is always to keep this to the minimum needed by any particular patient (e.g. on alternate days). Beclomethasone dipropionate ('Becotide') aerosol therapy can sometimes effectively replace systemic corticosteroids.

'Intal' and 'Becotide' must be taken regularly, whether the patient has any symptoms or not, and they must not be confused with drugs, such as isoprenaline, which are also administered by aerosol but only when a quick effect is needed. Some patients may need continuous systemic steroid therapy, e.g. prednisolone 10 mg daily by mouth, in order to live reasonable lives. Without it they would be chronic invalids, unable to work. Such treatment is mainly needed in intrinsic asthma. In patients below the age of 40 years everything possible should be done to avoid long-term systemic steroid therapy. Regular breathing exercises may be beneficial.

The pneumonias

The term pneumonia means inflammation of the alveoli of the lungs which become airless and solid with exudate. There are a number of different types, causes and possible methods of classification. Perhaps in the first instance the simplest way is to retain the old division into lobar and broncho-pneumonia, but at the same time to remember that there are a number of different organisms which can cause both types.

From the point of view of immediate treatment the sensitivity of the causal organism to an antibiotic is the most important fact. Pneumonia may be caused by:

pneumococcus (*Streptococcus pneumoniae*)
streptococcus
staphylococcus
influenza bacillus (*Haemophilus influenzae*)
viruses and mycoplasma etc.

Lobar pneumonia is usually an acute primary infection occurring in a previously healthy respiratory tract and the causal organism in most cases is the pneumococcus.

Broncho-pneumonia, on the other hand, is often secondary to other conditions such as bronchitis, aspiration of foreign or infected material, blockage of a bronchus causing airlessness and collapse of the affected part of the lung (atelectasis), or congestion of the lungs.

Lobar pneumonia, as its name implies, means that the whole of a lobe of the lung is involved and consolidated. In broncho-pneumonia the patches of solid lung may be scattered through one lobe or several lobes of either or both lungs.

Lobar pneumonia (pneumococcal pneumonia)

Definition. An acute infection most frequently caused by the pneumococcus and characterized by toxaemia, consolidation of one or more lobes of the lung, and pyrexia which, unless treated by antibiotics, ends by crisis.

Cause. The disease may occur at any age. Although the pneumococcus is usually the exciting cause, chill and exposure, general ill-health, over-fatigue and alcoholic excess are said to predispose to the condition which is now less common than formerly.

Pathology and morbid anatomy. The pneumocci reach the alveoli of the lung and their supporting tissue either as a result of inhalation or by the bloodstream. The process of inflammation commences in and around the alveoli, spreads throughout the whole of one or more lobes of the lung and, when it reaches the surface, involves the pleura. The bronchi, however, remain unaffected.

Symptoms. In typical untreated cases the onset is abrupt and consists of a rapid rise in temperature, often accompanied by a rigor or vomiting. The tongue is furred and the pulse and respiration rates increased, especially the latter, so that the pulse-respiration ratio is reduced from the normal of 4 : 1 to 3 : 1 or even 2 : 1 (e.g. pulse 120, respiration 40–60). A short dry cough is present which is later accompanied by the characteristic 'rusty' sputum and finally becomes looser when the exudate from the alveoli is coughed up. Pain in the chest, which is worse on coughing and deep breathing, is common and is due to the involvement of the pleura by the inflammatory process (pleurisy). The development of groups of small vesicles about the mouth and lips, known as herpes (p. 480), is frequently seen. Flushing of the cheeks, which is often more marked on the same side as the affected lung, together with cyanosis of the lips and ears may be present.

Course of the disease. The actual duration of acute symptoms is very variable; in the average untreated case the temperature remains high, never varying more than 0·6–1·2 °C (1–2 °F), for about 7 days and then ends by crisis in the course of 4 to 6 hours. Profuse sweating generally precedes the fall in temperature which may be followed by sleep and a general diminution in symptoms. The crisis may, however, be accompanied by signs of collapse. In some instances the illness may be shortened to 3 days and in others prolonged for 10 days before the crisis occurs, while occasionally the temperature subsides by lysis.

Sleeplessness is often a distressing symptom and is aggravated by the presence of pleuritic pain. Restlessness and delirium may occur, especially in patients who are the subjects of chronic alcoholism. Throughout the disease an added strain is thrown upon the heart which is weakened by toxaemia; consequently cardiac failure, terminating fatally in some cases, can occur, especially in elderly patients. The indications that the action of the heart is becoming weakened are increasing cyanosis together with a rising pulse rate and a fall in blood pressure.

When treated with antibiotics this clinical picture is not seen and the temperature may subside to normal by lysis in about 48 hours.

Complications. (*a*) Acute pleurisy is really part of the disease and always occurs when the inflammatory process reaches the surface of the lung.

(*b*) Empyema is an important complication but is less commonly seen now that cases are adequately treated by antibiotics. The inflammation of the pleura goes on to suppuration and pus collects in the chest between the visceral and parietal layers of this membrane. In most instances, this occurs after the crisis has taken place and is accompanied by a further rise in temperature. There is often a return of cough and sweating is common.

(*c*) Delayed resolution.

(*d*) Cardiac complications include cardiac failure as a result of damage to the myocardium by the toxins of the disease, and very rarely endocarditis or pericarditis.

(*e*) Pneumococcal septicaemia.

Prognosis. Unless promptly treated lobar pneumonia must be regarded as a serious disease, especially if it occurs at the extremes of life, and in chronic alcoholics. The modern treatment with antibiotics has, however, improved the outlook considerably.

Treatment. This is essentially the same both in lobar and broncho-pneumonia. Efficient nursing is an important factor. The main points to bear in mind are:

1. The patient is placed in bed in a well-ventilated room.

As a rule, he should be nursed in the most comfortable position, usually this is sitting propped up on pillows or a back-rest. A seriously ill case or elderly person should not be permitted to remain recumbent as there is a tendency for the bases of the lungs to become congested.

He should be disturbed as little as possible. Sponging may be carried out twice daily and may be repeated more frequently if the temperature exceeds 39·5 °C (103 °F).

2. In the early stages the diet consists of liquids and semi-solid foods, including milk, arrowroot, cornflour, fruit juice, eggs, broth, custard and junket. Sugar may be given in large quantities, up to 250 g ($\frac{1}{2}$ lb) of glucose being taken in 2–3 litres (4 or 5 pints) of water flavoured with lemons during 24 hours.

3. Usually, penicillin, to which the pneumococcus and many other organisms are sensitive, is given by intramuscular injection in the first instance. This may be followed by oral administration. If the infection fails to respond to penicillin, or if the bacteriological examination of a specimen of sputum indicates that the organism is resistant to these drugs, other antibiotics, including tetracycline, may be necessary.

Ampicillin may be required if influenza bacilli are present and a tetracycline is given in virus pneumonia. Erythromycin or cloxacillin ('Orbenin') may be needed for staphylococcal pneumonia.

In the majority of cases these drugs are very effective and considerably modify the course and symptoms of the disease.

Oxygen is administered when required and is especially valuable if cyanosis be marked. Other points in the general treatment include attention to the bowels which should be opened by salines, suppositories or enemata, but strong purgatives are avoided.

The relief of pain and cough are important in order that adequate sleep may be obtained. Pain is due to pleurisy and may be relieved by the application of a kaolin poultice.

Care must be taken that the weight of the poultice or tightness of the bandage, especially in children, does not embarrass breathing. A linctus may be given to relieve troublesome cough. Hypnotic drugs, such as nitrazepam or chloral are used to induce sleep, but if the insomnia is due to excessive pain, Dover's powder, nepenthe, pethidine or morphine may be necessary. Morphine, however, is administered very cautiously in pneumonia and is only given in the early stages. Alcohol may be helpful in elderly patients and infants. The diagnosis and progress of the disease is confirmed and observed by x-rays of the chest.

Broncho-pneumonia

This may be defined as inflammation of the terminal bronchioles and air-cells, due to various organisms.

It differs from lobar pneumonia in some ways. It has been seen that in the latter the whole of one lobe becomes solid as a result of the inflammation affecting the air-cells but not involving the bronchi. In broncho-pneumonia, however, the bronchioles are also inflamed and a number of areas of consolidation are formed throughout one or both lungs so that the lesion is a patchy one and not of entirely lobar distribution. The term pneumonia indicates inflammation of the lung tissue alone, whereas broncho-pneumonia suggests a combination of bronchitis and pneumonia.

The following are the circumstances in which it is most liable to occur:

1. In children under 5 years, when it resembles lobar pneumonia in its course and symptoms.

2. As a complication of infectious fevers such as measles, whooping-cough and influenza and as a result of downward spread of bronchitis.

3. Following (*a*) aspiration of septic material into the lungs in serious illness when the patient is semi-comatose and unable to keep the throat clean, or during anaesthesia, (*b*) a foreign body in a bronchus, (*c*) blockage of a bronchus by a plug of mucus such as may occur after an operation under general anaesthesia.

4. Following pulmonary embolism.

5. When the bases of the lungs are congested in heart failure or in a weak recumbent patient whose respiratory movements are poor.

The malady is most frequent in childhood and old age. In the former, measles and rickets and in the latter general debility and chronic disease, such as bronchitis or nephritis, are predisposing causes.

The symptoms, as a rule, are less abrupt in onset than in lobar pneumonia. There is generally an increase in the severity of pre-existing bronchial catarrh, rapid pulse and respiration rates, and a rise in temperature. Cyanosis and dyspnoea are common in severe cases, while cough and sputum are variable. The pyrexia is irregular and ends by lysis.

The prognosis is usually more serious than in lobar pneumonia, and cardiac failure may occur. Broncho-pneumonia may be followed by permanent damage to the lung tissue so that fibrosis of the lung is sometimes a sequel.

Treatment. The treatment is essentially the same as that of lobar pneumonia. Care must be taken to change the position of the patient from time to time in order to prevent congestion of the bases of the lungs which is specially liable to occur. It is for this reason that the sitting posture is advisable.

The following note indicates the various ages at which the different types of pneumonia are most likely to occur:

1. Infants under 2 years—primary broncho-pneumonia resembling lobar pneumonia.

2. Children 2–5 years—(*a*) broncho-pneumonia associated with rickets and the acute fevers.

   (*b*) aspiration of foreign bodies.

3. Adolescents and adults—(a) lobar pneumonia.

                                 (b) broncho-pneumonia following—

                                         (i) influenza,

                                         (ii) aspiration of foreign bodies and after operations.

4. Middle and old-age—broncho-pneumonia secondary to chronic disease such as bronchitis or nephritis. It may also occur in association with carcinoma of the lung and this may be suspected if resolution is delayed.

Pleurisy

The pleura is a serous membrane which covers the lungs and lines the thoracic cavity. The portion covering the lungs is called the visceral layer and that lining the chest-wall, the parietal.

Inflammation of the pleura is common and the pathological processes which occur are comparable with those seen in inflammation of other serous membranes such as the pericardium (p. 108). Thus, pleurisy may be acute or chronic in type and may be dry or with effusion, the latter being serous, purulent or haemorrhagic in character, i.e.:

1. Acute.   (i) Dry.

                (ii) With effusion (a) serous,

                                     (b) purulent (empyema),

                                       (c) haemorrhagic.

2. Chronic (adherent).

The condition may be localized to a small area or may be extensive and the anterior, posterior or diaphragmatic surfaces of the lung may be involved.

Cause. One cause of pleurisy is pulmonary tuberculosis. It also occurs as a complication of lobar pneumonia, in acute infectious fevers, after severe colds or bronchitis and as a result of cancer of the lung or other pulmonary conditions such as an infarct. The organisms most commonly responsible are tubercle bacilli, pneumococci, streptococci and sometimes a virus.

Morbid anatomy. When the pleura becomes acutely inflamed the following changes take place:

1. The membrane becomes red, swollen and engorged with blood.

2. An exudate of fibrin is poured out on the surface so that it becomes roughened. The visceral and parietal layers will then no longer glide smoothly over each other as respiration takes place.

Instead, a coarse grating sound, referred to as **pleural friction** or a rub, will be heard with the stethoscope. This friction is generally accompanied by pain in the chest.

3. In some cases there is a great outpouring of fluid into the pleural cavity which constitutes a pleural effusion. This may be clear in character but, if pus-producing organisms are present, it will be purulent and constitutes an abscess within the layers of the pleura known as an empyema.

4. Complete resolution with absorption of all exudate may take place. In some cases this may be followed by permanent thickening of the membrane the two layers of which are liable to become adherent in the same manner as the visceral and parietal pericardium.

Symptoms

(a) ACUTE DRY PLEURISY. The main symptom is pain in the chest of sudden onset, which is aggravated by coughing and deep breathing. The temperature and pulse-rate are generally increased, the cough is short and dry and a pleural rub can be heard with the stethoscope or, occasionally, felt when the hand is placed over the affected area.

The main principles of **treatment** are:

1. To prevent the spread of the process.

2. To relieve pain.

The patient should be kept in bed on a light diet until the temperature has subsided. His subsequent convalescence will depend on the cause of the condition.

Pain may be relieved in the following ways:

1. By application of a kaolin poultice.

2. Aspirin or other analgesics which may be given with a hypnotic can be used for the relief of pain and to induce sleep; occasionally morphine, pethidine or similar analgesic may be required.

3. A linctus or sedative lozenges to diminish the cough.

(b) PLEURAL EFFUSION. If an effusion of fluid occurs, the inflamed surfaces of pleura are separated and the pain disappears. There is frequently an increase in the severity of the cough and dyspnoea. The lungs are elastic in character and therefore compressible. It follows that, if the effusion is a large one, the surrounding lung will be compressed. In addition, pressure will be transmitted to the opposite lung. These mechanical changes result in the heart being pushed over to the side of the thorax opposite to the effusion, in order that the additional fluid may be accommodated on the affected side (see Fig. 61). The percussion note over an effusion is dull and the fluid appears as a dense shadow on x-ray.

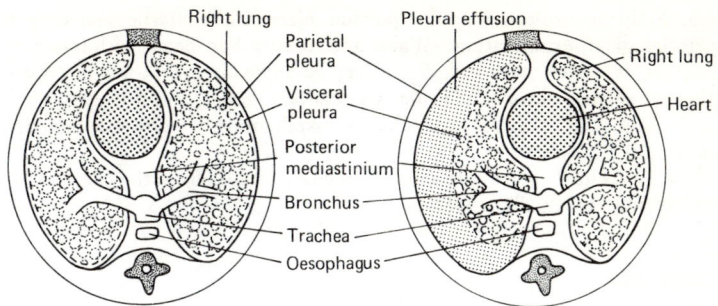

Fig. 61.

I. Horizontal section of the chest showing normal positions of the heart and lungs.

II. Horizontal section of the chest showing heart and mediastinum pushed over to the right by a left-sided pleural effusion, which is also compressing the left lung.

The common **causes of pleural effusion** are:
1. Chest Conditions.
> (a) Pulmonary tuberculosis (clear yellow fluid).
> (b) Cancer of the lung (clear or blood-stained fluid).
> (c) Lobar pneumonia (purulent fluid, i.e. empyema).
> (d) Pressure on the great veins in the thorax by tumours, etc. (clear fluid).
> (e) Pulmonary infarction.

2. General Causes.
> (a) Part of a general anasarca in (1) heart failure (clear fluid). (2) chronic nephritis (clear fluid).
> (b) In septicaemia or pyaemia, when organisms are carried to the pleura by the bloodstream (clear or purulent fluid).

Paracentesis thoracis. Removal of the fluid from the chest is frequently carried out both for diagnostic and therapeutic reasons. For the former, only a small quantity is withdrawn, while for the latter, as much as several pints may be aspirated or the whole of the effusion removed.

Exploration of the chest is carried out in the following way. The skin is cleaned, painted with iodine and surrounded with sterile towels. Procaine or lignocaine is injected into the skin and deeper layers of the chest wall between the ribs down to and including the parietal pleura. A needle of larger size attached to a 20 ml syringe is inserted through the anaesthetized area. Fluid is aspirated and a portion placed in a sterile test-tube for bacteriological examination. When the needle has been withdrawn the puncture is sealed with collodion. Very occasionally symptoms of collapse (**pleural shock**) occur while this is being carried out, and it is advisable to have a stimulant such as adrenaline or nikethamide at hand for immediate injection if necessary.

If it is decided to remove a large quantity of fluid from the chest a 'two-way' syringe is usually employed.

Empyema

When pus collects in the pleural cavity it is removed either by repeated aspiration or by allowing continuous drainage by inserting a polyethylene catheter between the ribs. Often, however, open operation (thoracotomy) and drainage is necessary.

Antibiotics may be injected into the cavity, a form of treatment which sometimes avoids the necessity for operation.

Subsequent breathing exercises are of great importance and help to expand the lung and obliterate the abscess cavity.

Empyema may occur as a result of pneumonia, lung abscess, cancer of the lung, tuberculosis and septicaemia.

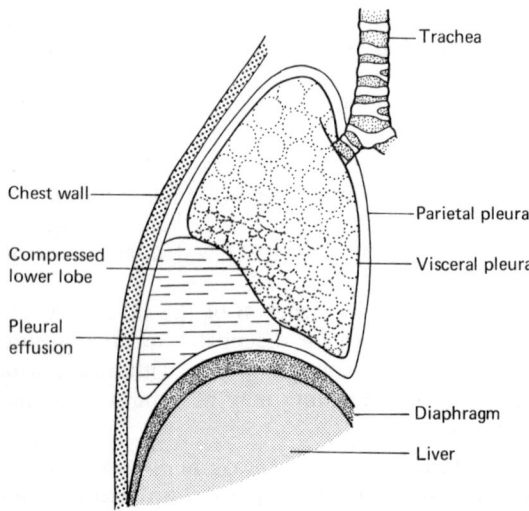

Fig. 62 Diagram illustrating compression of lower lobe of lung by pleural effusion (lateral view).

Pneumothorax

By pneumothorax is meant the separation of the visceral and parietal layers of pleura by air, i.e. the presence of air in the pleural cavity.

1. Spontaneous pneumothorax. This is a pathological process which may occur when a diseased or weakened area of lung is in close contact with the surface of the visceral pleura and rupture takes place, so that there is a direct path of communication between the

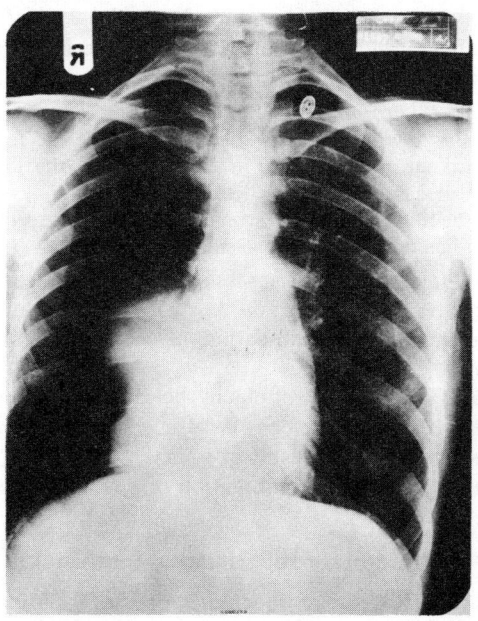

Fig. 63 Right-sided pneumothorax showing right lung collapsed and heart shifted to right.

pleural cavity and the air in the alveoli and bronchi. Emphysema, pulmonary tuberculosis, and injuries of the chest-wall involving the lungs may be responsible for this condition. In many instances there may only be a small localized area of emphysema, (a subpleural 'bleb') which has ruptured in an otherwise healthy individual.

The first symptom is acute pain of sudden onset in the affected side of the chest. In some cases, the ruptured area acts as a valve-like flap which permits air to enter the pleural cavity from the bronchi with each respiratory movement but which prevents its return. In these circumstances a large amount of air accumulates under increasing pressure, so that the affected lung becomes compressed and the heart is pushed over towards the opposite side of the chest (Tension pneumothorax). The symptoms then include increasing dyspnoea and cyanosis which may become very serious and constitute an acute medical emergency. In the absence of urgent symptoms, rest in bed for a time is required, but in those cases in which the pressure within the pleura produces increasing respiratory distress, it is necessary to insert a wide-bore catheter between the ribs in order to allow the excess of air to escape via tubing led under water (closed drainage). Sometimes a suction pump has to be connected to the closed drainage system. In some recurrent cases surgery may be indicated.

2. Artificial pneumothorax. In certain conditions, especially pulmonary tuberculosis, it was sometimes considered advisable to introduce air deliberately into the pleural cavity in order to allow the lung to collapse and so ensure adequate rest of the diseased part.

Following the introduction of streptomycin and other drugs, artificial pneumothorax has now become obsolete.

The following terms are sometimes used to describe various affections of the pleura:

Hydrothorax. The accumulation of clear watery fluid in the pleural cavity.

Pyothorax. The presence of pus in the cavity, i.e. empyema.

Haemothorax. When blood is effused between the layers of pleura—most commonly a result of injury.

Pyopneumothorax. A combination of pus and air in the cavity.

Pulmonary tuberculosis (phthisis)

Definition. A disease of the lungs due to the tubercle bacillus (of Koch).

Morbid anatomy. It has been seen (p. 24) that the tubercle bacillus produces a chronic inflammatory change (granulation tissue). Small areas of disease are referred to as tubercles, each of which consists of a central portion containing tubercle bacilli and tissue killed by their toxins, surrounded by inflammatory cells and a layer of fibrous tissue. A number of adjacent tubercles may run together and produce a large area of tuberculous disease. The process by which masses of cheesy material are formed by the death of the tissues is called *caseation.*

It has also been pointed out that, if the body resistance is sufficient, the disease may be prevented from spreading and ultimately be overcome by the processes of *fibrosis* and *calcification*. These changes take place when the lung becomes affected by tuberculosis. In addition to the primary focus in the lung tissue the infection may spread to the glands at the root or hilum of the lung (Fig. 64). The resistance of the individual may be feeble, in which case the process will spread rapidly throughout the lungs. This spread may take place either from the primary focus, the hilar glands or from a secondary focus which has developed in another part of the lungs. On the other hand, the progress may be slow or the disease may be arrested, the caseating areas becoming fibrosed and calcified.

The destruction of tissue associated with caseation often causes the formulation of *cavities* of varying size in the lung substance, and a blood vessel in the vicinity may become eroded by the disease. When this happens free haemorrhage followed by haemoptysis takes place.

An area of tuberculous disease on the surface of the lung will cause inflammation of the pleura (acute pleurisy) which may be accompanied by a clear (serous) pleural effusion. It has been seen that rupture of the pleura in a lesion of this type may also result in a spontaneous pneumothorax in which there is a direct communication between the pleural cavity and the air cells and bronchi.

In addition to the local damage to the lung, toxins formed by the bacilli are absorbed into the general circulation, producing a profound effect on the metabolic processes of the body. Pyrexia, rapid pulse, sweating and loss of weight are caused in this way. When the individual manufactures sufficient antibodies to limit the local activity of the disease and to neutralize the circulating toxins there is improvement in these general symptoms.

It must be remembered that bacilli are frequently present in the sputum in large numbers and that the malady is, therefore, infectious.

Three main types of disease process are seen in the lungs:

1. Acute miliary tuberculosis in which the lungs are riddled with minute tubercles. The disease progresses very rapidly and, unless arrested by treatment, death ensues before generalized caseation or fibrosis has time to occur. This condition is frequently associated with what may be described as a tuberculous septicaemia, for similar lesions may be found at the same time in the spleen, liver, kidneys and the meninges (tuberculous meningitis).

2. The caseous type. In this variety caseation is predominant and there is little fibrosis to limit the spread of the disease. Cavities are formed and toxaemia is severe. Unless the process is checked the patient goes downhill rapidly. Rarely a tuberculous pneumonia develops.

3. The fibrotic type. In this form, although some caseation is present, fibrosis predominates. The greater the amount of fibrosis, the slower the progress of the disease and the less the general toxaemia. Fibrosis may occur quite early so that a small healed area will result. On the other hand, one or both lungs may be seriously damaged by extensive areas of caseation which have produced cavities, before the resistance of the body is sufficient to limit the spread of the disease by the formation of fibrous tissue.

Modes of spread and sources of infection. The disease is rarely, if ever, transmitted from the mother to an unborn child, but a hereditary lack of resistance to the tubercle bacillus is liable to be present especially in primitive communities. A child may, however, be infected by a tuberculous parent during infancy.

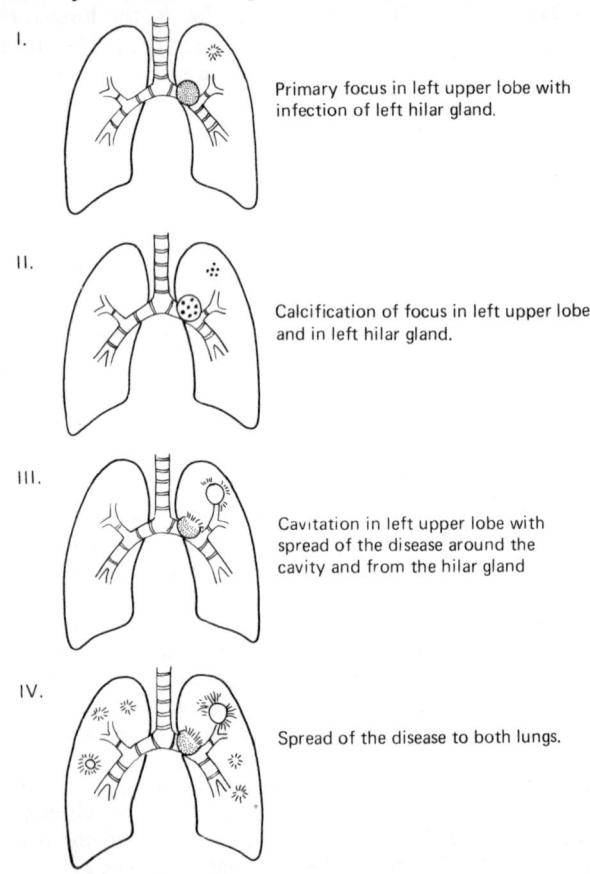

I. Primary focus in left upper lobe with infection of left hilar gland.

II. Calcification of focus in left upper lobe and in left hilar gland.

III. Cavitation in left upper lobe with spread of the disease around the cavity and from the hilar gland

IV. Spread of the disease to both lungs.

Fig. 64 Stages in the development of pulmonary tuberculosis.

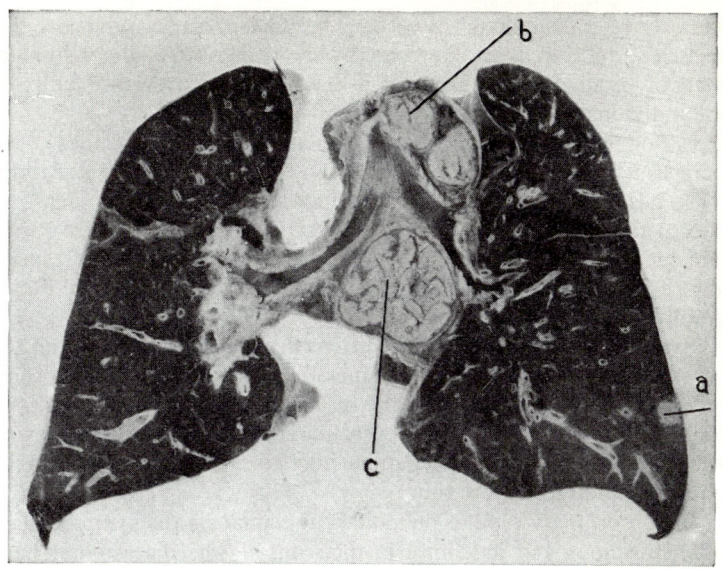

Fig. 65 (*a*) Primary lesion near the surface of right lower lobe. (*b*) and (*c*) Enlarged caseous tracheo-bronchial glands in relation to the lesion.

The disease is spread as a result of direct infection, the sources of which are:

1. Tuberculous sputum, which may be expectorated by careless individuals so that it becomes dried up and tubercle bacilli accumulate in the dust. Bacilli can also be inhaled by droplet infection or gain entrance to the alimentary canal from handling infected articles. Close contact with an infected individual is, therefore, the commonest source of infection.

2. Milk from tuberculous cows may cause the entrance of the tubercle bacillus into the body, especially in children, and in countries where hygienic control of milk is less strict.

Tuberculous infection may occur at any age, but in young children it is usually of the glandular type. The ordinary pulmonary tuberculosis of adults is not common before puberty, although the miliary type with diffuse spread throughout both lungs and elsewhere in the body may be found in infancy.

Many individuals living in a civilized community acquire a tuberculous infection before they reach the age of 25, and this is demonstrated by the presence of a positive Mantoux or Heaf test, but there is a great difference between minor tuberculous infection and active tuberculous disease. The fact that an infection has occurred, and has been overcome by the resistance of the individual without producing any signs of ill health, adds to the immunity of the individual.

Although the incidence of pulmonary tuberculosis has been dramatically reduced during the past 25–30 years in Great Britain there has been a tendency for it to increase recently. This is largely due to the influx of non-Europeans who may enter the country with undetected disease. Constant vigilance is therefore necessary, especially in patients entering general hospitals, by relying on radiography and repeated sputum tests.

Symptoms. The symptoms are very variable and depend on the type of disease present and whether drug treatment has been commenced at an early stage. In the miliary and rapidly caseating type the onset is acute with high fever, marked sweating, and increasing weakness and wasting. The patient may go rapidly down hill and die in a comparatively short time.

In the ordinary type of pulmonary tuberculosis the symptoms are often insidious and indefinite in their onset. The disease may have been active for weeks or months, spreading all the time, before medical advice is sought or the possibility of the diagnosis considered. The main ones are:

1. General symptoms, produced by toxaemia.

2. Pulmonary symptoms, produced by the disease process in the lung.

1. General symptoms. (*a*) LASSITUDE AND FATIGUE. Loss of energy, general fatigue, especially towards the end of the day, and sometimes a slight cough are often the first symptoms. Women may complain of amenorrhoea.

(*b*) LOSS OF APPETITE. This is usually an early symptom which may persist throughout the disease. It accounts for the fact that tuberculous patients are often difficult over matters of food and tend to complain a good deal when in institutions. Loss of morning appetite is particularly noticeable.

(*c*) LOSS OF WEIGHT. There is generally some loss of weight which in serious cases becomes extreme so that emaciation is very marked. A steady gain in weight is associated with improvement in the general condition and indicates that the patient is overcoming the toxaemia.

(*d*) FEVER. In the majority of cases, acute or advancing disease is accompanied by pyrexia. The temperature tends to be of the intermittent type, rising between 4 p.m. and 6 p.m. but falling to normal in the morning. It is high in the more serious cases and may be continued for many weeks. Exercise in excess of the individual's capabilities may produce a rise in temperature in an otherwise afebrile patient.

In association with pyrexia it is important to remember that the pulse rate is also increased.

(e) SWEATING. This is especially liable to occur while the patient is asleep, and 'night sweats' are characteristic of active and advancing disease. They may be very severe, the patient waking to find the night clothes drenched.

2. Pulmonary symptoms. (a) COUGH. This is almost always present and occurs early. At first it is dry and hacking but later becomes looser and is accompanied by sputum.

(b) SPUTUM. At first this is muco-purulent but later becomes nummular in character (p. 273); occasionally it is bloodstained. Haemoptysis may, therefore, be considered either as a symptom or complication.

(c) DYSPNOEA. Shortness of breath, especially on exertion, is common and may be noticed in the early stages.

(d) PAIN IN THE CHEST. This occurs as a result of pleurisy and is often the first indication of pulmonary disease. It may be associated with a clear pleural effusion especially in the young. In fact, some early cases present as a primary pleural effusion. The fluid may contain tubercle bacilli. In others they are never found and the patient makes a full recovery without any active disease in the lungs being proved.

Progress of the disease. It is clear that the progress of the disease depends upon the resistance of the individual and that great variability therefore occurs. Except in the miliary and very acute caseating types, improvement and even arrest in its progress may be expected if an early diagnosis has been made and efficient antibiotic treatment adequately carried out.

When fibrosis is sufficient to limit the spread of the disease the temperature becomes normal, the symptoms subside and the patient may gradually indulge in a useful life with perhaps only slightly restricted activity.

Complications. In a disease of this nature it is difficult to separate complications from symptoms, but the following may be regarded as the most important complications:

1. Haemoptysis.
2. Pleurisy, dry or with effusion.
3. Pneumothorax.
4. Laryngitis.

In addition, an anal fissure is sometimes present and tuberculous inflammation of the bowel (enteritis) may occur in the later stages.

Diagnosis. The diagnosis is made by considering the history and symptoms of the case together with the signs found in the chest on examination. It is confirmed by the x-ray appearance of the lungs and by the presence of tubercle bacilli in the sputum. The organism is not always found and cases with a negative sputum are sometimes referred to as 'closed' cases, while those with a positive sputum as 'open' ones. If sputum is not obtainable (e.g. in children and patients who swallow it), gastric lavage may be performed and the stomach contents examined for tubercle bacilli.

The Sedimentation Rate (ESR) is usually raised and may be very high when the disease is active. It tends to fall as improvement occurs.

Mass or miniature radiography, in which x-ray pictures are taken of the chest of large numbers of people on small films, may reveal shadows requiring further investigation. By this means previously unsuspected lung disease, including pulmonary tuberculosis, may be detected.

Tuberculin tests. The basis of the various tests for tuberculous infection is tuberculin. This is an extract obtained from tubercle bacilli and contains their toxins.

Mantoux test. This consists of the intradermal injection of 0.1 ml of 1 in 10,000 dilution of Old Tuberculin into the forearm. In a positive reaction an area of redness and swelling develops at the site of inoculation within a few hours and reaches its maximum in 24 to 48 hours. If negative, subsequent tests may be carried out with stronger solutions (1 in 1000 and 1 in 100).

This test is interpreted on a different basis to the tests for diphtheria and scarlet fever. Firstly, a distinction must be made between tuberculous infection and tuberculous disease. Sooner or later tubercle bacilli gain entrance to the body of almost every individual, but it is only in a few that active clinical tuberculous disease develops.

A positive reaction means that an individual has been infected by the tubercle bacillus at some time which may or may not have produced evidence of disease. By this infection he has been rendered sensitive or allergic to the toxins of the tubercle bacillus, and the positive Mantoux test is an allergic reaction in the skin to the proteins contained in these toxins.

A positive reaction in young children often indicates active tuberculous disease. Except in special circumstances, a negative reaction indicates that there has been no tuberculous infection. It is usual to exclude staff having a negative Mantoux reaction from tuberculosis wards and sanatoria.

Patch tests. These are similar in principle and consist of the application to the surface of the skin of a patch of material saturated with tuberculin.

This is left in position for 24 to 48 hours. Local redness and swelling indicate a positive reaction.

The Heaf test employs a multiple-puncture gun which is quick and efficient and gives easily-read results in the form of a ring of small papules, if positive.

BCG vaccine may be used to convert Mantoux negative individuals into Mantoux positive ones, who are less likely to contract tuberculosis. This consists of a single intradermal injection of 0·1 ml of vaccine, usually into the skin of the upper arm. A small papule develops after a few weeks and leaves a small local scar.

The lines of treatment to be considered are:
1. Prophylaxis.
2. General measures.
3. Special measures   (i) Antibiotic drugs.
                     (ii) Special procedures.
                     (iii) Major surgery.
4. Treatment of symptoms and complications.

1. Prophylactic treatment. The prevention of tuberculosis involves matters affecting public health, such as housing, sanitation, purity of the milk supply and the segregation of 'open cases', and it is for these reasons that cases are notified to the local District Community Physician (M.O.H.).

Chest clinics play an important part, not only in the domiciliary treatment of patients, but also in the follow-up of contacts.

Mass radiography, as already mentioned, is important in detecting unsuspected cases.

Immunization with BCG vaccine of infants, school children, nurses, doctors and other workers in tuberculosis who are Mantoux negative is of value in increasing immunity.

In addition, the patient must follow the necessary principles of personal hygiene. He should carry a sputum flask, the contents of which are disinfected before disposal. He must not spit into a handkerchief which, in any case, should be carried in a linen bag which can be boiled frequently, thus avoiding contamination of the pockets.

In a general hospital appropriate isolation is usually carried out, in a special tuberculosis ward. The nurse must wear a gown when attending to patients, and be most careful of her own personal hygiene, especially hand-washing before her meals. She must be careful to observe the rules laid down for the care, collection and disposal of sputum, bed linen, handkerchiefs, etc., and the routine instructions which are in operation in the unit in which she is working.

2. General measures. The aims of treatment are to increase the patient's resistance, thereby improving his general nutrition and abolishing the toxaemia, and to improve or cure the lung condition by drug therapy which now dominates the whole treatment of the disease. Treatment is best carried out initially in a hospital. This is advantageous in that infectious cases are removed from home surroundings where they may pass on the disease to others, and that the patient can be taught those rules of self-discipline which are subsequently of value to him. It also ensures that drug reactions are observed and dealt with promptly. Reactions (especially fever and rashes) to antituberculous drugs are not uncommon.

(a) REST. In febrile cases with marked toxaemia rest in bed is necessary. As the temperature settles he is gradually allowed to do more for himself. Other cases are confined to bed or get up for varying periods according to their progress and capabilities. In cases who are up all day, an hour's rest before lunch and tea is desirable.

(b) FRESH AIR. Plenty of fresh air is desirable but exposure during damp, cold or foggy weather is avoided in cases complicated by bronchitis. Sunbathing is harmful and may lead to spread of the disease.

(c) DIET. No special food is necessary in pulmonary tuberculosis, and three good, easily digested, palatable meals should be taken at regular hours. One or two pints of milk daily are generally given and plenty of cream and additional vitamins may be included. Alcohol, as a rule, is restricted or forbidden. It is a mistake to attempt to overfeed tuberculous patients for it will only result in indigestion.

(d) CLIMATE. This rarely plays any part in the treatment of the disease, except in those cases in which bronchitis is present. Such patients do better in warm, dry places.

(e) GRADUATED EXERCISE. An important aim in treatment is to get the patient sufficiently well to return to a useful life. The amount of exercise prescribed will depend upon the special features of each case. Provided the temperature and pulse remain normal and extensive disease is not present, exercise is allowed and gradually increased. Short walks are taken at first, the distance being increased by easy stages. Later, light manual work is undertaken. In suitable cases this is made harder but is never carried beyond the amount which the patient can perform without exhaustion and is always controlled by the temperature and pulse rate.

(f) OCCUPATIONAL THERAPY AND REHABILITATION. These are to some extent linked up with graduated exercise. The treatment of pulmonary tuberculosis may involve long periods in bed and it is important to avoid boredom. While in the early stages of treatment rest may be essential, there may be many weeks subsequently when the patient can be occupied for some hours a day with some light form of occupation such as embroidery, leather-work, weaving on a small loom, etc., even though confined partially or completely to bed.

Rehabilitation involves teaching the patient some craft or trade by which he can earn or contribute to his living when it would be unwise or impossible for him to return to his former employment. Special training centres are available for tuberculous patients.

Special measures

(i) *Drugs*   1. Streptomycin.
2. Para-amino-salicylic acid (PAS).
3. Isoniazid ('Rimifon', 'Pycazide', etc.) (INAH)
4. Prothionamide, ethionamide, ethambutol, rifampicin, pyrazinamide, capreomycin, thiacetazone, and cycloserine.

Drugs numbered 1 to 3 are the 'first-line' drugs in Britain. Drugs listed under 4 are the 'second-line' drugs, which are reserved for patients who cannot tolerate the 'first-line' drugs or whose organisms are resistant to them.

These are the most important antibiotic and chemotherapeutic agents used in the treatment of pulmonary tuberculosis. Each may have a lethal effect on the tubercle bacillus when tested in the laboratory. In the body, however, they are conveyed to the tuberculous lesion by the blood stream, and therefore cannot penetrate into the middle of caseous or very fibrotic lesions where the blood supply is defective or absent. They are peculiarly useful, however, in attacking new or spreading lesions and in miliary tuberculosis before either caseation or a fibrous tissue reaction has occurred.

Unfortunately, the tubercle bacillus has the power of developing partial or complete resistance to their action and after a period of administration their effect may be useless. This development of resistance is, however, prevented if two or three of the above-mentioned drugs are employed simultaneously.

Streptomycin is given by intramuscular injection. An average dose is 1·0 gram daily for at least three months.

In children, elderly patients and those with renal disease it may be necessary to give a lower dosage. The main toxic effect is damage to the 8th cranial nerve, causing vertigo.

PAS (sodium aminosalicylate) is given by mouth. 12 to 15 grams is given daily in cachets.

306 Diseases of the Respiratory System

Isoniazid is given by mouth in doses of 200 to 300 milligrams daily.

In a typical case combined drug therapy is maintained for up to two years.

(ii) *Special procedures.* With the advances in chemotherapy these are now rarely employed. Careful selection and timing is necessary before they are used. They include:

(*a*) Postural drainage.
(*b*) Postural retention.
(*c*) Artificial pneumothorax.
(*d*) Artificial pneumoperitoneum.
(*e*) Phrenicotomy.

(*a*) POSTURAL DRAINAGE is sometimes carried out in order to obtain free drainage of purulent sputum from a cavity. According to the situation of the cavity in the lung the patient is kept in an appropriate position in bed, e.g. the foot of the bed may be raised.

(*b*) POSTURAL RETENTION. In some cases which are not responding to ordinary treatment (especially those with apical cavities), a directly opposite procedure to that of postural drainage is carried out. If the foot of the bed is raised there will be no drainage from a cavity situated at the apex but the pressure of the abdominal contents will reduce the lung movements and probably the blood supply to the apex of the lungs will be increased.

(*c*) ARTIFICIAL PNEUMOTHORAX (p. 296). This is now rarely if ever performed.

(*d*) PNEUMOPERITONEUM, or the injection of air into the peritoneal cavity, with the object of raising the diaphragm, has been carried out.

(*e*) PHRENICOTOMY. Crushing of the phrenic nerve or its injection with alcohol, causes paralysis of the diaphragm on the same side. This results in partial collapse of the lung and permits additional local rest. It was only performed in selected cases and was combined with pneumoperitoneum.

(iii) *Major Surgery.*

(*a*) THORACOPLASTY. In those cases in which it was considered desirable to cause partial collapse of the lung, especially if a large cavity was present and when artificial pneumothorax was not possible on account of the pleural adhesions present, removal of portions of several ribs allowed the chest-wall to fall in. This operation resulted in local collapse of the lung and is referred to as thoracoplasty.

(*b*) LOBECTOMY, which may be partial (i.e. local excision) or complete, is occasionally carried out when the disease is limited to one lobe and will not respond to other methods of treatment.

Even with all these therapeutic weapons, it is usually more correct to speak of 'arrested disease' than of cure.

Treatment of symptoms and complications. Suitable cough mixtures or a linctus are given when cough is troublesome. Night sweats generally cease after a few days of open-air treatment at a sanatorium. Patients liable to suffer from them should wear flannel night clothes, and it is the duty of the nurse to see that these are changed if they become damp.

The treatment of pleurisy is referred to on p. 292 and of haemoptysis on p. 279.

In every case of pulmonary tuberculosis the nurse must encourage the patient and, at the same time, see that rules are strictly carried out. The patient must learn that if he wishes to get well his treatment will entail self-discipline, self-denial and endurance of some discomfort.

Other chronic affections of the lungs

Emphysema

This condition tends to occur in elderly patients and is frequently associated with chronic bronchitis and asthma. The alveoli of the lungs become over-distended with air and degenerative changes take place in their walls which lose their elasticity. In severe cases the expansion of the chest with respiration is poor and it is fixed in the inspiratory position, with the result that it becomes rounded and barrel-shaped. The diameter from the back to front then measures almost as much as from side to side.

The symptoms are mainly due to the associated chronic bronchitis and consist of cough, shortness of breath, especially on exertion, and occasional cyanosis. The strain on the heart may result in cor pulmonale (p. 121). Pure emphysema causes dyspnoea as the sole symptom, which is at first experienced only on exertion but is ultimately present also at rest.

Emphysema of the lungs must be distinguished from 'surgical' or subcutaneous emphysema, which occurs after injuries of the chest or air-passages and consists of air escaping from the lungs into the cellular tissues of the chest wall, often spreading up into the neck and down to the abdomen. The affected areas impart an elastic sensation when palpated and gas can be felt crackling under the examining fingers.

Fibrosis of the lungs

Any acute or chronic inflammatory condition occurring in the lungs may be followed by the formation of a varying amount of scar tissue in the connective tissue framework of the organs. Depending on the extent and severity of the original inflammation, this may be localized to one lobe or may involve both lungs extensively.

It has been seen that the process of fibrosis may follow pneumonia and is common in pulmonary tuberculosis. Cases are, therefore, divided into two main groups, non-tuberculous and tuberculous. Extensive fibrosis interferes with the circulation of blood through the lungs and may cause an increased strain to fall upon the right side of the heart which terminates in cor pulmonale.

In addition, the contraction of the scar tissue produces a pull on the wall of the bronchi which become dilated in various places—a condition known as bronchiectasis.

In very severe unilateral cases the area may be so extensive and the contraction so marked that the heart and mediastinum are pulled over towards the affected side.

Pneumoconiosis

This is a chronic lung condition caused by the inhalation of various dusts in industrial workers. It results in diffuse pulmonary fibrosis and emphysema which may not only resemble tuberculosis in an x-ray but may also predispose to the development of this condition, e.g.

(a) Silicosis from sand-blasting, etc.
(b) Anthracosis in coal miners.
(c) Siderosis in iron, tin and lead miners.
(d) Asbestosis.
(e) Byssinosis.

Symptomatic treatment is required for cough, sputum and dyspnoea but most important is the prevention by good working conditions, proper ventilation and the use of respirators when appropriate.

Bronchiectasis

This condition consists of localized dilatation of the bronchi which become fusiform in shape, together with damage to their epithelial surface in the affected parts. As a rule, the condition is confined to one or both lower lobes.

Causes. It has been pointed out that fibrosis of the lungs from any preceding inflammation is liable to cause bronchial dilatation on account of the pull on the walls of the tubes produced by the contraction of scar tissue. It follows that bronchiectasis may be caused by pneumonia, bronchitis, the presence of foreign bodies in the bronchial tubes, and empyema or may occur as a result of pulmonary tuberculosis.

The main **symptoms** are cough, which is worse in the morning, accompanied by foul-smelling, purulent sputum and foetor of the breath. Sputum stagnates in the bronchiectatic cavities, micro-organisms multiply in it and produce putrefactive changes which account for the vileness of its odour. Changes of posture, such as occur on rising in the morning, result in some of the sputum reaching other parts of the bronchial tree, where they set up the cough reflex. After the tubes have been emptied purulent material again accumulates and is expectorated some hours later when it reaches the healthy tubes. As much as 350 ml (12 ounces) of sputum may be produced in 24 hours.

Other symptoms include loss of weight, sweating, occasional fever and haemoptysis. A special feature of bronchiectasis and fibrosis of the lungs is the occurrence of changes in the shape of the fingers, the distal ends of which become enlarged and bulbous. This produces a 'drumstick' appearance and the nails tend to curve over the extremities. The condition is referred to as **clubbing of the fingers.**

Bronchiectasis may be complicated by recurrent attacks of broncho-pneumonia, pleurisy or an abscess in the lung tissue. Occasionally an abscess develops in the brain as a result of septic emboli.

The **diagnosis** may be assisted by x-ray of the chest, especially after the injection of 'Dionosil' (p. 269), which outlines the dilated bronchi (Bronchogram).

The **treatment** consists of improving the general health and securing efficient drainage of the cavities at frequent intervals in order to lessen the putrefactive changes which occur when purulent material accumulates within them. The simplest method of doing this is to place the patient with the head low and the rest of the body raised so that sputum may drain away by gravity. This is called **postural drainage.** The patient may lie across the bed with the hands on the floor or low stool, or adopt the 'knee-elbow position' at regular intervals during the day. Special beds are obtainable which can be adjusted for postural drainage. The cavities may also be emptied by suction after the passage of the bronchoscope. Antibiotics may be given to control infection, according to the sensitivity of the organisms present.

In suitable cases surgical treatment is adopted, viz. removal of the whole lung (Pneumonectomy) or an affected lobe (Lobectomy).

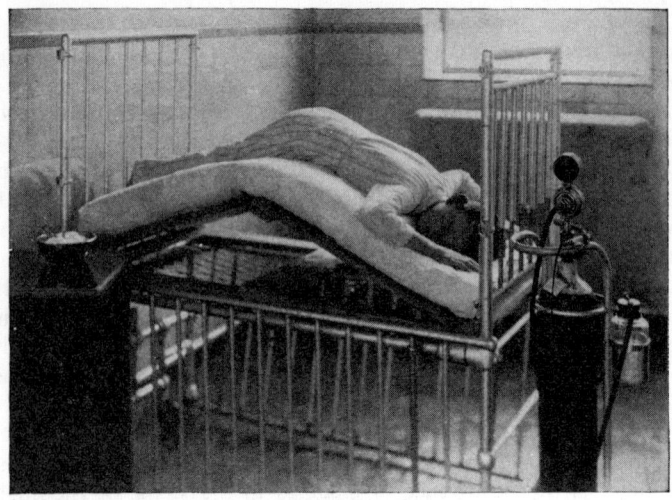

Fig. 66 Postural drainage

Atelectasis (pulmonary collapse)

In this state the whole, or part, of a lung becomes airless and solid. It may be acute or chronic. The chief cause is some type of bronchial obstruction, e.g.

1. Within the lumen of the bronchus: foreign body, plug of thick mucus.
2. Disease of the bronchial wall: inflammation, tumours.
3. Pressure on the lung from outside: pleural effusion.
4. Paralysis or impairment of respiratory movements: poliomyelitis, injury, tight dressings.

Fetal atelectasis is failure of the lungs to expand at birth, among the causes of which may be over-sedation of the mother.

Post-operative pulmonary collapse, especially after operations on the upper abdomen, may be associated with heavy sedation which suppresses the cough reflex, excessive oxygen administration and tight dressings.

The results of untreated atelectasis are:

(*a*) Infection of the collapsed area.

(*b*) Later, fibrosis and bronchiectasis.

Symptoms depend on the extent and rate at which collapse occurs. In some instances they may be minimal and the condition only demonstrated by x-ray. In others cough, dyspnoea, cyanosis and shock may predominate.

Treatment. Post-operative collapse can largely be prevented by avoiding heavy sedation, turning the unconscious patient, oxygen and CO_2 inhalations, breathing exercises and early ambulation. Other cases may require bronchoscopy or bronchial suction and treatment of the primary cause. Antibiotics are required for any infection.

Lung abscess

A single abscess may develop in the lung substance as a result of local septic inflammation or multiple abscesses may occur as part of a general pyaemia. The condition is always serious and is accompanied by cough, fever, sweating and progressive emaciation. Single abscesses may result from pneumonia, from bronchiectasis, aspiration of septic material following tonsillectomy or tooth extraction, from the presence of a foreign body or a carcinoma.

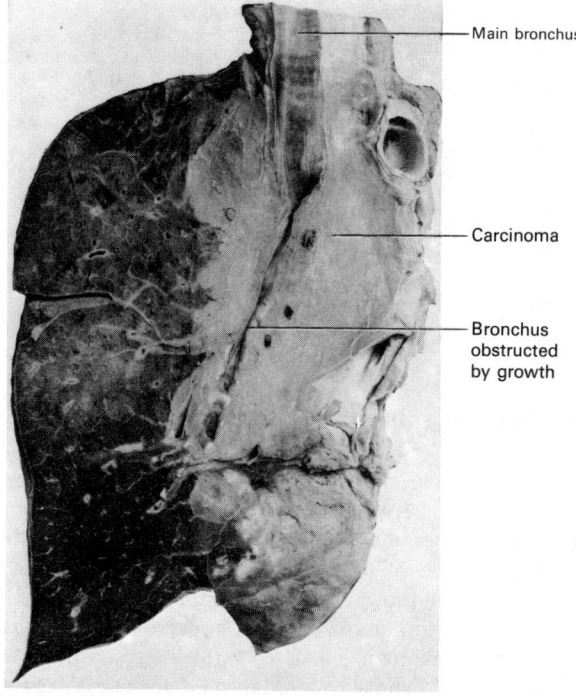

Fig. 67 Primary carcinoma or bronchus.

Treatment in the acute stages is similar to that employed for bronchiectasis, viz. postural drainage and bronchoscopic aspiration supplemented by chemotherapy and penicillin injections. In chronic cases surgical measures are usually adopted, e.g. drainage through the chest wall. Thoracoplasty or lobectomy may occasionally be required.

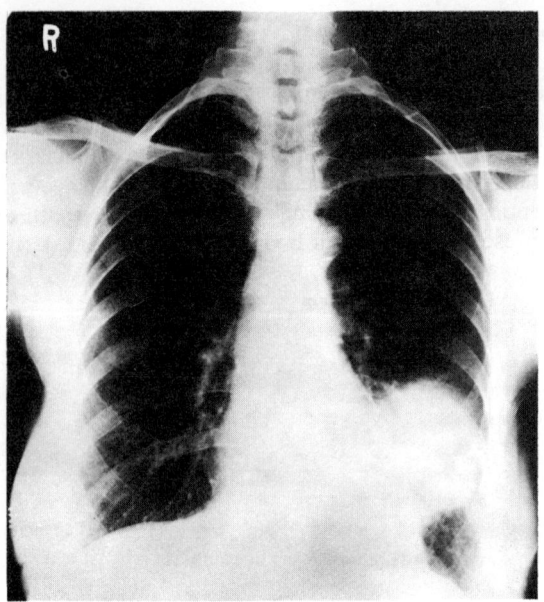

Fig. 68 Cancer of the lung.

Cancer of the lung (bronchial carcinoma)

Secondary deposits of cancer arising from other organs are common but primary cancer arising from a bronchus is also frequently seen, especially in males between 45 and 60. The commonest cause is smoking, usually twenty or more cigarettes a day for twenty to forty years. The incidence of bronchial carcinoma is less in people who stop smoking than in those who continue the habit. Adenocarcinomas are as common in non-smokers as in smokers and the cause of this type of cancer is unknown.

Uranium miners, exposed to radon gas, are at risk of developing bronchial carcinoma and the risk is increased by smoking.

The symptoms are variable and include shortness of breath, cough, dry and irritating at first but later with sputum which may be bloodstained. Pleurisy either dry or with effusion, which is also sometimes bloodstained, may develop. Loss of weight may be delayed. The diagnosis may be confirmed by x-rays, bronchoscopy and occasionally by finding cancer cells in the sputum. Secondary deposits may occur in the brain, liver or other organs.

Sometimes it is possible to remove the affected lung (pneumonectomy). Occasionally deep x-ray therapy may produce some temporary improvement.

Innocent tumours (e.g. adenoma) of the bronchi occasionally occur and may produce bronchial obstruction and haemoptysis.

7 Diseases of the Urinary System

Introduction. The anatomical structures included in the urinary system are the kidneys, the ureters, the bladder and the urethra. The two kidneys are the excretory organs, the remaining portions being the channels through which the urine passes in order to leave the body.

The kidneys are situated behind the peritoneum on either side of the spinal column, and extend from the twelfth dorsal above, to the third lumbar vertebra below. A fibrous capsule surrounds the secreting tissue which consists of glomeruli and tubules. The latter open into the pelvis which is the expanded upper end of the ureter.

The ureter is the duct from the kidney and conveys its secretion from the pelvis to the bladder where the urine is stored and evacuated from time to time via the urethra by the act of micturition.

One of the functions of the kidneys is to keep the composition of the blood more or less constant. In addition to excreting water, the excess of salts and other substances taken in the diet but not required by the body for purposes of metabolism, toxins, drugs and the waste products of metabolism are also removed from the circulation. Among the most important of the latter is the nitrogen-containing material derived from broken-down proteins which leaves the kidneys in the form of a compound known as urea.

The normal kidney only excretes certain substances from the blood when their concentration reaches a definite level. Thus, in health the sugar content of the blood remains fairly constant, but if for any reason it rises, as in diabetes, the excess of sugar will be excreted by the kidneys until blood sugar returns to normal.

If the kidneys are damaged, however, they may fail to excrete a substance (e.g. urea) which will therefore accumulate in the blood and produce toxic symptoms. On the other hand, they may allow various materials (e.g. protein in the form of albumin) to pass through them more easily and the blood will consequently become depleted of a normal constituent. In other words, there is a standard level of concentration or *threshold value* for various substances in the blood and, until this is reached, the normal kidney will not excrete them. In disease, however, the threshold value may be either increased or decreased.

The glomerular filtrate is very dilute and, in order to conserve water in the body, resorption must occur in the renal tubules. Tubular

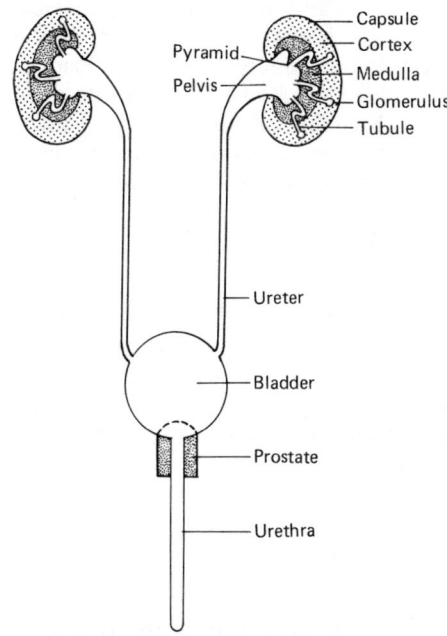

Capsule
Cortex
Pyramid
Medulla
Pelvis
Glomerulus
Tubule

Ureter

Bladder

Prostate

Urethra

Fig. 69 Diagram of the Renal Tract.

resorption of water is promoted by the antidiuretic hormone (ADH) which is secreted by the posterior lobe of the pituitary gland. Other valuable substances may be conserved by tubular resorption. Aldosterone, secreted by the adrenal gland, promotes resorption of sodium.

Most of the common conditions affecting the renal tract can be included in the following scheme, bearing in mind that the individual anatomical structures of the tract may be separately or collectively involved.

(1) *Congenital*   Single or horseshoe-kidney. Polycystic disease. Hypospadias.

(2) *Traumatic*   Crush or penetrating injuries of the kidney, bladder (e.g. in fractured pelvis), urethra.

(3) *Mechanical*   Renal, ureteric or bladder stones (calculi). Aberrant renal artery, Hydronephrosis. Enlarged prostate. Urethral stricture.

(4) *Inflammatory*   Nephritis. Pyelitis and pyelonephritis. Cystitis. Urethritis. Renal tuberculosis.

(5) *Circulatory*   Renal infarcts. Atheroma of renal arteries.

(6) *New growths*   Carcinoma of kidney or bladder. Pipilloma of bladder. Adenoma or carcinoma of prostate.

(7) *Miscellaneous*   Neurological disturbances of micturition. Urinary retention and incontinence. Enuresis.

(8) *Haematuria*   Many of the above conditions. Anticoagulant overdosage. Sulphonamide crystals. Blood diseases, e.g. leukaemia, purpura.

Methods of investigating disease of the urinary system

A. Examination of the urine. (Chemical, microscopic and bacteriological.)

B. Cystoscopy.

C. X-ray of the renal tract and pyelography.

D. Renal function tests.

E. Chemical examination of the blood.

F. Renal biopsy.

G. Isotope renography.

A. Examination of the urine

The Collection and testing of specimens and its significance

Owing to variations in the composition of the urine which occur during the day it may be necessary to obtain a specimen from the total quantity collected during 24 hours. As a routine measure, however, the early morning specimen is usually tested. This is a most important examination which should never be omitted. In particular, tests for albumin and sugar must always be done.

In collecting specimens from male infants it is often convenient to insert the penis into a test-tube, while baby girls may be placed on a suitable receptacle during and just after a feed.

If a bacteriological examination is required it is essential that a sterile, mid-stream specimen of urine be obtained, remembering that occasionally catheterization may be a very undesirable necessity.

The following observations are made:

1. The odour. Freshly passed normal urine has an aromatic or slightly ammoniacal smell. In some cases of diabetes the odour of acetone can be detected. In infection of the urinary tract it may be 'fishy' in character.

2. Colour. Normal urine is described as 'straw-coloured,' amber, or resembling pale sherry. Concentrated urines of high specific gravity tend to be more deeply coloured than dilute specimens. (An exception is the pale urine of high specific gravity passed in diabetes.)

The following abnormalities in colour may be found:

PINK OR RED: due to blood or drugs such as rhubarb and senna: also after sweets coloured with eosin.

ORANGE-RED: due to phenindione ('Dindevan').

BLACK OR BROWN: due to bile; also after poisoning with phenol or lysol and in associated with a special variety of cancer known as melanotic sarcoma in which a black pigment, melanin, is excreted in the urine.

BLUE OR GREEN: after drugs such as methylene blue.

3. Quantity. In the adult 1100 to 1500 ml (40 to 50 fl oz). This may be increased (**polyuria**) if large quantities of fluid are taken, in diabetes, and in certain cases of chronic nephritis. It is diminished (**oliguria**) when the fluid intake is small, if sweating is excessive, in febrile conditions and in acute nephritis. Actual suppression of urine (**anuria**), when none or very little is secreted by the kidneys, occasionally occurs in acute shock from blood loss or fluid depletion, acute nephritis, in certain cases of bilateral renal calculus, severe crush injuries and following the administration of sulphonamide drugs (p. 516). Severe diminution of urinary output should always be reported.

4. Specific gravity. This is ascertained by means of the urinometer, the level to which the instrument sinks being read off on the scale when it is floated in a specimen glass full of urine.

The specific gravity of water is taken as 1000. The normal figure for urine, which has a higher specific gravity than water on account of the dissolved salts which it contains, is between 1015 and 1025. In other words, if a given volume (1 litre) of water weighs 1000 g, the same volume of urine would weigh 1015 to 1025 g.

The specific gravity of urine is raised in diabetes and concentrated urines but is low in certain forms of nephritis and dilute urines.

5. Reaction to litmus. The reaction is usually slightly acid (turns blue litmus red), but may be alkaline (red litmus turns blue) if the patient is having a vegetarian diet or taking alkaline drugs, such as potassium citrate.

N.B.—it is not necessary to render alkaline urine acid before commencing routine tests.

6. Deposits. After normal urine has been standing for a short time a woolly cloud, which tends to settle to the bottom, may be seen. This is due to mucus. In alkaline urine a heavier white deposit consisting of phosphates is often present. This dissolves when acetic acid is added. If the urine is acid, urates are commonly seen and are light pink in colour.

Abnormal deposits may be due to blood which has a reddish or chocolate appearance, or pus which is creamy in character.

7. Chemical abnormalities. Six abnormal constituents may be discovered by the routine chemical tests employed, viz. albumin, sugar, ketone bodies, blood, pus and bile.

(1) Albuminuria

The presence of protein in the urine is usually indicative of some disturbance of renal function but not necessarily permanent organic disease of the kidneys or renal tract. The commoner causes of albuminuria may be classified in the following way:

(a) Due to minor kidney lesions

FEBRILE ALBUMINURIA. Any acute febrile condition may be accompanied by slight albuminuria due to toxic changes in the secreting cells of the kidneys which recover when the fever has subsided.

CONGESTIVE ALBUMINURIA. If the kidneys become congested in heart failure, albumin frequently occurs in the urine.

(b) Due to gross kidney lesions

Acute and chronic nephritis.
Nephrotic syndrome.
Acute and chronic pyelonephritis.
Malignant hypertension.
Tuberculosis of the kidneys.
Cancer of the kidneys.
Toxaemia of pregnancy and eclampsia.
Poisoning, by phenacetin, lead, mercury of cantharides.

(c) Due to lesions of the renal tract

Pyelitis (which may also occur during pregnancy).
Cystitis.
The above is a list of the more important conditions in which

albuminuria may occur. It must be remembered also that blood contains protein so that when haematuria is present it is accompanied by albuminuria.

Tests for albumin. One of the following tests is employed:

(a) The albustix test. This test is simple and quick but may give false results if the urine is not fresh or the containers are contaminated with soap or detergents. A positive test should be an indication for testing by some other method (see below).

(b) The boiling test. If the urine is cloudy it should be filtered into a test-tube until it is $\frac{2}{3}$ full. Holding the lower end so that the test-tube is slanting away from the body, the upper half of the column of urine is heated in a spirit lamp or Bunsen burner until it boils.

If no cloud is seen in the boiled portion, albumin is absent. When a cloud appears a few drops of dilute acetic acid are added. If the cloud persists it is due to the presence of albumin, but if dissolved by acid it is caused by phosphates. (This test is time-consuming but is reliable and is the only one which detects Bence-Jones protein.)

(c) The salicyl-sulphonic acid test. Add ten drops of 25% salicyl-sulphonic acid to 2·5 cm (1 in) of urine in a test-tube. The presence of a haze or cloud denotes the presence of protein.

(d) The quantitative test. Esbach's Albuminometer consists of a glass tube marked with the letters U and R and graduated from 0 to 7. Filtered urine to which two drops of acetic acid have been added is poured in to the U mark. Esbach's reagent, which consists mainly of a solution of picric acid, is added up to R. The tube is corked with a rubber stopper, inverted in order to mix its contents, and allowed to stand in the upright position for 24 hours.

The quantity of albumin present is indicated by the level which the precipitate reaches on the graduated scale and is expressed as grams of albumin per litre of urine.

N.B.—If the urine contains more than 7 g per litre it may be diluted with an equal quantity of water before it is placed in the urinometer. In order to obtain the result the fine scale reading is doubled.

(2) Glycosuria

The occurrence of sugar in the urine (glycosuria) is characteristic of **diabetes** but may occasionally occur in other conditions (see p. 439).

(a) The *'Clinitest'.* This test consists of a simple outfit which the patient may use himself to test for sugar without boiling.

(i) Five drops of urine are placed in the test-tube supplied and ten drops of water are added.

(ii) One of the special test tablets is placed in the tube. The reaction is watched until 'boiling' stops and for a further 15 seconds.

(iii) Shake the test tube gently and compare at once with the colour scale.

The tablets are poisonous and should be kept away from children. These tablets are also strongly caustic and should not be touched by hand.

(b) The *'Clinistix'* test shows the presence or absence of glucose but does not indicate the quantity. If the end of the strip moistened with urine turns blue in one minute glucose is present.

(c) Benedict's Test. 5 ml of Benedict's reagent, which is an alkaline solution of copper sulphate, is placed in a test-tube. Eight drops of urine are added and the mixture is boiled for 2 minutes. If sugar is absent no change occurs in the blue colour of the mixture: a small quantity of sugar causes the reagent to turn green, while larger amounts give a yellow or red colour.

(3) Ketone bodies

The two substances described as ketone bodies which occur in the urine are aceto-acetic (diacetic) acid and acetone.

They appear when the intake or utilization of carbohydrate in the body is insufficient for the complete metabolism of fat and are therefore seen in diabetes, starvation, and excessive vomiting, especially in children. (The condition is sometimes described as acidosis or ketosis, p. 440.)

(a) Acetest. 1. Put one drop of urine on the special tablet. 2. Compare the colour with the chart provided after 30 seconds. 3. Record result as negative, weak, moderate or strong positive.

(b) Rothera's Test. A teaspoonful of ammonium sulphate crystals is placed in the bottom of a test-tube and 5 to 10 ml of urine added. The mixture is shaken thoroughly and some of the crystals should remain undissolved (i.e. the urine is saturated with ammonium sulphate). Five drops of a freshly made, dilute (5%) solution or one or two small crystals of sodium nitroprusside are added, followed by 1 to 2 ml of strong ammonia.

The mixture is allowed to stand for a few minutes. If the reaction is positive a mauve colour develops. The amount of diacetic acid present can to some extent be estimated by the depth of colour and the rapidity with which it develops.

(c) Gerhardt's Ferric Chloride Test. Urine to the depth of 2–5 cm (1–2 in) is placed in the test-tube and 10% ferric chloride solution (liquor ferri perchloridi) is added drop by drop. If diacetic acid be present the urine turns a port-wine colour, which disappears on heating. This test is also positive if the urine contains phenol or salicylates, e.g. aspirin, which may be present after treatment with these drugs.

Note—Rothera's test is the more delicate. If it is negative, the ferric chloride test will also be negative. When Rothera's test is positive it should be followed by Gerhardt's test which, if positive, indicates the presence of a large amount of ketone bodies.

Rothera's test detects the presence of ketone bodies in the dilution of 1 in 250,000; the ferric chloride only when the concentration is 1 in 7,000 and is, therefore, much less sensitive.

(4) Haematuria

Bleeding may occur from any part of the renal tract (i.e. the kidneys, ureters, bladder or urethra) and may be caused in the following ways:

(*a*) Trauma: direct injury to any part of the tract, e.g. ruptured kidney, rupture of the bladder associated with fractured pelvis, injury to the urethra.

(*b*) Mechanical: the presence of a calculus or stone in the kidney, ureter or bladder.

(*c*) Acute or chronic inflammation, e.g. nephritis, pyelitis, cystitis and tuberculosis of the renal tract.

(*d*) Tumours: (i) innocent, e.g. papilloma of bladder. (ii) malignant, e.g. carcinoma of kidney or bladder.

(*e*) Overdose of anticoagulants, e.g. heparin, 'Dindevan'.

(*f*) Sulphonamide crystals.

(*g*) General diseases: Blood diseases (e.g. leukaemia and purpura), poisons, embolism affecting the kidneys. Blood may also get into the urine during menstruation.

The treatment of the condition depends on the cause.

The presence of blood in the urine is detected by:

The *Occultest.* One drop of urine is placed on a piece of filter paper, and the occultest tablet put in the centre of the wet area. Two drops of water are added to the tablet. If blood is present a blue colour develops around the tablet within 2 minutes.

A quick test for blood is to dip a 'Hemastix' strip into the urine. Alternatively, pH, glucose, protein and blood can all be detected with one strip of 'Hema-Combistix'. For detection of blood, orthotoluidine and an organic peroxide are incorporated in the strip.

Small amounts of blood are detected by finding red corpuscles on microscopic examination.

(5) Pyuria

Pus in the urine occurs in suppurative conditions affecting the renal tract. The commonest causes are pyelonephritis, pyelitis, cystitis and urethritis. Pus cells are detected in the urine by microscopic examination.

(6) Bile in the urine

The causes of bile in the urine have been discussed in connection with jaundice (see p. 249). Both bile pigments, which produce a greenish-brown discoloration, and bile salts may be present.

Tests for bile pigments. One of the following tests is employed:

(a) The ictotest tablet. Five drops of urine are placed on a test mat and a test tablet is put in the centre of the moist area. Two drops of water are placed on the tablet. If bile is present a bluish-purple colour develops on the wet mat. (Pink or red is not significant.)

(b) The iodine test. If an alcoholic solution of iodine (10%) is poured on top of a layer of urine in a test-tube an emerald-green ring forms at the junction of the liquids when bile is present.

Hay's sulphur test for bile salts. Sprinkle some powdered sulphur on the surface of urine in a specimen glass. With normal urine it floats. If bile salts are present it will sink.

(This test is dependent on the fact that the salts lower the surface tension of the urine.)

(7) Chlorides in urine

This test may be of importance in connection with the administration of saline. There is often severe loss of chlorides from the body in cases of vomiting and diarrhoea, and chlorides are either diminished or disappear from the urine. The following test indicates the presence and amount of urinary chlorides.

Measure 10 drops of urine into a test-tube with a pipette. Rinse pipette with distilled water. Add 1 drop of 20% potassium chromate. Rinse pipette again.

Add 2·9% silver nitrate, a drop at a time, until the colour turns from yellow to brown. Count the number of drops.

One drop represents 1 g of sodium chloride per litre, and so on, but an immediate colour change is regarded as indicating absence of chloride from the urine.

(8) Phenylpyruvic acid in urine

Phenylpyruvic acid is present in the urine of infants with phenylketonuria, a rare condition due to an inborn error of metabolism. It may be detected by testing the urine, or wet napkin, with 'Phenistix' which turns green. If treated early enough, by dietary restriction of the amino acid, phenyl-alanine, mental deficiency may be prevented.

(9) Microscopic abnormalities

Microscopic examination of a catheter specimen of urine may show the presence of blood cells, pus, bacteria and other parasites. In addition what are known as **casts** of the renal tubules may be found in cases of nephritis.

(10) Bacteriological examination

The bacteriological examination of urine is usually undertaken by pathology laboratories. If no laboratory is available, however, or if delay in transit to the laboratory is anticipated, another method for detecting bacteriuria must be used. Delays in the transit of urine specimens allow contaminant organisms to grow in them, giving false positive results.

The dip-slide method for the detection of bacteriuria is rapidly and easily performed by a nurse. It gives few false positive results and practically no false negative results.

The dip-slide ('Uricult') method for the detection of bacteriuria. A glass slide is supplied coated on one side with one culture medium (MacConkey's agar) and on the other side with another (e.g. nutrient agar), neither of which must be touched. This dip-slide is dipped into a freshly voided mid-stream specimen of urine in a sterile container so that the coatings are completely immersed. The excess urine is drained off and the slide is replaced in its tube, which is labelled with the patient's name and with the date and time. The tube is placed in an incubator at 37 °C for 16–24 hours. The dip-slide is then removed and examined with the naked eye. If colonies of bacteria have grown, their density is compared with standard density models to obtain the bacterial count of the urine, this count being proportional to the number of bacteria which were caught on the culture media. A count of 10,000 (10^4) or less bacteria per ml is regarded as negative and a count of 100,000 (10^5) or more per ml is regarded as positive. If the count is between 10^4 and 10^5, the test should be repeated.

Unused dip-slides, in unopened containers, are best kept in a refrigerator (at 4 °C) but must not be frozen.

Summary. In the routine examination of urine, the nurse is expected to carry out the following observations:

1. The general characters, including the quantity, colour, odour and presence of deposit.
2. The reaction.
3. The specific gravity.
4. The boiling test for albumin or 'Albustix' test.
5. 'Clinitest' or Benedict's test for sugar.
6. 'Acetest' or Rothera's test for ketone bodies.
7. 'Occultest' test for blood.
8 'Ictotest' or the iodine test for bile pigments.
9. 'Labstix', for reaction, protein, sugar, ketones and blood. Each item shows if positive, its respective change on one or more of five separate areas on the strip.

B. Cystoscopy

This is an important means of investigating disease of the urinary tract. An illuminated instrument, the cystoscope, is introduced into the bladder via the urethra. The walls of the bladder can be seen and the openings of the ureters inspected. It is sometimes possible to see blood or pus coming from one or both ureters. In other cases, an intramuscular injection of a dye (indigo-carmine, or methylene blue) is given. This colours the urine and is normally excreted by the kidneys in a few minutes. If one kidney is affected by disease, dye may be seen coming only from the opposite ureter.

When necessary a fine catheter can be passed into one or both ureters so that the urine coming from each kidney can be collected separately and examined for chemical or microscopic abnormalities.

C. X-ray examination

X-ray plates are frequently taken of the renal tract and the presence of calculi may be confirmed in this way.

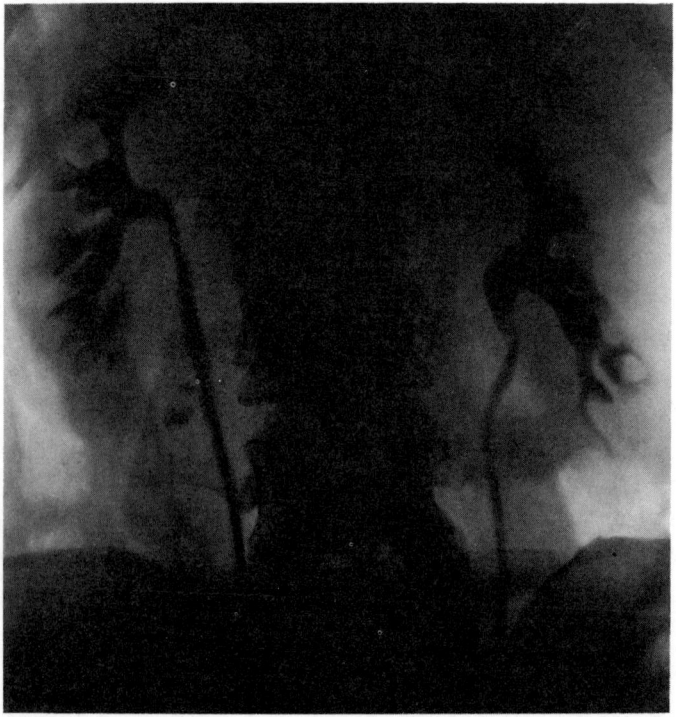

Fig. 70 Normal pyelogram showing opaque catheters in each ureter and the pelvis of the kidney filled with sodium iodide solution.

It is important that the colon should, as far as possible, be empty of gas before the examination is made. For this purpose an aperient is given two nights before and vegetables are excluded from the diet until the plates have been taken. Enemata and colon lavage should be avoided.

Urography (Pyelography). This is a type of x-ray examination in which special measures are adopted to outline the renal tract. There are two methods which may be employed:

1. Excretion or intravenous pyelography.
2. Instrumental or retrograde pyelography.

1. Excretion urography (Intravenous pyelography). A suitable drug such as 'Hypaque', which is rapidly excreted by the kidneys and is opaque to x-rays, is given by intravenous injection. Pictures are taken at intervals of 2, 5, 15 and 25 minutes.

The outline of each kidney, its pelvis, ureter and the bladder can then be seen.

2. Instrumental or retrograde urography (Pyelography). A cystoscope is passed and the orifices of the ureters determined. After ureteric catheterization 5 to 10 ml of a sterile 20% solution of sodium iodide or 'Hypaque' (25%) is injected, the injection ceasing when the patient complains of discomfort in the loins.

The solution is opaque to x-rays and in this way a shadow of the outline of the pelvis of the kidney is obtained.

D. Renal function tests

In addition to the estimation of the blood urea there are a number of tests designed to estimate the excretory powers of the kidneys. Those in common use may be divided into 2 types:

(*a*) Water excretion tests:
   The water elimination test;
   The water concentration test.
(*b*) Urea excretion tests:
   The urea concentration test;
   The urea clearance test.

The water elimination test. The patient passes urine on waking in the morning and immediately drinks 1 litre of water within half an hour. Specimens are collected at half-hourly or hourly intervals for 4 hours. The volume and specific gravity of each specimen is measured and recorded. If the kidneys are excreting water normally, 80% of the 1 litre taken will be excreted in 4 hours and the specific gravity of at least one specimen will not exceed 1005.

The water concentration test. The intake of fluid is restricted to 500 ml (20 fl. oz.) in 24 hours, but normal meals may be consumed. All the urine passed is collected, measured, and the specific gravity of each specimen recorded. If the kidneys are functioning normally the total volume of urine should not exceed 500 ml (20 fl oz) and the specific gravity of one specimen should not be less than 1025.

The urea concentration test. The following test is sometimes employed in order to estimate the capacity of the kidneys to excrete a dose of urea given by mouth.

No fluid is given for several hours, the bladder is then emptied and 15 g of urea dissolved in 100 ml of water are taken.

Two or three specimens of urine are collected at intervals of an hour and sent for chemical analysis. If the kidneys are functioning normally the second- and third-hourly portions should contain at least 2% of urea.

The urea clearance test. There are several methods of performing this test, which depends on comparing the blood urea with the output of urea in the urine.

The creatinine clearance test. Creatinine is a normal constituent of plasma and urine. Its clearance is calculated from its concentration in these two fluids and from the volume of urine collected over a period of 24 hours. It is a better test of glomerular function than the urea clearance, which it has largely replaced. The normal creatinine clearance exceeds 100 ml/min/ 1·73 sq m of body surface area. Damage to the glomeruli reduces the creatinine clearance.

E. Chemical examination of the blood

Blood urea. If the kidneys are failing to excrete this nitrogen-containing by-product of protein metabolism, the normal figure of 40 mg per 100 ml of blood will be exceeded.

F. Renal biopsy

By inserting a special needle into the kidney and withdrawing a specimen of tissue it may be possible by microscopic examination to determine the type and degree of renal damage present, thus assisting in the diagnosis and prognosis of the condition.

G. Radio-isotope renography

[131]I-hippuran injected intravenously is taken up by the kidneys and excreted in the urine. A suitably positioned detector can detect the gamma rays emitted from the compound in the kidney and a graph

can be drawn. A normal renogram yields a curve with a sharp peak, since all the nephrons function simultaneously.

Isotope renography is used to detect renal ischaemia (due to renal artery stenosis), when this is suspected as a cause of hypertension, and in the investigation of obstructive nephropathy (e.g. kidney disease due to obstruction by stones).

Micturition and its disorders

Normally the act of emptying the bladder, or micturition, is under the control of the nervous system and is, in many ways, comparable with defaecation (p. 238).

The bladder is supplied with afferent and efferent nerves in the same manner as the rectum. When the muscle of the bladder becomes stretched by distension of the organ, impulses pass along the afferent nerves to the spinal cord whence they travel upwards to the brain in order to reach consciousness. The act of micturition is initiated by motor impulses passing down the cord and entering the bladder and associated muscles via the efferent nerves. When the motor impulses reach the bladder its musculature contracts, but at the same time the sphincter muscle at its urethral opening relaxes and allows the urine to escape.

In the infant the act is a reflex one and in certain cases of nervous disease when impulses are unable to travel up the spinal cord to the brain, it is no longer governed by voluntary control. In these circumstances sensory impulses pass from the bladder to the spinal cord, whence they travel directly to the muscles associated with micturition via the efferent nerves. It follows, therefore, that when the spinal cord is severely damaged or there is loss of consciousness, the voluntary act of micturition is abolished.

Micturition may also be disordered as a result of local lesions in the urinary tract.

The common alterations in this function may be classified in the following way:
1. Incontinence.
2. Retention:
    (*a*) acute,
    (*b*) with overflow.
3. Frequency.
4. Difficult or painful micturition (dysuria).

1. Incontinence of urine. If the voluntary impulses from the brain are cut off, either by damage to the spinal cord, or impairment of consciousness as in coma or an epileptic fit, urine will be passed at intervals because, by reflex action, distension will cause afferent impulses to pass to the spinal cord and initiate motor impulses which pass to the bladder.

In many cases this is associated with incontinence of faeces because the reflex nervous mechanisms of the two acts are similar and closely connected. In true incontinence the bladder is empty and this condition must be carefully distinguished from 'retention with overflow'.

There are a number of causes of incontinence apart from the reflex type just mentioned, e.g.:

(a) Stress incontinence in which the sphincter muscle and the muscles of the pelvic floor are weakened, as they may be after repeated pregnancy.

In this condition any sudden contraction of the diaphragm raising the intra-abdominal pressure, such as may occur in laughing, sneezing, coughing or lifting a heavy weight, will cause a distressing leakage of urine from the bladder.

(b) Nocturnal enuresis or 'bed wetting', a troublesome condition which occurs mainly in young children and adolescents.

This is by no means an easy condition to treat and requires much patience. Pathological conditions must first be excluded. Psychologically it is most important for the child to establish confidence in himself. Observation of the time enuresis occurs and waking to empty the bladder beforehand may be helpful. Ephedrine is a useful drug. A course of imipramine ('Tofranil') taken at bedtime for 6 to 8 weeks, then gradually withdrawn, may succeed.

A 'buzzer device' which wakes the child immediately urine commences to be passed on to a special blanket is often useful.

2. Retention of urine. Among the common causes of retention of urine are:

1. Mechanical.
> Urethral stricture.
> Enlargement of the prostate gland.
> Tumours of the bladder.
> Pressure on the bladder by pelvic tumours including the pregnant uterus and uterine fibroids.

2. Nervous.
> Hysteria and functional states.
> Tumours and injury of the spinal cord.
> Reflex spasm of the sphincter after operations in the neighbourhood, e.g. rectum.

Postoperative retention.

Tabes dorsalis, disseminated sclerosis and other organic diseases of the nervous system.

'Retention with overflow' is a combination of retention and incontinence. In this condition, unless relieved by catheterization, the bladder becomes more and more distended until the sphincter muscle which closes its outlet is finally forced open by the pressure inside. Small quantities of urine then escape from time to time. The distended bladder can be felt as a rounded tumour above the pubis and extending upwards towards the umbilicus.

It is of the utmost importance to distinguish retention with overflow associated with a distended bladder from simple incontinence. In the former condition the bladder must be emptied very slowly after catheterization so that the over-stretched muscle can contract gradually and regain its tone.

It is also important to distinguish between retention of urine in the bladder and suppression of urine (anuria) in which no urine is being secreted by the kidneys (p. 339).

3. Frequency of micturition. Increased frequency of micturition may be due to the fact that a large amount of urine is being excreted (polyuria) in such conditions as excessive fluid intake, diabetes and certain cases of chronic nephritis. It may also be caused by local conditions of the bladder or urethra, such as a calculus, cystitis, urethritis or by pressure on the parts by a pregnant uterus or pelvic tumour, where the quantity of urine excreted is normal but the bladder is abnormally irritable. It may also occur in anxiety states.

4. Difficult or painful micturition (dysuria). Difficult micturition is caused by stricture of the urethra, enlargement of the prostate and diseases of the nervous system. The act may be painful in inflammation of the bladder and urethra.

Treatment of the disorders of micturition

The main points of treatment may be summarized in the following way:

1. Incontinence. Great care must be taken of the back and surrounding parts in order to prevent the development of a urine rash or bed-sores.

The parts must be dried, treated with spirit and powder and the wet linen changed frequently. 'Water repellent' creams may be applied to the affected skin, e.g. 'Conotrane', 'Siopel'.

2. Acute retention. In acute retention every effort should be made to induce the patient to pass urine naturally before resorting to a catheter. Any of the following methods may be employed:

1. By suggestion, i.e. turning on a tap and allowing the patient to hear the sound of running water.
2. An enema.
3. Altering the position of the patient (if possible) by allowing him to sit over the edge of the bed, to adopt the knee-chest position or, failing this, to turn on his side.
4. A drink of hot tea, or hot lemon.
5. An injection of carbachol in some cases.
6. In suitable cases a hot bath, the patient being directed to micturate into the water.

If these methods fail a soft rubber or polythene catheter is passed, but in no case should retention be allowed to continue for more than twelve hours.

Retention with overflow. This is specially liable to occur in states of unconsciousness. With careful observation a patient should not be allowed to get into this condition. The bladder being over-distended, the urine must be withdrawn slowly by catheterization.

The bladder must not be emptied all at once. As a rule about $\frac{1}{2}$ litre (20 fl oz) is withdrawn. A similar quantity is removed at intervals of two hours until the bladder is empty and the patient is able to control micturition himself. This condition is treated under the direction of the doctor.

In all disorders of micturition it is of the utmost importance to discover whether or not the bladder is distended.

Nephritis

The term nephritis or Bright's disease (Richard Bright, 1789–1858) is applied to a number of conditions in which the kidney is affected by disease. The pathology of some of these processes is not fully understood and it is not possible to give an exact classification of renal disease.

It must be remembered that structurally the kidney consists of two main elements:

1. The glomeruli and secreting tubules which are described as the parenchyma.
2. The fibrous and connective tissue framework (interstitial tissue) which supports the parenchyma and contains the blood vessels.

When a lesion occurs the glomeruli and the tubules may be more or less equally affected, or the damage may predominate in one of these elements. Likewise, fibrosis (or sclerosis) of the interstitial tissue may be the main feature of some types of chronic renal disease.

Glomerular disease may present as any of the following conditions:

Acute nephritis.

The Nephrotic Syndrome.

Chronic nephritis.

Acute nephritis

Definition. Acute inflammation of the kidney substance, especially the glomeruli and secreting tubules.

Cause. Acute nephritis of this type generally follows an attack of tonsillitis or other streptococcal infection (e.g. scarlet fever) after an interval of 1–3 weeks. Why this should happen in some cases only, when streptococcal sore throats are so common is not fully explained, but it appears to be, in part, the result of some impairment of the immunity mechanism. The disease usually is seen in children and young adults.

Circulating **antigen-antibody complexes** may combine with **complement,** a normal constituent of plasma, and be deposited in the glomeruli, where they cause a thickening of the basement membrane visible under the ordinary light microscope (renal biopsy specimens are also examined by electron microscopy).

The glomerular basement membrane may itself act as an antigen. Antibodies become attached to it and the antigen-antibody complex so formed attracts complement from the plasma. Again, thickening of the basement membrane results.

The deposit on the basement membrane attracts polymorphonuclear leucocytes which release proteolytic enzymes and damage or destroy the glomeruli.

A nephritogenic strain of group A streptococci has been found to possess an antigen in common with human kidney. Antibodies formed against the streptococcus can react not only with the bacterium but with the basement membrane of the glomeruli.

Occasionally other bacteria (e.g. staphylococci) and viruses may induce the changes leading to acute nephritis.

Pathology and morbid anatomy. The kidneys are red and enlarged. Small haemorrhages appear on their surface and in their substance. The glomeruli and tubules are swollen and the protoplasm of their cells is damaged. The lumen of the tubules tend to become blocked by the products of the inflammation and the interstitial tissue as oedematous.

Symptoms. The onset is acute. The patient complains of headache, aching in the loins, vomiting with diarrhoea or constipation.

There is usually some rise in temperature and the pulse rate is increased. Puffiness of the eyelids may be the first sign noticed. Subsequently there is **oedema** of the rest of the face, the ankles and legs, and sometimes of the scrotum, of varying degree, and usually most marked in the morning. (This should be contrasted with the oedema of chronic heart failure which affects the most dependent parts of the body and in which the face is not affected, and is worse towards the end of the day.) In very severe cases the oedema may be accompanied by more extensive effusion of fluid into the subcutaneous tissues, the peritoneal cavity (ascites) and pleural cavities (hydrothorax) and dyspnoea may be marked. The oedema, however, is not usually as marked as that seen in the nephrotic syndrome. The blood pressure is raised and the blood urea is increased above the normal figure of 40 mg per 100 ml.

The urine is scanty in amount (*oliguria*), about $\frac{1}{2}$ litre or less (8 to 12 oz) being passed in 24 hours, while in very severe cases suppression of urine may occur. The specific gravity is raised (1025–1035). Its dark 'smoky' appearance is due to **blood** which, in many cases, is present in sufficient quantity to be obvious and to colour the urine red. **Albumin** is present in moderate amounts (Esbach's test up to 10 grams per litre).

Microscopic examination shows the presence of **cellular casts**.

Progress of the disease. The acute disease may be followed by:

1. Complete recovery in the course of several weeks, which may be anticipated in over 90% of children and in over 50% of adults. In a favourable case, after one to three weeks, the urinary output increases (diuresis), often quite rapidly, and the oedema disappears. The blood pressure also falls to normal.

2. Death from renal or heart failure. These are fortunately rare in the acute stages.

3. A form of chronic nephritis. This will ultimately shorten the life of the patient, although there may be an interval or latent period of many months or even years, during which there are no special symptoms and all that can be found is some albuminuria and possibly some rise in the blood pressure. Finally, there will be oedema, hypertension, raised blood urea and death from renal failure.

Complications. (1) RENAL FAILURE. The power of the kidneys to excrete urea may be impaired and if the concentration of this substance in the blood becomes excessive the state of **uraemia** (p. 338) will develop. Complete suppression of urine may prove fatal.

(2) CEREBRAL ATTACKS ASSOCIATED WITH HIGH BLOOD PRESSURE. The blood pressure is raised in acute nephritis and in the

latest stages of chronic nephritis. Occasionally attacks of a cerebral nature associated with hypertension may occur and are referred to as hypertensive encephalopathy. The main features of this condition are headache, temporary loss of sight, various type of paralysis, convulsions and coma. In some respects these symptoms resemble uraemia, but there is no marked rise in the blood urea and they are probably due to a lack of blood supply to the brain caused by a spasm of the cerebral arteries (p. 143) or may be associated with cerebral oedema.

(3) PROGRESSIVE OEDEMA. The occurrence of ascites and pleural effusion has been mentioned. The lung tissue itself may also become oedematous (pulmonary oedema), producing serious dyspnoea which may be associated with cardiac failure.

(4) SECONDARY INFECTION. Oedematous tissue is easily infected by micro-organisms and conditions such as pleurisy and pericarditis may occur.

(5) ANAEMIA due to loss of blood and toxaemia affecting the blood-forming organs.

(6) HEART FAILURE. This may supervene and will cause the oedema to increase. It is marked by breathlessness, cough, and weakness of the pulse.

Diagnosis. The diagnosis is made on the history, symptoms, and the appearance of blood, albumin, and casts in the urine, associated with oedema. A raised anti-streptolysin (ASO) titre in the serum helps to confirm the diagnosis.

Treatment. The main principles of treatment are:
1. To rest the kidneys as much as possible by dieting.
2. To treat symptoms and complications as they arise.

General measures. The patient is kept in bed in a warm room. Pulmonary oedema will, if present, necessitate a sitting posture. The patient is usually kept in bed until diuresis has occurred, albuminuria has diminished and macroscopic haematuria has disappeared.

Diet. Protein is excluded from the diet as far as possible in the acute stages, for it has been seen that urea is excreted with difficulty by the damaged organs and tends to accumulate in the blood. At the same time an adequate carbohydrate intake is important in order to prevent the patient utilizing his own tissue proteins.

The oedema is due to the retention of water and salt in the body and, therefore, the fluid intake is restricted and a salt-free diet given until diuresis has occurred and the oedema has disappeared. An accurate intake and output chart must be kept.

Moderate quantities of fluid only are, therefore, allowed. The amount in each case is adjusted to the urinary output, allowing 500 ml more than the previous day's excretion. An extra allowance is made for water lost by sweating, vomiting and diarrhoea.

1. During the first few days simple fluids such as soda water, barley water, orange juice, lime water or weak tea are given. Benger's food and arrowroot may be used instead of milk. Milk is unsuitable since it contains too much protein and salt. Toffee, being composed of sugar and fat, may be taken in large quantities (500 g, ½ lb daily), if there is no nausea.

Some physicians institute a 'starvation' period of 2 or 3 days or longer at the commencement of treatment. In the patient who has severe diminuation of urinary output this may take the form of a fluid intake of 500 ml plus the volume of the previous day's urinary output and containing at least 500 g of carbohydrate.

2. After the 'starvation' period of a few days, when the acute condition is subsiding, more carbohydrate and starchy foods, such as bread and butter, potatoes, vegetables, fruit, milk puddings, cream and jam are added gradually.

3. After 2 or 3 weeks, 1 or 2 eggs may be given.

4. After about 3 to 5 weeks, fish, chicken and rabbit are gradually introduced, i.e. a gradual increase in the protein allowance up to 40 g daily.

5. Later, provided progress is satisfactory, a full diet may be allowed (protein up to 90 g). The actual rate at which the diet is increased depends on the progress of the case and in some instances may be more rapid than that suggested.

The onset of diuresis must be carefully watched for so that excessive fluid and electrolyte loss can promptly be made good.

Treatment of any residual infection with antibiotics, e.g. penicillin, is necessary but does not affect the actual course of the disease.

The bowels are kept comfortably open but excessive purging is avoided and diuretic drugs are not usually employed.

Treatment of special symptoms

1. VOMITING. Ice may be given to suck. Metoclopramide ('Maxolon') 'Avomine', promazine or 'Fentazin', are sometimes effective.

2. HYPERTENSIVE ENCEPHALOPATHY. Hypotensive drugs are used, e.g. diazoxide 100–300 mg intravenously in adults, or reserpine 1–2·5 mg i.m. (0·05–0·1 mg/kg b.w. for a child). Diazepam, 2–10 mg is injected intravenously to control convulsions. If fits recur, phenytoin is given intramuscularly (dose: 100 mg twice daily).

3. OEDEMA. If the routine treatment of restricting fluids and a salt-free diet fail to control oedema, large doses of frusemide may be effective. If they are not, peritoneal dialysis can be used to remove water from the body. A pleural effusion may be aspirated.

4. ANAEMIA. Iron is given in full doses.

5. ANURIA or severe oliguria—see p. 339.

The nephrotic syndrome

The nephrotic syndrome may result from damage to the glomeruli in a variety of different conditions including diabetes mellitus, systemic lupus erythematosus (SLE), renal vein thrombosis, syphilis, troxidone toxicity, quartan malaria and allergy to a bee sting. It may occur at any age, even in young children, and is characterized by severe oedema which usually starts in the legs and which may progress to a general anasarca. There is gross albuminuria and a low blood albumin concentration. The serum cholesterol level is raised. Blood is rarely detected in the urine except occasionally on microscopic examination. The condition may remit spontaneously or persist for many months or years, and only in the late stages does the blood pressure rise and the patient die from chronic renal failure (uraemia), or a complicating infection such as pneumonia or pericarditis.

Treatment is given to reduce the oedema. This is due to the accumulation of water in the tissues as a result of salt retention and a diminution of the blood proteins. The constant loss of large amounts of albumin in the urine causes this fall in blood proteins which lowers the osmotic pressure of the blood and allows fluid to collect in the tissues instead of being absorbed into the blood and carried to the kidneys for excretion.

The treatment, therefore, consists of:

1. Raising the blood proteins by giving a high protein diet. e.g. up to 100 g daily. There is usually no risk in this because the blood urea is not raised until the latest stages of the disease. Salt-free human albumin is sometimes given intravenously to raise the osmotic pressure of the blood.

2. In some cases attempting to raise the osmotic pressure of the blood by giving intravenous infusions of dextran or salt-free human albumin.

3. A salt-free diet, including the use of salt-free bread, is necessary.

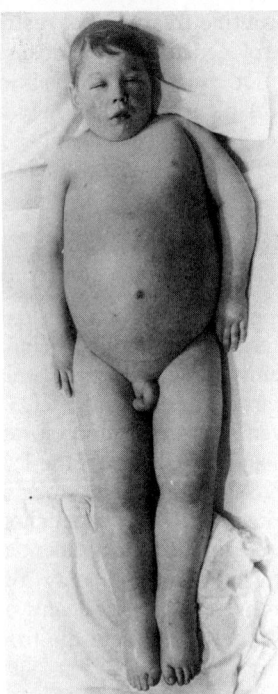

Fig. 71 General anasarca showing oedema of limbs and face with distension of the abdomen due to ascites, in the nephrotic syndrome.

4. Removal of excess of fluid from the tissues if this is considered to be essential by:
   (*a*) Diuretics, e.g. thiazides or frusemide, and spironolactone or rarely by
   (*b*) Paracentesis of abdomen or chest.
   (*c*) Removal of fluid from the legs either by incisions of the skin on the dorsum of the feet or by Southey's tubes.

For this purpose the patient should be placed with the legs low for a day or two beforehand in order to allow the fluid to gravitate to the dependent parts. Great care must be taken to sterilize the skin and to maintain strict asepsis as the oedematous tissues are particularly liable to infection. Should this occur it may be treated with antibiotics.

5. Periodic estimation of the blood electrolytes and urea is necessary and daily weighing helps to indicate the response to treatment.

6. Prednisolone or similar steroids may induce remissions, especially in children. Cyclophosphamide may be used in steroid-dependent or steroid-resistant cases. Cyclophosphamide is an immunosuppressive drug which interferes with antibody synthesis.

   These drugs are given when the glomeruli in a renal biopsy specimen appear normal or show only 'minimal change' under the light microscope. More advanced changes do not respond.

7. Methyldopa or other antihypertensive drugs may be required for hypertension. The blood pressure should be taken regularly.

8. Antibiotics are given for intercurrent infections, to which nephrotic patients are prone.

Chronic nephritis

Chronic nephritis may be a sequel to acute nephritis but often there is no history of this condition. There may at first be no symptoms

	Acute nephritis	Nephrotic syndrome	Chronic nephritis
Age	Children and young adults	Children and young adults	Any age
Blood pressure	Raised	Normal or slightly raised	High
Oedema	Moderate	Marked	Rare
Urine	Diminished	Diminished	Increased (polyuria)
	High specific gravity	High specific gravity	Low SG
	Albumin	Albumin	Albumin, trace
	Blood	Blood (? trace)	No blood
Blood Urea	Raised	Normal or slightly raised	Raised
Termination	1. Recovery 2. Chronic nephritis 3. Death from uraemia or heart failure	1. Recovery 2. Death from: (a) General anasarca (b) Uraemia (c) Pneumonia or pericarditis	Death from: 1. Uraemia 2. Heart failure 3. Cerebral haemorrhage

and the disease may be discovered when albuminuria or hypertension is found during a routine medical examination. Oedema is usually absent. Polyuria is a common complaint and the ability of the kidneys to concentrate or dilute the urine is impaired. The specific gravity of the urine becomes fixed at 1·010. Chronic uraemia ensues and the patient eventually dies of this or of one of the complications of hypertension—e.g., cerebral haemorrhage.

Treatment. There is no cure for the disease. The patient must lead a regular life. A moderate diet in which protein is reduced is allowed, while beer is avoided. Careful attention is given to the bowels and special symptoms and complications are treated as they arise. When end-stage renal failure occurs, regular intermittent haemodialysis is a possible treatment.

Renal failure (uraemia)

Failure of the kidneys to function may be either acute or chronic in character, and the term **uraemia** is often used to describe the condition. Uraemia may be defined as the accumulation of toxic substances in the blood which are normally excreted by the kidneys. It is associated with a raised blood urea, urea being an end-product of nitrogen and protein metabolism. Actually, urea itself is not a toxic substance and can be given therapeutically as a diuretic in certain cases but the term uraemia is used to describe the syndrome which results from a number of biochemical disturbances, of which a raised blood urea is one which can be easily estimated.

It is possible to recognize three types of uraemia, viz.:
1. Uraemia with acute renal failure.
2. Uraemia with chronic renal failure.
3. 'Extra-renal' uraemia.

'Extra-renal' uraemia (which means that it is caused by something outside or away from the kidneys) is due to kidney failure caused by diminished blood supply or conditions which disturb the functions of the kidney by upsetting the general metabolism of the body and the composition of the body fluids without there being any actual kidney disease. This may occur in such conditions as intestinal obstruction, severe diarrhoea and vomiting with marked dehydration, diabetic coma and acidosis, and shock from injury or severe haemorrhage. In shock the blood pressure may be so low that there is little blood flow through the kidneys and urinary excretion is reduced to a minimum.

Acute renal failure

This is usually associated with the suppression of urine (anuria) when the urinary output is reduced to nothing or else very markedly diminished (oliguria). This state may continue for a week or more and the patient may still recover. But if the re-establishment of urinary secretion does not then take place a fatal result must be expected in the absence of special treatment.

The **symptoms** observed are those of the primary condition causing the renal failure to which may be added general drowsiness.

Causes. It may occur as a result of acute nephritis, anuria due to bilateral renal calculus, overdosage with sulphonamides causing blockage of the renal tubules by crystals of the drug and incompatible blood transfusion in which the wrong blood group is used.

Certain operations (e.g. those on jaundiced patients) carry a special risk of acute renal failure. The risk may be reduced by giving 50 ml of 25% mannitol intravenously early in the operation.

With appropriate **treatment** of established acute renal failure many cases recover. Since the kidneys are not excreting, it is important not to overload the tissues with water or salts, for this may result in pulmonary oedema and cardiac failure. Treatment in the first instance is directed to the primary cause, e.g. ureteric obstruction and 'extra-renal' conditions. The next points are to regulate the fluid intake and to exclude salts and protein until diuresis is established and the kidneys are excreting 1000 ml (35 oz) in 24 hours.

Repeated investigation of electrolytes and blood chemistry is necessary.

Up to 300 g lactose are given daily in 500 ml of water by mouth or by a Ryle's tube. If the patient is vomiting, this therapy is replaced by an intravenous infusion of 50 g fructose in 500 ml of water. The total quantity of fluid administered during a period of anuria must not exceed 500 ml per 24 hours unless there are abnormal losses (e.g. in sweating and diarrhoea). The patient is weighed daily to detect fluid retention. High doses of frusemide (up to 2 g per day) may be given by intravenous infusion.

Excess of potassium in the body can cause serious disturbances of cardiac rhythm and death. If there is hyperkalaemia (an abnormally high serum potassium level), a cation exchange resin, e.g. 'Resonium-A' orally (15 g tds) or rectally is often effective in treating it.

If anuria continues, these measures will not be sufficient. Urea and excess electrolytes must then be extracted from the circulating blood by dialysis. Peritoneal dialysis is effective if time is available. In the crush syndrome, however, where anuria is due to crushing trauma of limbs, uraemia tends to increase so rapidly that haemodialysis is imperative.

Dialysis

Substances accumulating in the blood in toxic quantities in renal failure can be removed by diffusion through a membrane. This membrane may be a natural one—the peritoneum, or a man-made one—cellophane. The unwanted substances (e.g. urea, potassium and acid) diffuse through from the blood on one side of the membrane to the dialysing fluid (dialysate) on the other side.

Peritoneal dialysis

A suitable glucose-electrolyte solution is introduced into the peritoneal cavity via a nylon catheter (e.g. 'Dialaflex') inserted through the abdominal wall. The blood flowing through the capillaries of the peritoneum exchanges constituents with the dialysate, which is then run out of the peritoneal cavity into a receptacle. The effluent fluid carries with it the waste products and electrolytes extracted from the blood.

The nurse must remember that
1. the patient's bladder must be emptied prior to insertion of the dialysing catheter;
2. dialysing solutions vary in their glucose content (e.g. 1·36% and 6·36%) and the nurse should ensure that the intended one is used. Failure to do this may result in serious, possibly fatal, water deprivation or intoxication;
3. the bags of dialysing fluid should be warmed to 40 °C in a water bath before use.

Haemodialysis

This utilizes an 'artificial kidney' or haemodialyser. Blood is tapped from the radial artery, fed through the machine, and returned to the basilic vein. An arteriovenous shunt or fistula is established between the two vessels to provide ready access to the bloodstream for frequent dialysis.

In the machine, the blood flows over a cellophane membrane of large area, in the form of tubing around which is pumped the dialysing fluid.

Chronic renal failure

As the name implies, this is a more gradual process. It occurs in the late stages of the nephrotic syndrome, chronic nephritis and in those cases of acute nephritis which are progressive; also in the later stages of other chronic kidney disease, such as hypertensive renal disease, chronic prostatic enlargement and other conditions causing hydronephrosis.

The main symptoms are headache, nausea, vomiting, hiccough, shortness of breath, a dry furred tongue together with cramps and twitching of the muscles. Sometimes a uriniferous odour can be detected in the breath. Actual fits or convulsions followed by coma may occur. These fits are probably due to the associated high blood pressure and some oedema of the brain rather than the actual uraemia.

Treatment is primarily conservative but suitable patients may go on to **regular haemodialysis** or to **renal transplantation.**

Conservative treatment is

(a) dietary;

(b) pharmacological.

(a) Dietary management. Protein restriction is the first consideration in keeping the blood urea down. In early cases, 55–60 g of protein may be allowed daily (about 90 g would be a normal daily protein intake in the UK). When the glomerular filtration rate (or creatinine clearance) falls to 5 ml/min, protein intake has to be restricted to 45 g daily. At a glomerular filtration rate of 3 ml/min or less, a selected low protein diet—the Giordano-Giovanetti diet—giving only 20 g of protein daily is needed. A high calorie intake (3,000–4,000 calories daily) is advised but is made difficult by the fact that a strict low protein diet does not permit the patient to eat ordinary bread and cakes. Special low-protein bread (e.g. Rite Diet bread) and low-protein pasta, macaroni and biscuits are obtainable. 'Caloreen', a glucose polymer, is a very high calorie food which is free of protein and electrolytes; it may be used to replace milk in coffee, to thicken soups, to add to cake flour and to make ice cream. 'Hycal' is less well tolerated because of its high free glucose content but is available in several flavours as a food drink.

Distilled spirits, such as whisky, brandy, gin and vodka, are permissible sources of calories but beer and wine are not, because of their protein and electrolyte content.

(b) Pharmacological management. 1. The glomerular filtration rate and hence the urinary output can often be increased by

prescribing large doses of frusemide orally—up to 1·5 g daily. Sodium restriction will not then need to be so severe. Patients whose chronic renal failure is being treated with frusemide should be encouraged to take fluids by mouth.

2. Ion-exchange resins (e.g. calcium resin) may be needed to combat hyperkalaemia (an excess of potassium in the serum).

3. Aluminium hydroxide may be prescribed to bind phosphate in the gut and thus to prevent its absorption. Phosphate is one of the undesirable substances which accumulate in the blood in renal failure.

4. The anaemia of chronic renal failure may partially respond to iron, vitamin B_{12} and folic acid, all of which may be deficient in the patient's restricted diet.

5. Large doses of vitamin D may be needed to treat renal bone disease (renal osteodystrophy).

6. Patients with chronic renal failure are prone to urinary tract infection and this should be sought by microscopy and culture of mid-stream specimens of urine. Infection should be treated with an effective and safe antibiotic, e.g. ampicillin.

In **end-stage renal failure**, the maintenance of life can only be ensured by dialysis or renal transplantation.

Dialysis

For details, see p. 340.

Patients on a chronic intermittent dialysis programme are able to eat a less restricted diet than patients on the conservative regime because the excess urea and electrolytes are being removed by the procedure, which is usually performed twice a week.

To be suitable for chronic intermittent haemodialysis, a patient must have a stable personality and be free of serious cardiovascular disease and generalised diseases such as systemic lupus erythematosus (SLE).

Self-dialysis by patients in their own homes is generally encouraged because it is often more convenient for the patient, makes him feel less dependent, relieves the pressure on hospital beds and staff and has a lower incidence of complications.

Renal transplantation

The body rejects any tissue which it recognizes as foreign. What are recognized are antigens on the surface of the foreign cells. These are known as transplantation antigens (T-antigens) and their measurement is called **tissue typing**. The tests are done on blood samples and a donor and recipient should have compatible ABO blood groups and similar leucocyte antigens. A perfect match is rarely obtainable and is unnecessary providing continuous drug therapy is given to suppress rejection. The drugs most often used for this **immuno-suppressive therapy** are azathioprine ('Imuran') and prednisolone.

In the UK, nearly all transplanted kidneys are from fresh cadavers. The permission of the next of kin and of the coroner is required before the organs are removed from the cadaver.

Successful renal transplantation releases patients from the restrictions of diet, fluid and machines. Even if enough donor organs were available, however, not all patients with chronic renal failure would be suitable recipients. Examples of conditions which render a patient unsuitable are diabetes mellitus, glomerulonephritis, and abnormalities of the bladder and urethra.

Diseases of the renal tract

Pyelitis. Pyelonephritis

By pyelitis is meant inflammation of the pelvis of the kidney without involvement of the renal tissue. However, there is usually some involvement of renal tissue which may be relatively minor and which does not usually interfere with urinary excretion in acute cases. Therefore, the term pyelonephritis is frequently used. The condition may be acute or chronic in type and is frequently caused by the colon bacillus (*Esch. coli*). Next in frequency are infections by *Proteus mirabilis* and 'coliforms', in that order. Occasionally streptococci or staphylococci are responsible.

It is common in children and young adults and is seen more often in females than in males.

It may commence in a previously healthy renal tract. It may follow catheterization or may complicate already existing lesions such as renal calculus, enlarged prostate and cystitis. Pressure on the ureters by the pregnant uterus causing stagnation of urine in the pelvis of the kidney, a condition which predisposes to the multiplication of bacteria, is a common cause of the malady.

Symptoms. The main symptoms in acute pyelitis are pyrexia, often associated with rigors, pain and tenderness in the loins and frequency of micturition accompanied by the appearance of albumin, pus cells and sometimes blood in the urine. The diagnosis is confirmed by the bacteriological examination of a midstream or catheter specimen of urine.

Residual infection may result in chronic pyelonephritis with perhaps recurrent acute attacks.

The presence of organisms in the urine is referred to as **bacilluria.**

An excess of white blood cells in the urine is referred to as pyuria (pus in the urine).

Treatment. The patient should have rest in bed while pyrexia is present. In contrast with acute nephritis large quantities of fluid are administered, for the undamaged kidneys have no difficulty in excreting water which, in this instance, flushes out the urinary tract and helps to remove the inflammatory products and bacteria. Barley water, weak tea or lemonade may be used.

The bowels are kept open comfortably by giving mild aperients as required, but strong purgatives should be avoided.

The urine is, as a rule, acid in reaction, but endeavour may be made to render it alkaline by potassium citrate in doses of 4 g (30 to 60 grains), every 3 or 4 hours (unless streptomycin or mandelic acid are used in treatment). At the same time an antibacterial drug, which is excreted by the kidneys and therefore helps to sterilize the renal tract, is given. The following drugs are used, depending on the sensitivity of the infecting organism:

   (*a*) Sulphonamide drugs, e.g. sulphatriad, sulphadimidine, sulphamethizole ('Urolucosil') (p. 516).
   (*b*) Co-trimoxazole, trimethoprin in combination with a sulphonamide as in 'Septrin' and 'Bactrim'. Most of the organisms which infect the urinary tract are sensitive to this drug.
   (*c*) Ampicillin, 500 mg, 8 hourly.
   (*d*) Nitrofurantoin ('Furadantin'), 100 mg 4 times daily.
   (*e*) Nalidixic acid ('Negram').
   (*f*) The cephalosporins e.g. cephalexin.
   (*g*) Preparations of mandelic acid are occasionally used.

Chronic pyelonephritis. Recurrent attacks of urinary infection are strongly suggestive of pyelonephritis and require full investigation of the urinary tract and renal function. Surgical treatment may be needed to remove calculi etc. but the above drugs are also essential. The destructive effect of chronic pyelonephritis on the kidney ultimately causes hypertension.

Cystitis

Inflammation of the bladder may be acute or chronic and is of bacterial origin. The infection may reach the bladder from above, e.g. pyelitis, or may be the result of organisms introduced by catheterization. It occurs also in cases of nervous disease when there is delay in emptying the bladder.

The main symptoms are pain and tenderness above the pubis and in the perineum, frequent and painful micturition with the passage of blood and pus in the urine.

The treatment is similar to that of pyelitis: i.e. large quantities of fluid, alkaline drugs, which may be followed by urinary antiseptics. In addition, heat to the suprapubic region may give relief from pain. In chronic cases the bladder may be washed out through a catheter with noxytiolin ('Noxyflex S') or 'Betadine' solutions.

Hydronephrosis

If the outflow of urine from one or both ureters or the bladder is partially obstructed, the pelvis of the kidney will become dilated above the obstruction in order to accommodate the unpassed fluid. This condition of dilatation of the pelvis of the kidney is called hydronephrosis.

It usually affects one side, but if it is caused by lesions of both ureters or if the obstruction is situated at the outlet of the bladder it will be bilateral.

The common causes are:

1. Obstruction to the lumen of the ureter, e.g. renal calculus.
2. Disease of the walls of the urinary tract, e.g. growth of ureter or bladder.

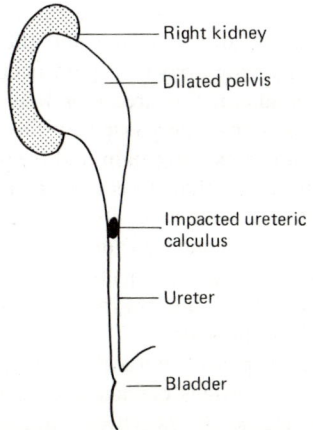

Fig. 72 Diagram illustrating the production of a hydronephrosis by a calculus impacted in the ureter.

3. Pressure on the ureter from outside, e.g. tumours or an abnormally placed renal artery which causes a kinking of the duct.

The main symptoms are attacks of pain together with the development of a swelling in the loin. If the pelvis of the kidney becomes infected and pus forms, the condition is called pyonephrosis.

The treatment of both is surgical.

Complete and permanent obstruction of the ureter leads to atrophy of the kidney.

Renal calculus

Renal stones may consist of any one of the following substances derived from the urine or a mixture of them: calcium oxalate, urates or phosphates. They are sometimes the result of overactivity of the parathyroid glands (hyperparathyroidism), which causes elevated blood and urine calcium levels. More commonly there is simply too much calcium in the urine (idiopathic hypercalciuria).

Calculi may be single or a number may be present and they may be found in any part of the urinary tract. A stone may sometimes remain in the kidney without producing symptoms but, when it enters and passes down the ureter, it will give rise to acute pain, referred to as **renal colic**, often combined with haematuria. Renal colic is of sudden onset and consists of paroxysms of pain in the loin which shoots round into the abdomen and into the groin. It is frequently associated with vomiting and sweating and the patient may roll on the ground in agony as each spasm of pain occurs.

The stone may remain in the ureter or may eventually reach the bladder. It it is small it may be passed by the urethra, otherwise it will remain in the bladder causing pain and frequency of micturition.

It has been pointed out that a renal calculus may cause hydronephrosis and that its presence may often be demonstrated by x-rays.

Treatment. For renal colic morphine (15 mg, gr $\frac{1}{4}$) combined with atropine (0·6 mg, gr $\frac{1}{100}$) is injected or pethidine may be used. A hot bath may also relieve the spasm. The patient may remain in bed while haematuria is present.

Small stones may be passed naturally, and with this end in view medical treatment is sometimes carried out. It must be remembered, however, that there are no drugs which will cause the usual type of stone to dissolve. A high fluid intake and sometimes a low-calcium diet are advised. Idiopathic hypercalciuria may be treated with

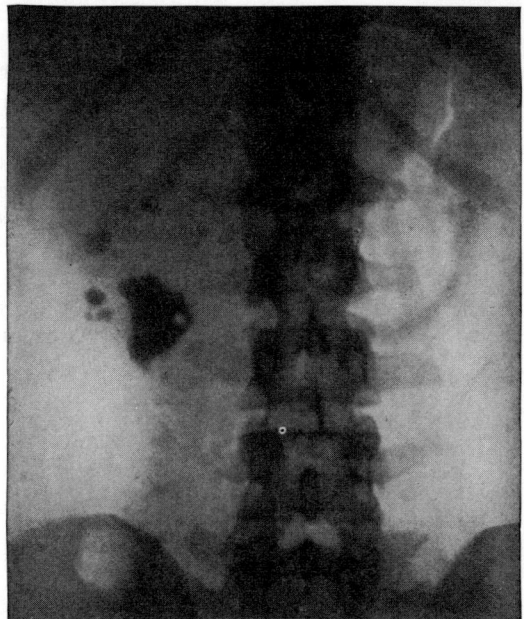

Fig. 73 X-ray showing calculi in right kidney.

sodium cellulose phosphate (5 g 3 times a day, with meals), which exchanges sodium for calcium in the gut.

Parathyroidectomy is performed in cases of hyperparathyroidism.

Calculi may be removed by operative means.

Other renal conditions

The kidney is sometimes the site of a **tumour** which may be malignant and in most cases the treatment is surgical.

N.B.—Provided one kidney is normal removal of a diseased one (nephrectomy) is not in itself detrimental to the health of the individual.

Tuberculosis may also affect one or both kidneys. The main symptoms are frequency of micturition, pain in the loin, haematuria and pyrexia. Tubercle bacilli may be found in the urine, a 24-hour specimen being necessary for this investigation. A non-functioning kidney may be removed by operation, but cases are treated with anti-tuberculous drugs and on the general lines employed in pulmonary tuberculosis.

Congenital cystic disease (Polycystic kidney) of the kidneys is an uncommon hereditary and often familial condition in which the kidneys become converted into large cystic masses like bunches of grapes. Cysts may be present in the liver and other organs. The disease tends to be slowly progressive and usually terminates with uraemia. Some cases may be suitable for renal transplantation.

Urethritis. Urethritis, inflammation of the urethra, causes scalding pain on micturition. It may be caused by the organisms which commonly cause urinary tract infections (see pyelitis, p. 343). In two instances, however, it is a venereal disease—gonococcal urethritis and non-specific urethritis. The association of non-specific urethritis with arthritis and conjunctivitis is known as Reiter's syndrome.

8 Diseases of the Nervous System

Introduction. Neurology is the study of organic nervous diseases and, to understand its principles, it is essential to correlate the anatomy and physiology of the nervous system with the common symptoms of its disorders.

Nervous tissue consists of cells which constitute the grey matter and fibres which form the white matter. Each nerve cell with its own fibres is called a **neurone.**

The important anatomical parts of the system are:

The cerebrum, the cerebellum, the brain-stem consisting of the mid-brain, pons and the medulla, the cranial nerves, the spinal cord, the peripheral nerves, the cerebrospinal fluid, the meninges.

The main points concerning each will be recapitulated.

The cerebrum. This portion of the brain, situated within the skull, is formed by the two cerebral hemispheres connected by the corpus callosum. Each hemisphere is described as having frontal, parietal, temporal and occipital lobes.

The surface of the cerebrum consists of grey matter containing nerve cells—the cerebral cortex. The interior is made up of nerve fibres and is referred to as the white matter.

The important activities of the cerebrum may be divided into psychic, motor and sensory, and the areas in which these functions are controlled have, to some extent, been localized.

It will be recalled that each motor and sensory area sends and receives impulses from the **opposite side** of the body.

One of the most important parts of the grey matter is the motor cortex, or precentral (Rolandic) area, situated just in front of the central sulcus (fissure of Rolando), which separates the frontal from the parietal lobes.

Among the important masses of grey matter buried deep in the white matter of each cerebral hemisphere are:

1. The **thalamus**, the cells of which register pain and also relay sensory

impulses (touch, heat, cold and muscle sense) from the spinal cord to the cerebral cortex.

2. The **hypothalamus**, lying below the thalamus in the base of the brain. In it are centred important functions, e.g.:

(*a*) Metabolic control of carbohydrate, fat and water.

(*b*) Regulation of body temperature.

(*c*) Control of pituitary hormones.

(*d*) Some personality and emotional reactions.

The cerebellum is situated behind and below the cerebral hemispheres. Among its important functions are the maintenance of posture and muscle tone.

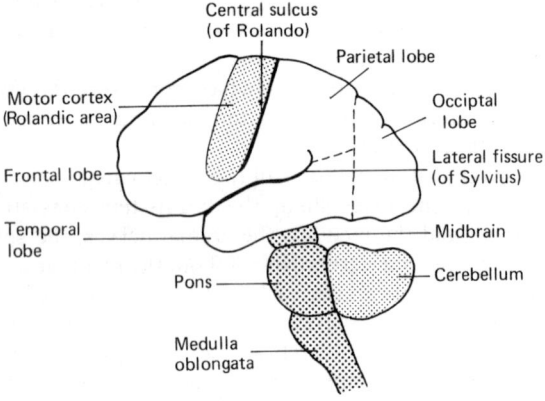

Fig. 74 Diagram illustrating the outer surface of the left cerebral hemisphere, the cerebellum and the brain stem.

The brain stem. The mid-brain, pons and medulla connect the cerebrum and cerebellum with the spinal cord. In addition to the important tracts of nerve fibres, passing up and down in their substance, they contain groups of nerve cells, among which are the respiratory centre, the vasomotor centre, the vomiting centre and the nuclei of various cranial nerves.

The cranial nerves are 12 in number on each side, and with the exception of the first two, they arise from the brain stem.

1st, the olfactory nerve, conveys the sensation of smell from the nose to the cerebral hemisphere.

2nd, the optic nerve, transmits vision from the retina to the brain.

3rd, 4th and 6th are concerned with movements of the eye.

5th, the trigeminal, is the sensory nerve of the face and front of the scalp but also supplies motor fibres to the jaw muscles.

7th, the facial nerve, supplies the muscles of the face.

8th, the auditory nerve, is the nerve of hearing and is also concerned with balance.

9th, the glosso-pharyngeal, is mainly the nerve of sensation to the mucous membrane of the pharynx.

10th, the vagus nerve, supplies the palate, pharynx, larynx, heart, oesophagus and stomach.

11th, the (spinal) accessory nerve, supplies the trapezius and sterno-mastoid muscles in the neck.

12th, the hypoglossal nerve, is the motor nerve of the tongue.

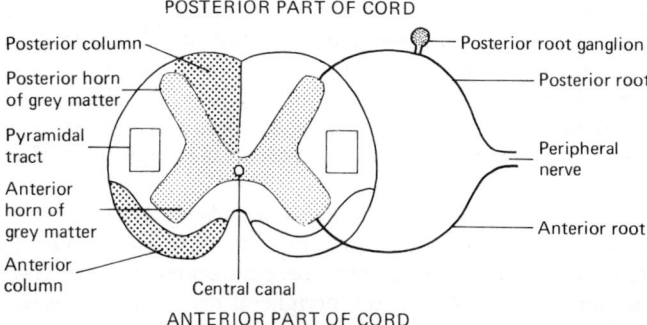

POSTERIOR PART OF CORD

Posterior column — Posterior root ganglion
Posterior horn of grey matter — Posterior root
Pyramidal tract — Peripheral nerve
Anterior horn of grey matter
Anterior column — Anterior root
Central canal

ANTERIOR PART OF CORD

Fig. 75 Diagram illustrating a cross-section of the spinal cord and showing the relative positions of the grey matter and various tracts of white matter.

The spinal cord. This extends from the first cervical to the level of the first lumbar vertebra and is enclosed within the spinal canal.

It consists of grey matter, arranged in an **H**-shape, surrounded by white matter. In this respect it differs from the brain in which the grey matter is situated on the surface. The white matter is made up of a number of important tracts of nerve fibres which convey impulses to and from the brain.

Reference to the diagram will show the arrangement of the grey matter and the important tracts. The portion of the cord situated towards the front of the body is called the anterior part; that behind, the posterior part; while the sides are referred to as the lateral parts. Thus, the grey matter is divided into anterior and posterior horns, and the white matter into anterior, lateral and posterior columns.

The motor path. The impulses which initiate voluntary muscular movement commence in the cells of the motor cortex (pre-central or Rolandic area). The fibres of these cells are collected together in the pyramidal tracts which descend through the internal capsule and the brain stem. In the lower medulla the majority of the fibres on each side cross over (decussate) and continue down the spinal cord in the lateral columns. These fibres end round the cells of the anterior horn of grey matter. New fibres arise from these cells and carry motor impulses to the muscles via the peripheral nerves.

The sensory path. Sensory impulses pass from the peripheral nerves to the posterior horn of grey matter in the spinal cord. Fibres carrying the sensations of position, vibration and touch travel upwards in the posterior columns and cross over in the medulla. Fibres conveying the sensations of pain and temperature, however, cross over at once in the cord and travel in the opposite lateral and anterior columns (spinothalamic tracts). Both these sensory columns become united in the upper brain stem and in the internal capsule are very close to the motor fibres.

It can be seen that each side of the brain receives the sensory impulses and controls the movements of the opposite half of the body.

The peripheral nerves. The motor impulses leave the spinal cord by the anterior nerve roots, while the sensory impulses enter by the posterior roots. These two roots become united as they leave the spinal canal and constitute the peripheral nerves which pass to all parts of the body.

Reflex action. The nurse learns about reflex action in physiology, but since this function plays an important part in the examination of the nervous system and disorders frequently occur in nervous diseases the main principles will be illustrated.

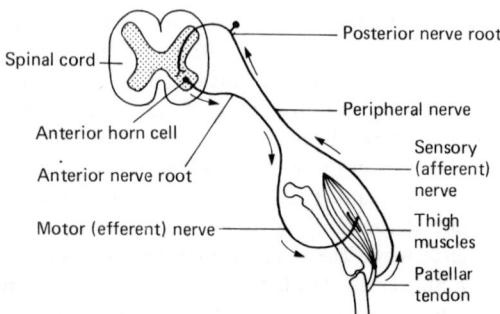

Fig. 76 Diagram illustrating reflex action (knee jerk).

When a stimulus reaches a sensory nerve, for example a sharp tap applied to the patella tendon, an impulse passes up its fibres and enters the posterior horn of grey matter in the spinal cord. In addition to passing up the sensory tracts to the brain, the impulse is conveyed directly to the motor cells in the anterior horn, whence it is passed on via the anterior nerve root and motor nerve to the thigh muscles which contract and move the knee-joint, without any conscious effort on the part of the individual. This reflex, the knee jerk, is commonly employed in testing the functions of the nervous system.

The cerebrospinal fluid. This is a clear fluid secreted within the ventricles of the brain by the choroid plexus. The fluid also fills the subarachnoid space which surrounds the outer surface of the brain and spinal cord. In order that it may pass from the ventricles to the subarachnoid space there is a small opening called the foramen of Magendie situated in the roof of the brain stem. If this opening becomes blocked, as it may in some cases of meningitis, fluid accumulates within the ventricles producing the condition of hydrocephalus (p. 375).

Owing to the intimate association of the cerebrospinal fluid with the nervous tissues and the meninges, disease of these structures is often associated with changes in the fluid which may be removed for examination by the procedure known as lumbar puncture.

The following are some of the changes which may occur in the cerebrospinal fluid as a result of disease:

1. It may be turbid or purulent in cases of meningitis.
2. A smaller increase in the number of cells occurs in poliomyelitis.
3. Blood is present in cerebral haemorrhage, subarachnoid haemorrhage due to intra-cranial aneurysm and some cases of head injury.
4. The pressure and amount of protein are often raised in cerebral tumours.
5. The Wassermann reaction is positive in cerebral syphilis and tabes dorsalis.

The meninges. The brain and spinal cord are covered by membranes, called the dura mater, the arachnoid mater and the pia mater. The dura mater or outer layer is closely applied to the skull and bony walls of the spinal canal. The cerebrospinal fluid circulates in the subarachnoid space, between the arachnoid and pia mater. Inflammation of the meninges is called meningitis.

Examination of the nervous system

Routine examination of the nervous system includes estimation of the cerebral functions, and testing of the cranial nerves, the motor and sensory systems.

The following accessories may be required:
1. Electric torch, in order to test the reaction of the pupils to light.
2. Patella hammer. This is used in the examination of the tendon reflexes.
3. Ophthalmoscope. By means of this instrument it is possible to examine the retina, its blood vessels and, especially, the entrance of the optic nerve.
4. A pin, cottonwool and test-tubes containing hot and cold water for testing sensation. In addition, a tuning fork for estimating the sense of vibration may be needed.

Special methods of examination include: x-ray of the skull and spine, lumbar puncture, cistern puncture, arteriography, ventriculography, encephalography and electroencephalography.

Lumbar puncture. Lumbar puncture consists of passing a special needle between the spines of the lumbar vertebrae into the subarachnoid space for the purpose of withdrawing cerebrospinal fluid.

It must be emphasized that this can only be done with ease when the patient is correctly placed and that the task of arranging and maintaining the position is frequently allotted to the nurse. He should lie on one side (preferably his left) close to the edge of the bed. The back must be at right angles to the floor and care must be taken that the uppermost shoulder does not fall forwards.

The spine is then arched, the neck being bent forwards and the knees drawn up until they almost touch the chin. The ideal posture is obtained if the nurse, standing opposite to the doctor, places one hand on the nape of the neck and the other behind the knees and draws them as closely together as possible without hurting the patient.

The head may be supported on a low pillow, while blanket and night clothes are removed from the operation site and the iliac crest. The latter is used as a landmark to determine the level at which the puncture is to be made.

The skin over the lumbar region and the uppermost iliac crest is cleaned with ether, sterilized with iodine and the area surrounded with sterile towels. The point generally chosen for inserting the needle is between the spines of the 3rd and 4th lumbar vertebrae which corresponds to a line joining the iliac crests. At this point the skin is anaesthetized by a local anaesthetic. A lumbar puncture needle is introduced until it reaches the subarachnoid space and cerebrospinal fluid flows after the withdrawal of the stylet. Fluid is collected in a sterile test-tube and sent for examination. After the removal of the needle, the puncture is sealed with collodion or covered with a sterile dressing secured by strapping.

The pressure of the cerebrospinal fluid may be measured by attaching a glass manometer tube to the needle.

Withdrawal of cerebrospinal fluid may be followed by severe headache. In order to avoid this the patient should be kept lying flat, preferably prone, for a period of 6 to 12 hours after the operation. If headache occurs owing to the lowered intracranial pressure,

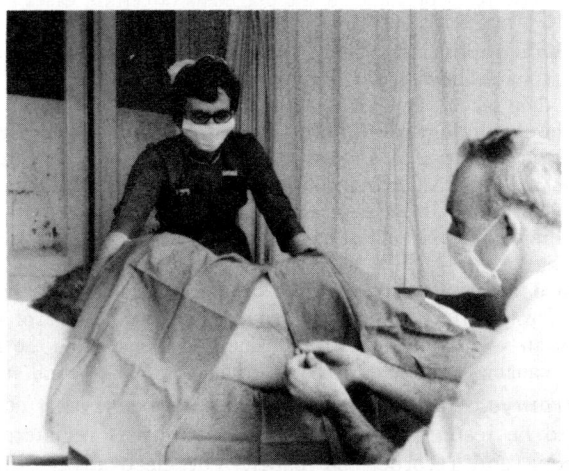

Fig. 77 Lumbar puncture: the position of the patient.

the foot of the bed is raised on blocks, plenty of fluids should be given and aspirin or similar analgesic drugs administered.

Lumbar puncture is performed for the following purposes:

1. Withdrawal of cerebrospinal fluid for examination in the diagnosis of nervous disease.
2. For the purpose of injecting drugs, e.g. streptomycin or penicillin, in the treatment of certain types of meningitis.
3. To produce spinal anaesthesia, special drugs being injected when the needle is in the epidural space.
4. For the injection of 'Myodil' or radio-opaque solution in order to ascertain by means of x-rays the presence and level of a tumour pressing on the spinal cord.

Cistern puncture. This is a special operation for withdrawing cerebrospinal fluid used only in selected cases. The needle is introduced into the subarachnoid space at the base of the brain by inserting it between the occiput and spine of the axis vertebra.

Radio-opaque solutions and other drugs may also be introduced by this route.

Ventriculography. The scalp is shaved and sterilized; procaine is injected and a short incision made. A small hole is drilled in the skull and a needle is then inserted through the brain substance until it reaches the ventricles. Cerebrospinal fluid is withdrawn and air introduced. An x-ray picture shows the outline and size of the ventricles.

This procedure is of value in the diagnosis of certain cases of cerebral tumour.

Encephalography. After lumbar puncture, air is injected with a syringe into the subarachnoid space and allowed to rise to the skull. An x-ray picture is then taken.

Electroencephalogram (EEG). This is a record of electrical waves obtained from the brain by the use of a special apparatus. Variations from the normal may be of value in the diagnosis of epilepsy and cerebral tumour. An 'alpha' rhythm of 10 cycles per second is the normal wave-form obtained from the brain when the subject has his eyes closed and is not concentrating on anything.

Cerebral arteriography. A radio-opaque substance may be injected into the carotid artery in order to render the blood vessels of the brain visible on an x-ray plate. This is of value in demonstrating the site of an aneurysm causing subarachnoid haemorrhage, and in cerebral tumours.

Electromyography. A special needle-electrode is inserted into the muscle to be tested and its electrical activity is registered on an oscilloscope and recorded on paper. The electromyogram (EMG) so obtained may be used, for example, to distinguish between lesions of the lower motor neurone and of muscle (myopathy).

The **conduction time** of a nerve may be measured by timing the response to an electrical stimulus. It is prolonged if the nerve is diseased (neuropathy).

Echo-encephalography. Ultra-high frequency sound waves, which are inaudible to the human ear, are transmitted into the skull and are reflected from some of the structures, producing echoes. These are registered on an oscilloscope and photographed. Displacement of the brain (by a space-occupying lesion) may thereby be detected and the side of the lesion may be deduced. The procedure has no ill-effects on the patient.

Brain scanning (gamma-encephalography). The brain may be scanned after the intravenous injection of a tracer dose of a radioactive isotope, e.g. technetium. Tumour tissue concentrates the isotope more rapidly than does normal brain tissue and therefore shows up as an area of increased gamma-ray emission.

The signs and symptoms of organic nervous disease

Symptoms due to diseases of the nervous system may be considered as those due to:
1. Intra-cranial disorders.
2. Spinal cord disorders.
3. Disorders of special senses.
4. Peripheral nerve disorders.

1. Disorders of cerebral function

Alterations in the functions of the brain commonly result in disturbances of consciousness, behaviour, memory, speech, movement and sensation. These may take place as a result of organic disease of the brain due to injury, tumour, degeneration or inflammation or may depend on toxic states or disorders of the ductless glands. In many cases of mental disease, however, the actual cause of alteration in behaviour is unknown.

The important conditions associated with organic disease will be considered.

Loss of consciousness

Loss of consciousness may be partial **(stupor)** or complete **(coma)**. In some cases it is associated with convulsions. Unconsciousness due to sudden lack of blood to the brain has already been referred to in connection with fainting attacks. This is usually of a transitory nature.

The common **causes** of loss of consciousness are:

1. Alteration in the blood supply to the brain resulting in lack of oxygen (cerebral anoxia), e.g. fainting attacks, Adams-Stokes disease (p. 107), asphyxia.

2. Gross damage to the brain substance by injury (fractured skull), cerebrovascular accident (i.e. cerebral haemorrhage, embolism or thrombosis), subarachnoid haemorrhage, cerebral tumour, concussion.

3. Inflammation of the brain (meningitis, encephalitis, brain abscess).

4. Epilepsy.

5. Poisoning, especially by alcohol, anaesthetics, opium, morphine, coal gas (carbon monoxide) and hypnotic drugs, such as barbiturates.

6. General metabolic disturbances producing a toxic effect on the brain, e.g. uraemia (p. 338), eclampsia, diabetic coma (p. 450), hypoglycaemia (p. 448), liver failure (hepatic coma, p. 255).

7. Shock due to injury, electric shock.

N.B.—In many respects this list is similar to that given for the causes of convulsions and fits. The main additions are the poisons, diabetic coma and electric shock.

'Aide Memoire' for common causes of coma:

A. Apoplexy, alcohol, asphyxia, anoxia, anaesthetics, Adams-Stokes syndrome.

E. Epilepsy, electric shock, eclampsia, encephalitis.

I. Injury, insulin.

O. Opium and Other Poisons!

U. Uraemia.

D. Diabetes, drugs.

Cerebral compression

In some cases of head injury, cerebral haemorrhage and tumour **(space-occupying lesions)** the loss of consciousness is accompanied by a rise in the pressure within the skull which is followed by compression of the brain substance. This takes place because the skull is like a rigid box and if, for example, haemorrhage occurs the effused blood can only occupy space at the expense of the brain matter which in consequence becomes compressed. A similar state will be present if the brain becomes oedematous and therefore increased in volume. The condition of raised intracranial pressure is accompanied by increasing headache and later by coma, with stertorous breathing, a slow pulse and vomiting.

In the other conditions causing loss of consciousness the nerve cells are poisoned by the action of toxic substances and cease to function.

Convulsions or fits

It has been seen (p. 22) that irritation of the brain at the onset of febrile disorders in children may result in loss of consciousness accompanied by involuntary muscular movements.

The following is a summary of the factors most commonly met in clinical work which may be regarded as being liable to produce convulsions.

1. Organic disease of the brain: Injury, inflammatory conditions such as encephalitis and cerebral abscess, syphilis of the brain (GPI), tumours of the brain, both primary and secondary.

2. Circulatory disorders: Hypertensive cerebral attacks.
   Adams-Stokes syndrome (p. 107).

3. Metabolic disorders: Excessive water retention.
   Asphyxia.
   Cerebral anaemia.
   Hypoglycaemia.
   Tetany (disordered calcium metabolism).

4. Toxic causes: Acute infections in childhood.
   Uraemia.
   Eclampsia (Toxaemia of pregnancy).
   Drugs, such as ether, lead, cocaine. Withdrawal of drugs such as barbiturates and tranquillizers in patients accustomed to large doses.

5. Idiopathic epilepsy: The cause of which is not fully explained.

Fits are generally sudden in onset and often unexpected, although in some cases of epilepsy the patient may have a warning of their approach which is called an aura. The individual, if standing, will fall down and may injure himself. In addition, the violent involuntary movements or spasms may result in further damage. The teeth are clenched and foaming at the mouth may occur. Not infrequently the tongue is bitten and urine and faeces may be passed.

Hysterical fits. Another type of fit is that seen in hysteria (p. 405). In this condition, although the patient appears to be unconscious the movements are more purposeful. He takes care not to hurt himself and, if held, the movements tend to get more violent and he struggles deliberately to get away. Incontinence of urine does not occur, the tongue is not bitten although occasionally the lips and cheeks may be injured. If the patient is left alone the movements tend to subside.

The treatment of coma and fits. The nurse is often the first person to observe sudden loss of consciousness or the onset of a fit, and these are, therefore, matters of great importance to her.

In the first place she should send for medical assistance and at the same time observe carefully the state of the patient and any changes which occur, in order that she may inform the doctor on his arrival. She should also know what to do during the interval.

(a) Coma

In a case of coma the following facts should, if possible, be ascertained from relatives:

1. Previous history of disease, e.g. high blood pressure, nephritis or diabetes.
2. Previous history of similar attacks, e.g. epilepsy.
3. The mode of onset of coma, i.e. sudden or gradual.
4. The presence of any drugs or poisons on or near the patient.

GENERAL EXAMINATION OF THE PATIENT. The presence or absence of cyanosis, stertorous breathing, injury about the head, and bleeding from the nose, ears or mouth should be noted.

Acetone or alcohol may be detected in the breath, although the presence of the latter does not necessarily indicate intoxication as it may have been administered by a well-meaning onlooker. The staining caused by corrosive poisons may be seen about the mouth or lips.

EXAMINATION FOR PARALYSIS. The state of the limbs should be compared with each other. In cases of hemiplegia it will be found that those of the affected side are either limp or abnormally stiff. One half of the face may be paralysed and the corresponding cheek puffed out with each expiration.

The eyes must be examined for the presence of squints and the state of the pupils and their reaction to light ascertained. In cases of coma the pupils may be dilated or contracted and are often unequal in size and fail to react to light. (Contraction of the pupils to 'pinpoint' size is a constant feature of morphine poisoning, while in overdosage with atropine and belladonna they are widely dilated.)

OTHER POINTS. The pulse and respiration and the temperature should be recorded. A specimen of urine must be obtained, by catheterization if necessary, and tested in the routine manner, special note being made of the presence of albumin, sugar or acetone.

In cases of suspected poisoning all vomitus must be carefully collected and saved together with any bottles which may have contained poison.

Further investigation by the doctor may include examination of the eyes with an ophthalmoscope, estimation of blood pressure, and lumbar puncture, so that the necessary apparatus for these procedures should be at hand.

Treatment of coma. The nurse can only carry out 'First Aid' treatment herself.

Whenever possible the patient should be placed prone or semi-prone with the head turned to one side because in this position the tongue is less liable to fall back and obstruct the airway to the larynx and, if vomiting takes place, the chance of food being aspirated into the larynx is diminished. The foot of the bed may also be raised. A sucker should be available.

It may be necessary to pull the tongue forwards with forceps, but care should be taken not to bruise the organ. False teeth must be taken out, the clothing about the neck should be loosened and the shoes removed. Cold water may be applied to the face but on no account should stimulants be given unless ordered by the doctor, as harm may be done in certain cases.

The patient should be kept warm with blankets in order to prevent loss of heat from the body, which occurs rapidly in unconscious patients. Serious burns have resulted from the misuse of hot-water bottles. They should therefore be avoided in unconscious or paralysed patients.

If coma is prolonged, the nursing of the case is of utmost importance. The actual treatment will to some extent depend on the cause of the condition. The patient is nursed flat in bed or with one pillow. His position is changed every 2 to 4 hours in order to avoid congestion of the lungs, while great care must be taken of the skin of the back and over pressure points. Feeding with a nasal tube is generally necessary and may be supplemented by intravenous fluids or subcutaneous saline with 'Hyalase'.

Prolonged unconsciousness is associated either with retention or incontinence of urine and faeces. The bladder must, therefore, be watched carefully and over-distension avoided by catherization. Enemata may be required for constipation. When incontinence is present the patient must be kept scrupulously clean and changed frequently or the condition of the skin will deteriorate rapidly.

(b) Fits

The nurse should observe the nature of the movements, how they start and whether both sides of the body are affected.

The important point in treatment is to prevent the patient from injuring himself. He should, therefore, be laid upon the ground or prevented from falling out of bed, and objects which he might knock over should be removed. The clothing about the neck should be loosened. A piece of wood, a cork, handkerchief, or the handle of a spoon wrapped in lint should, when possible, be placed between the teeth in order to prevent the tongue being bitten. When this is being done, care must be taken that teeth are not dislodged and swallowed or aspirated into the air passages. It is often possible to slip a suitable gag into position when the muscles of the jaw relax momentarily but force should not be used.

The severity of movements may be modified by gentle restraint, but great force should not be used.

Epilepsy

The true nature of this disease is usually unknown (hence the term idiopathic epilepsy) but it appears to be due to irritation of the cerebral cortex by some toxic or metabolic factor. Occasionally there is a familial tendency and it may have its onset at any age. In severe cases mental deterioration necessitating confinement to an institution may eventually develop.

Two types are described, the minor and major. In **minor epilepsy** (petit mal) there is momentary loss of consciousness without convulsions, which the patient may describe as a 'black out'.

Major epilepsy is characterized by loss of consciousness accompanied by fits, the main features of which have already been described, viz.:

1. A warning or **aura**, such as giddiness, noises in the head, or a tingling sensation, is felt in a number of cases.
2. Convulsions of sudden onset.
    (*a*) The **tonic stage**, i.e. general rigidity with the muscles firmly contracted lasting about half a minute.
    (*b*) The **clonic stage**, i.e. rhythmic twitchings of the muscles, which contract and relax alternately. Frothing at the mouth occurs, urine and faeces may be passed and the tongue bitten.
    (*c*) The **stage of coma**, i.e. the limbs are limp (flaccid): the patient remains unconscious for a varying period and may gradually pass into a deep sleep.

Sometimes on recovery from a fit an epileptic will perform actions or carry out work of which he is unaware. He may, for example, start to undress in public, presumably because in his clouded state of consciousness he feels drowsy and wants to go to bed. This may have unfortunate legal consequences.

Crimes of violence are sometimes committed in this state of **post-epileptic automatism.**

A succession of fits may occur rapidly one after the other without the return of consciousness, a condition known as **status epilepticus.**

Focal or jacksonian epilepsy. This consists of attacks of local muscular spasms or twitchings without loss of consciousness and are usually due to some local damage to the brain, e.g. following head injury. Sometimes sensory symptoms occur.

Treatment. 1. The management of the patient during an attack is described above.

The medical attendant may order anticonvulsant drugs. Deep intramuscular injections of paraldehyde, 5 to 10 ml (not more than 5 ml in one injection site), or soluble phenobarbitone, 200 mg (3 grains), may be given. These may have to be repeated in status epilepticus, which may also require intravenous pentothal, or whiffs of chloroform. A drug which may be effective is intravenous diazepam ('Valium'). If status epilepticus fails to respond to intra-muscular paraldehyde etc., and unconsciousness is prolonged, electrolyte disturbances and pulmonary congestion may require treatment.

2. Between attacks: Epilepsy may be largely controlled by the use of special anti-convulsant drugs. The dose of each is adjusted to the patient, but it is of the greatest importance that they should be taken regularly over a long period, e.g. at least two to three years after the occurrence of the last fit.

They include (doses are approximate):

Phenobarbitone ('Luminal'). Dose: 30 to 120 mg.
Phemitone ('Prominal', methyl phenobarbitone). Dose: 200 mg.
Phenytoin ('Epanutin', 'Dilantin'). Dose: 50 to 200 mg daily.
Methoin (Mesontoin). Dose: 100 mg.
Primidone ('Mysoline'). Dose: 250 to 500 mg.
Ethosuximide ('Zarontin'). Dose: 250 to 1500 mg daily.

Troxidone ('Tridione') is liable to produce toxic reactions. Like Ethosuximide it is only used in the treatment of petit mal.

'Epanutin' sometimes produces toxic symptoms such as rashes, giddiness and double vision.

In many instances a combination of two or more drugs is used.

3. GENERAL POINTS. The patient should, as far as possible, lead a normal life but alcohol should be forbidden. He should avoid working with machinery, swimming, car driving, and give up any occupation or pastime which is likely to be dangerous to himself or others if a fit should occur. A bath should only be taken when he can be under observation and open fires should be heavily guarded.

In doubtful cases the diagnosis may sometimes be confirmed by the electroencephalogram (EEG).

Fits or convulsions, with or without complete loss of consciousness, are relatively common occurrences in medical practice.

It has been seen (p. 22) that irritation of the brain at the onset of febrile disorders in some children may result in loss of consciousness accompanied by involuntary muscular movements. It has also been mentioned that epileptic fits, uraemic twitchings and cerebral seizures should be regarded as convulsions of a special type. In fact there are a number of conditions, one of the characteristic features of which is the occurrence of fits. It is not always easy to explain why these fits should occur in some individuals and not in others.

Some light has, however, been thrown on the subject by the use of the **electroencephalogram** (p. 356). This apparatus shows that in a normal individual a regular series of smooth waves are being constantly transmitted from the nerve cells of the brain. These waves represent a regular discharge of nervous impulses or nerve 'energy' which is produced by the nerve cells and stored within them. The fact that these waves are rhythmic and regular in appearance indicates that this discharge of energy is carefully controlled by the cells and only allowed to escape in this regular manner.

In patients who suffer from epilepsy, and also in some other cerebral conditions, such as cerebral tumour, the electroence-phalogram shows that these regular waves are interrupted at times by irregular waves of larger size. This indicates that there is an abnormal and improperly controlled discharge of nervous energy from the brain cells of these subjects and that their nerve cells are less stable than those of normal individuals. During an actual epileptic fit such waves are grossly exaggerated, suggesting that there is then a sort of explosive discharge of energy which is quite uncontrolled.

Definite but less-marked abnormality of these waves may be observed in relatives of epileptics and other persons who have never had any fits. In other words, the presence of these abnormal waves indicates that the individual is a potential epileptic who is liable to have fits if the explosive type of discharge of nervous energy happens to be brought on by a sufficiently strong stimulus.

The occurrence of fits will, therefore, depend on two factors:

1. The stability of the nerve cells normally is such that only small, regular and controlled discharges of nervous energy take place. As might be expected, there are varying degrees of stability and instability. As instability increases there will be a certain threshold or level at which the discharge will become so irregular and excessive or liberated with such explosive force that a fit will be produced.

2. Although an individual has unstable nerve cells of this type which are discharging irregular and improperly controlled impulses some stimulus is necessary to produce the explosive variety of

discharge which results in an actual fit. Such stimuli or epilepsy-producing agents are quite numerous and different ones may operate in individual cases. Some are unknown and are responsible for the cases which are described as 'idiopathic epilepsy' in which recurrent fits may occur at longer or shorter intervals throughout a patient's life. Others occur as a result of actual organic disease of the brain, e.g. cerebral tumour, cerebral syphilis (GPI) or following head injuries. Another type of fit-producing stimulus is toxic in nature, e.g. acute infections in childhood, uraemia and eclampsia. Artificial stimuli are also available. These will be mentioned later.

It follows, therefore, that a fit is produced by a combination of these two factors. In one instance, it may be the result of a relatively minor agent acting on particularly unstable cells. In another, the reverse may operate and a very potent epilepsy-producing agent may be acting on cells which are only slightly if at all abnormal in their discharge of energy.

Another point which will help to explain some of the features observed in different types of fits is the following. The normal discharge of energy from a cell or group of cells tends to follow a normal route of distribution throughout the nervous system. The abnormal explosive type of discharge, however, spreads to other cells in the vicinity and may cause them to discharge their energy in the same way, and so on over large areas of the brain. This results in the generalized convulsions so commonly observed in epilepsy. If, on the other hand, the spread is limited, only localized twitchings without loss of consciousness may occur.

This theory may be illustrated by certain tests which are sometimes carried out to prove the presence of epilepsy. For example, giving a large quantity of water and a dose of pituitary extract, which temporarily prevents its normal excretion, causes water retention. This is an epilepsy-producing agent and if the epilepsy threshold is low, that is if the individual is an epileptic or a potential one, a fit will be produced which would not occur in a normal person. Similarly drugs such as cardiazol (leptazol) and overdosage with insulin (producing hypoglycaemia) are capable of producing fits.

In some epileptics external stimuli such as a shock, a loud noise or a sudden blow may bring on this abnormal discharge of nervous energy which will terminate in a fit. As has been indicated, if the spread of this abnormal discharge is localized only minor or local symptoms will occur; if it extends widely over the cerebral cortex, generalized convulsions with loss of consciousness may be expected.

The effect of the drugs used in the treatment of epilepsy is to lessen the instability of the nerve cells and to diminish the abnormal impulses arising from them. At the same time the spread of an explosive eruption may be limited so that even if a fit does occur it is less severe and less prolonged.

Insomnia or sleeplessness

An adequate amount of sleep is essential for bodily and mental health and it is of great importance in the treatment of all forms of disease.

Insomnia or sleeplessness is a problem which is frequently presented to the nurse and she should be thoroughly familiar with its types, causes and treatment.

Inability to acquire sufficient sleep implies not only an inadequate amount but also failure to obtain sound and restful sleep. Three main types of insomnia may be described:

1. Difficulty in getting to sleep.
2. Sleep is normal in onset but the patient awakes early and is unable to fall off again.
3. Sleep is interrupted by disturbing dreams.

The causes may be divided into two main groups:

1. Those due to physical disorders.
2. Those due to psychological disorders.

1. Insomnia due to physical disorders. Organic disease is responsible for many cases of sleeplessness by the production of pain or physical discomfort. Pain may result from inflammation, injury or the involvement of nerves in disease processes.

Discomfort sufficient to prevent sleep may also be due to gastro-intestinal disorders, cardiac conditions, frequency of micturition, dyspnoea, cough and itching of the skin (pruritis) and is present in various toxic states and in febrile disorders.

2. Insomnia due to physchological disorders. Depression, anxiety concerning private or business matters, emotional disturbances, nervous exhaustion, hysteria and insanity may all be causes of insomnia.

In many instances of insomnia due to physical disorders, the psychological factor is superimposed and therefore the latter must be considered in the treatment of all cases.

Many people suffer more from worrying about the lack of sleep than from the insomnia itself.

3. Organic disease of the brain.

Treatment of insomnia. The patient should be made as comfortable as possible and his surroundings should be conducive to sleep.

The bedroom must be quiet, warm and well ventilated. Clocks should be removed and windows and doors wedged to prevent rattling. Lights should be turned off or carefully shaded. The bedclothes must be adequate but not heavy—additional warmth, if required, being supplied by hot-water bottles or an electric blanket.

A warm bath on retiring promotes sleep in some individuals.

A light meal consisting of soup, Bovril, cocoa, milk or a preparation such as Ovaltine tends to produce drowsiness, but great care should be taken not to overload the stomach, while stimulants such as tea or coffee are avoided. The effect of alcohol varies; in some patients hot whisky or brandy in water is of great value, while in others it produces wakefulness. It must be remembered that alcohol increases the effect of barbiturates and many other drugs.

An attempt must always be made to treat the cause of the condition. For example, in flatulence a drink of hot water, a little peppermint or a carminative mixture may bring relief by the expulsion of gas. The pain of duodenal ulcer is relieved by an additional feed and a dose of magnesium trisilicate or similar antacid. A linctus or cough lozenge may be required. The application of hot-water bottles, poultices or electric pads to painful areas is useful.

Drugs. These may be used in insomnia either for their effect in relieving pain and, thereby, permitting natural sleep (analgesics) or by their action in depressing the sensitivity of the nervous system (hypnotics). Some drugs such as morphine combine both properties.

In no case must they be given without the instructions of the medical attendant, and they should not be repeated or continued without his advice for, in many instances, drug habits are commenced by their injudicious administration.

The following drugs are used as pure hypnotics and have little effect on pain:

1. Barbiturates, e.g. butobarbitone ('Soneryl'), quinalbarbitone ('Seconal'), amylobarbitone ('Amytal'), phenobarbitone (luminal).
2. Chloral, 'Welldorm' (dichloral phenazone), and paraldehyde.
3. Other non-barbiturate sedatives such as carbromal, 'Doriden', 'nodular', methaqualone and diphenhydramine ('Mandrax') nitrazepan ('Mogadon').
4. 'Tranquillizing' drugs, e.g. Meprobamate ('Equanil').

Morphine and various preparations of opium, e.g. nepenthe, combine analgesic with hypnotic effects, while aspirin or paracetamol ('Panadol') is of value in relieving minor degrees of pain. Pethidine may also be given for severe pain.

The nurse should keep a careful record of the number of hours sleep and should do everything possible to induce sleep before administering a drug.

Delirium

Delirium is a mental disorder of a transitory nature. It is frequently an accompaniment of the febrile state, but may occur in seriously ill patients without pyrexia or as a result of poisoning by certain drugs (e.g. belladonna); i.e. it may be due to the effect of toxins or drugs upon the brain.

Three types are seen:

1. Maniacal delirium, in which the patient is noisy, violent and irrational.

2. The low muttering delirium of the later stages of exhausting febrile illnesses such as typhoid fever (i.e. the typhoid state, p. 43), in which the patient lies curled up in bed and mutters incoherently.

3. Delirium tremens, a special type occurring in patients who habitually take large quantities of alcohol. It may come on after a drinking bout, during a febrile illness such as pneumonia or following an injury. The characteristics are a furred tongue, restlessness, shaking of the limbs (tremor) associated with delusions, hallucinations and disorders of behaviour. **Delusions** are false beliefs not amenable to reason, the patient imagining that people are talking about him, that he is being persecuted by some secret society, that the doctor or nurse are relatives or old friends and so on (see also p. 397). **Hallucinations** are false perceptions of the senses, commonly those of hearing or sight. The patient may state that he hears voices, bells or wireless messages, or that he can see someone under the bed or hiding in the corner of the room. In severe cases of delirium tremens he imagines he can see snakes gliding on the floor, mice or rats running about the room or over the bed and spiders crawling on the wall, etc. and he is acutely terrified.

Delusions and hallucinations, in addition to occurring in delirium, are also found in many cases of mental disorder.

In delirium tremens the patient is often abusive, violent and restless. He may spit about the room, be dirty in habits and refuse food. He tends, however, to become progressively weaker and, unless sleep can be obtained and nourishment administered, the condition may prove fatal.

Treatment. In acute maniacal delirium efforts must be made to keep the patient in bed and to prevent him from causing injury to himself and others. Persuasion tends to be more effective than coercion. In severe cases, some form of mechanical restraint may be necessary until sedative drugs have been administered and taken effect. Those frequently employed are haloperidol, diazepam, paraldehyde and chlormethizole. In severe cases morphine or hyoscine may be required. If delirium is due to pyrexia, tepid sponging and applications of cold compresses or an ice-bag to the head are valuable.

Low muttering delirium may require treatment with stimulants and efforts are made to maintain the strength of the patient by administering frequent small liquid feeds.

Careful nursing is necessary in delirium tremens. Drugs are given to induce sleep and if the patient refuses to take chloral or similar sedatives by mouth, 'Librium,' morphine, hyoscine, phenobarbitone or paraldehyde must be given by injection. Chlorpromazine ('Largactil') is particularly useful. As a rule, alcohol is absolutely forbidden, but in some cases it is found easier to withdraw it gradually.

Corticotrophin (ACTH) and steroids are of value in this condition. Injections of vitamin B are also given.

Fluid nourishment should be given freely and in a few instances nasal feeding is necessary.

The nurse should be careful to watch for the early signs of this condition in any patient who is known to have been a heavy drinker, especially in cases of pneumonia or injury. If the doctor is informed and treatment commenced early it is more likely to be successful than in the advanced stages.

There is a liability to heart failure, so that the attendants should endeavour to avoid struggling with the patient. It is often possible to humour him and he may then be kept under control by occupying his mind by means of writing materials, paper to tear up or by suggesting that, by some childish form of 'make-believe', he is carrying on his normal occupation.

Headache

Headache is a common symptom of many disorders and although usually of trivial importance, in a number of cases it is associated with serious organic disease.

It may be due to increased intra-cranial pressure and to local lesions of the brain, including cerebral tumour, cerebral abscess, meningitis, also nasal sinusitis, and is then persistent and severe.

It also occurs as a result of toxaemia in acute infections, especially typhoid fever and influenza; anaemia, alcoholism and lead poisoning. Some cases are due to cardiac disease, hypertension or eye disease, e.g. iritis. Headache is often complained of in anxiety states.

Migraine is a condition in which headaches recur at intervals and are frequently associated with vomiting and disturbances of vision. The headache usually affects only one side of the head and may last for many hours. Transient hemiplegia or visual loss occasionally occurs (hemiplegic migraine and hemianopic migraine).

Heredity is often a factor. Otherwise little is known about the causes of migraine. Allergy and reactions to tyramine (as in cheese) are among the causes suggested to be operating in some individuals. It is thought that a spasm of the cerebral arteries, followed by dilatation, accounts for the symptoms. It tends to occur in intelligent, perfectionistic personalities.

For the treatment of severe headache the patient should be placed in a dark, quiet room. In addition to dealing as far as possible with the cause of the condition, relief may be obtained by cold compresses to the head, attention to the bowels and the administration of drugs such as aspirin, codeine, paracetamol and caffeine either alone or in combination with each other. **Ergotamine tartrate** ('Femergin') is commonly used in migraine. Preparations containing ergotamine may be given by injection, by aerosol inhalation, by suppository and by mouth. It must be used with great caution in patients with arteriosclerosis, during pregnancy and in the presence of hepatic or renal disease.

Attacks regularly associated with menstruation may be relieved by progesterone.

Clonidine ('Dixarit'), 0·025 mg to 0·075 mg twice daily, taken regularly, may prevent or reduce the frequency of migraine attacks in some patients.

Another drug used on a long-term basis for the prevention of attacks is methysergide ('Deseril') but unfortunately this drug may cause retroperitoneal fibrosis which, by obstructing the ureters, can lead to renal failure.

Disorders of speech

Speech is a complicated function of the brain which is closely connected with the powers of reading, writing and hearing. Thus, a patient may be unable to express himself in spoken words, he may lose the power of understanding written words (word-blindness) or may fail to interpret what is said to him (word-deafness).

Loss of the ability to comprehend the ideas conveyed by words or the power to express ideas in words is called **aphasia.**

On the other hand, he may know exactly what he wants to say but owing to a defect in the nerves or muscles of the tongue and larynx, he is unable to articulate the words properly and to produce the normal sounds: this type of speech defect is called **dysarthria.** It should always be remembered that patients with speech defects may fully comprehend what is said in their hearing.

The function of speech in right-handed individuals is controlled by the left side of the brain, and aphasia is frequently seen accompanying paralysis of the right side of the body (hemiplegia) as a result of lesions of the left cerebral hemisphere.

2. Disorders due to defective function of the cerebrum, spinal cord or peripheral nerves

Disorders of movement

Disorders of movement may occur as a result of disease of the brain, spinal cord or peripheral nerves. In fact, a lesion in any part of the path from the precentral (Rolandic) area in the cerebral cortex to the endings of the motor nerves in the muscles will, depending upon its extent and severity, cause either weakness or complete abolition of muscular power. When some voluntary movement of a group of muscles is possible we speak of **paresis** or partial paralysis. When there is complete absence of movement it is called **paralysis**.

Almost any muscle or group of muscles in the body may become paralysed, but commonly the condition is confined to one or more limbs.

The following terms are used:

(a) Monoplegia—paralysis of one limb.

(b) Hemiplegia—paralysis of the arm and leg on one side of the body only.

(c) Paraplegia—paralysis of both legs. (The lower half of the body is frequently involved including the sphincter muscles of the rectum and bladder, so that incontinence is a common accompaniment of paraplegia.)

Among the causes of paraplegia are:

(i) Injury to the spinal cord; fracture of vertebrae, gunshot wounds.

(ii) Tumours of the spinal cord and pressure from adjacent tumours, including a tuberculous abscess arising from a vertebra.

   (iii) Inflammation of the spinal cord:
            Myelitis—e.g. due to a virus or to syphilis.
   (iv) Degeneration of the spinal cord:
            Disseminated (multiple) sclerosis.
            Subacute combined degeneration (p. 179).
            Cervical myelopathy due to cervical spondylosis.
            Motor neurone disease.
            Syringomyelia.
   (v) Thrombosis of the anterior spinal artery.

If the paralysed limb is examined it may be found to be rigid and difficult to bend at the joints. This is spoken of as **spastic paralysis** and the tendon reflexes are found to be exaggerated.

On the other hand, the muscles may be quite limp and the joints flail-like in character so that, when the elevated limb is dropped, it falls lifelessly to the bed: this is called **flaccid paralysis** and the tendon reflexes are absent.

The type of paralysis present depends on whether the upper motor neurone (i.e. the cells in the precentral (Rolandic) area and the pyramidal tracts), or the lower motor neurone (i.e. the motor cells in the anterior horn of the spinal cord and the peripheral nerve) are affected. In the former case a spastic paralysis results, in the latter a flaccid one. The conditions listed above all cause a spastic paralysis. Poliomyelitis differs in causing a flaccid paralysis, since it affects anterior horn cells and not the pyramidal tracts.

Other disorders of movement include spasms, tremor and ataxia. A **spasm** is an involuntary contraction of a muscle, of which there are two types, tonic and clonic. During a tonic spasm the muscle remains contracted for a varying period. **Tonic spasms** are seen in tetanus and strychnine poisoning and at the onset of epileptic fits. In some cases the whole body may pass into a state of tonic spasm. The stronger muscles of the back produce arching of the spine so that the back of the head and the heels are the only parts touching the bed. This state is called opisthotonos (see also p. 383).

Clonic spasms consist of a series of rhythmic movement which are due to alternate contraction and relaxation of muscles. These are also seen in epilepsy after the tonic state has passed off (p. 362).

Tremor

Shaking of the limbs may be continuous or only occur when a deliberate movement is made. Tremor may be seen in various disorders of the nervous system, common examples being paralysis agitans (Parkinson's disease), multiple sclerosis, cerebral arteriosclerosis and chronic alcoholism. A fine tremor of the hands occurs in thyrotoxicosis.

Ataxia or inco-ordination

Every voluntary movement is a complicated response of various muscles to nervous impulses. In order to move a joint, one or more groups of muscles must contract while others relax. If smooth, accurate movement is to be obtained delicate nervous control and exact co-ordination of the muscles is essential. In some cases of nervous disease this power of co-ordination is defective with the result that movements become coarse and inaccurate, the patient being unable to carry out simple actions in an orderly and efficient manner. Ataxia in walking is a symptom of tabes dorsalis (locomotor ataxia) and also occurs in various forms of disease of the cerebellum, and is characteristic of the movements of alcoholic intoxication.

Chorea, see p. 167.

Disorders of sensation

The conscious sensations may be divided into the special ones of smell, hearing and taste reaching the brain via the cranial nerves, and general ones including those of pain, touch, temperature and position which enter the spinal cord via the peripheral nerves.

Various alterations in general sensation occur. Loss of sensation is called **anaesthesia**. If the acuteness of sensation is increased it is referred to as **hyperaesthesia**, while an abnormal sensation, such as 'pins and needles', is spoken of as **paraesthesia**.

As in the case of motor disorders it is clear that alteration in sensation may occur as a result of lesions involving the peripheral nerves, the spinal cord or the brain itself.

Types of disease affecting the nervous system

The nervous system may be subject to any of the following types of disease, but **the symptoms produced will depend upon the situation in which the lesion occurs rather than on its cause.**

For example, a lesion of the optic nerve will result in blindness whether the cause be direct injury, inflammation or pressure upon the nerve from a neighbouring tumour.

1. Congenital conditions. Because of its complicated structure and mode of development the central nervous system is liable to a number of congenital defects, some of which may be hereditary and involve several members of a family. (These conditions include maldevelopment of the brain, mental deficiency and rarer diseases, such as Friedreich's ataxia and muscular dystrophies.)

2. Injury. Injury to the brain as a result of concussion or fractured skull is common: the spinal cord may be damaged in fractures of the vertebrae and peripheral nerves may be severed in wounds of the limbs.

Symptoms are often produced by the **mechanical effects** of pressure upon any part of the nervous system. Thus, a tumour of the brain or the accumulation of blood within the skull may cause a rise in intracranial pressure. (See cerebral compression, p. 358.) A tumour in the neighbourhood of a peripheral nerve may press upon it causing pain and loss of function.

3. Inflammation. Inflammation of the nervous system may be acute or chronic in type and may be caused by ordinary bacteria or by viruses. Organisms of the latter type, having a special affinity for nervous tissue and causing diseases such as poliomyelitis and various types of encephalitis, are called neurotropic viruses.

> Inflammation of the brain in called encephalitis.
> Inflammation of the spinal cord is called myelitis.
> Inflammation of the nerves is called neuritis.
> Inflammation of the meninges is called meningitis.

It has been seen that temporary changes in function may result from the action of toxins, drugs and disorders of metabolism and the ductless glands. Those affecting the brain many cause symptoms such as convulsions or coma, depending upon whether they irritate or depress the actions of the cerebrum.

The peripheral nerves may also be affected by diphtheria toxin (p. 57) and poisons such as arsenic, alcohol and lead.

It is important to remember that syphilis may be a cause of chronic inflammation of the nervous system and is responsible for tabes dorsalis and general paralysis of the insane.

4. Degeneration. Degenerative changes sometimes take place in the nerve cells or fibres. They may follow inflammatory or toxic conditions, but in many instances the actual cause of the process is unknown.

Subacute combined degeneration of the spinal cord, a complication of pernicious anaemia (p. 179), is an example.

5. Tumours. Tumours affecting the brain may be innocent or malignant, and of the latter some commence in the nervous system itself (e.g. gliomas) while others are secondary deposits from distant parts, e.g. from a bronchial carcinoma.

6. Circulatory disturbances. Temporary diminution of the blood supply to the brain (cerebral anoxia) may be due either to a rapid fall in blood pressure, to kinking of the carotid or vertebral arteries or to spasm of the cerebral or basilar arteries and will result in faintness (syncope).

More serious disturbances, however, are not uncommon. One of the cerebral arteries may become blocked by an embolism, or a clot may form in it as a result of disease of its walls. Rupture of an artery may occur, giving rise to haemorrhage into the brain substance, causing extensive and often fatal damage. These three conditions of cerebral embolism, thrombosis and haemorrhage cause the state known as apoplexy or cerebro-vascular accident.

There are numerous diseases which may affect the nervous system, many of which are rare, and the nurse cannot be expected to know the clinical details about them. Some of the more common ones, however, should be understood.

1. Congenital, traumatic and mechanical states

A number of conditions may be briefly referred to under these headings.

Hydrocephalus

This is frequently a congenital condition but may also follow meningitis and is due to blockage of communication between the

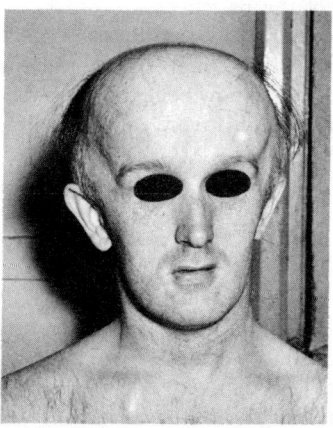

Fig. 78 Hydrocephalus.

ventricles of the brain in which the cerebrospinal fluid is secreted, and the subarachnoid space surrounding the brain and spinal cord from which it is absorbed (see p. 353). The mechanical effects of this produce great dilatation of the ventricles and enlargement of the skull. The latter can take place in infants because the sutures between the bones are not united. In many instances the convolutions of the brain become flattened as a result of the increased pressure. The cranium becomes enlarged out of proportion to the face. Death usually occurs within a few years in severe cases, but others may survive for considerable periods with or without the impairment of mental efficiency.

Sometimes surgical measures (shunt operations) are attempted in order to relieve the condition.

Microcephaly is a form of mental deficiency associated with a very small imperfectly developed brain and skull.

Cerebral diplegia (Little's disease)

Cerebral diplegia, a form of cerebral palsy, may be due to defective development of parts of the brain or possibly to injury at birth.

The limbs are stiff and spastic; the legs, as a rule, being more affected than the arms. In many cases walking is impossible, but in others a typical spastic or 'scissors' gait is present. Peculiar involuntary movements of a writhing nature may be seen and are referred to as **athetosis**. Such movements tend to be slower than those seen in chorea. It is often accompanied by mental deficiency. Contractures of muscles develop, causing deformities of the limbs. Epilepsy occurs in a small proportion of the patients.

Operations are occasionally performed to correct deformities and nerves may be divided in order to reduce the spasm.

Considerable thought is now being given to the care, education and rehabilitation of **spastic children.**

Acute inflammatory conditions

Encephalitis

Inflammation of the cerebral substance is not very common but may occur in the following conditions:
  1. In acute poliomyelitis, i.e. polioencephalitis.
  2. As a complication of certain fevers, e.g. measles, chicken-pox and whooping-cough.
  3. After vaccination.
  4. Certain virus infections.

Little is known of the viruses which produce encephalitis. On account of their special affinity for nervous tissue they are called neurotropic viruses.

The characteristic features of encephalitis are restlessness followed by increasing drowsiness and coma. There is usually some pyrexia. In milder cases recovery may be complete; in others permanent damage is done to the nervous tissues, while severe cases terminate fatally. There is no specific treatment which is, therefore, symptomatic.

Poliomyelitis (infantile paralysis)

Definition and cause. This is an acute infectious disease caused by a virus (of which there are several sub-types) which attacks and often destroys cells in the nervous system. Those most often affected are the motor nerve-cells situated in the anterior horns of the spinal cord. Depending on the extent of the inflammation, various muscles in one or more limbs may become paralysed. Paralysis occurs because voluntary impulses from the brain, reaching the anterior horns via the pyramidal tract, can no longer be passed on through the damaged anterior horn cells to the motor nerves. If the cells are completely destroyed, permanent paralysis of the affected part will follow. As a rule, however, a number of the injured cells recover and some improvement takes place.

Occasionally the virus may involve parts of the brain, including the brain stem and medulla (polioencephalitis).

The disease tends to occur in epidemics, but small groups or single cases may be seen. Unvaccinated children are more commonly affected than adults. The virus, which enters the body either through the nasal mucous membrane or the alimentary tract, and is present in the faeces, can be conveyed in a number of ways, including droplet infection, infected food and water, especially small streams, canals and possibly swimming-baths. Carriers may also play a part in its dissemination. There appears to be a fairly high degree of immunity among the population as a whole so that the infectivity rate is not as great as in some other infectious diseases.

The average incubation period is seven to fourteen days, but may be either shorter or longer in some instances. Fatigue due to strenuous muscular exercise, tonsillectomy and prophylactic inoculations (e.g. for diphtheria etc.), during this period, appear to pre-dispose to a serious attack.

Symptoms. There are three main groups of symptoms which may be observed in poliomyelitis and which tend to occur in definite

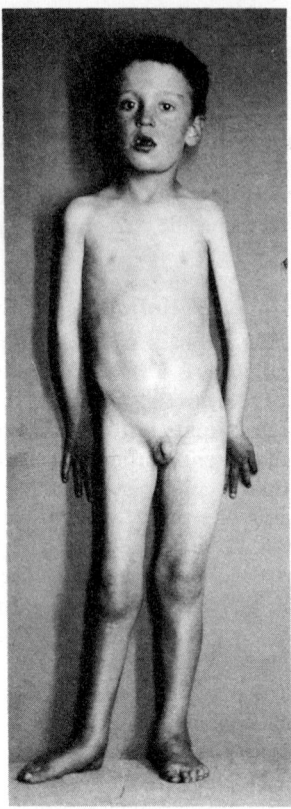

Fig. 79 Poliomyelitis showing wasting of muscles of right thigh and calf, also flat
   foot.

clinical stages. The first two groups constitute the preparalytic stage
of the disease during which it is not always possible to make the
diagnosis, and the third group the paralytic stage, viz.:

   1. Pre-paralytic stage.   (*a*) general symptoms.
                              (*b*) meningeal symptoms.
   2. Paralytic stage.   (*c*) paralytic symptoms.

In some cases, however, the disease does not progress beyond the
the first or second stages and paralysis does not develop.

   (*a*) GENERAL SYMPTOMS. There is sometimes a preliminary sore
throat or upper respiratory catarrh, but the onset is usually abrupt
with a rise in temperature, headache, malaise and muscular pains in
the limbs and back (which may be at first mistaken for rheumatism

but the joints do not become swollen). There may be drowsiness, constipation and general weakness. This stage (viraemia) may last from one to seven days.

(b) MENINGEAL SYMPTOMS. The symptoms of meningeal irritation which are observed in poliomyelitis include severe headache, stiffness of the muscles at the back of the neck which prevents full flexion of the head so that the chin cannot be made to touch the sternum, and a positive Kernig's sign (p. 383). Lumbar puncture may reveal an increase in the number of cells in the cerebrospinal fluid. During this stage also the bladder may be affected and retention of urine is not uncommon.

(c) PARALYTIC SYMPTOMS. As has already been indicated, some cases of poliomyelitis never develop any actual paralysis, but in those in which the disease becomes fully developed the paralysis may result from involvement of the following parts of the nervous system:

(i) The spinal cord. Any part of the spinal cord may be involved, causing paralysis of a group or groups of muscles in any of the limbs. In addition, the muscles of respiration and the diaphragm may be affected, which will result in death from asphyxia if appropriate treatment in an artificial respirator is not instituted without delay.

(ii) The brain stem. This is sometimes known as the bulbar type of the disease in which the muscles of the pharynx and palate are paralysed so that there is difficulty in swallowing and coughing and mucus accumulates at the back of the throat. The respiratory centre in the medulla may also be involved. Facial paralysis may occur or other cranial nerves may be affected.

Course. After the general and meningeal symptoms have been present for a few days they either subside completely or else paralysis develops rapidly and usually reaches its maximum within about 24 hours. The tendon reflexes in an affected limb are lost. After a while some recovery may take place, movements begin to return and continue to improve for a period of a year or more. Some muscle groups are likely to remain permanently paralysed or markedly weakened. In addition to this residual paralysis, the muscles become atrophied, and, in growing children, the neighbouring bones fail to develop normally. The limb, therefore, remains smaller than normal and deformities may occur at the joints owing to the pull of unaffected muscles.

Treatment

1. GENERAL. During the acute stages the patient is confined to bed. Strict isolation must be maintained for at least three weeks on the

lines laid down for typhoid fever. The nurse must wear a gown and a mask is advisable. She must pay particular attention to washing her hands after attending to the patient during this period. Disinfectant should be applied to all soiled linen and excreta before disposal and bedpans should be sterilized. The diet will depend on what the patient can take, but at first will be light with plenty of fluids. The patient should not be nursed in a general ward during the acute stages but in a cubicle or special poliomyelitis unit, preferably in a hospital for infectious diseases.

2. LOCAL TREATMENT. In many cases it is desirable to nurse the patient on a firm mattress with fracture boards. The paralysed limbs must be supported and removable splints or sandbags may be applied in such a way as to prevent deformities occurring from the active pull of muscles which are not involved and from the effect of gravity. In particular, it is important to prevent foot-drop, wrist-drop, contraction of the fingers and over-stretching of the deltoid muscles at the shoulder.

Muscular pain and spasm may be relieved by frequent hot packs, or the application of properly protected hot-water bottles or electric pads. Aspirin or similar analgesics may be required. Barbiturates or diazepam may be given for restlessness.

When the patient is free from pain and fever, usually in 1 to 2 weeks, the paralysed part is put through a full range of movement twice daily. Physiotherapy is then commenced; active movements are encouraged and aided by re-education exercises, massage and electrical treatment.

At a later stage, special orthopaedic appliances such as surgical boots, irons or walking calipers may be required, or operations performed to correct shortening of tendons and deformities of joints in order to get the best possible function.

Finally, occupational therapy and special training at a rehabilitation centre may be desirable. It is remarkable how many victims of poliomyelitis are able to adjust themselves to lead a useful and happy life even when their residual paralysis is severe.

3. SPECIAL TREATMENT is required for cases with respiratory failure. Artificial respiration must be commenced without delay and the patient later placed in an artificial respirator ('iron lung'). When pharyngeal paralysis is present secretions accumulate in the throat. The foot of the bed is raised and a tracheostomy combined with a positive pressure respirator may be required. A suction apparatus must also be available. Such patients should not be left unattended.

Lumbar puncture may be performed during the acute stages for diagnostic purposes if the diagnosis is in doubt.

The circulation in an affected limb may be defective and the part tends to become cold and blue. This is helped by the provision of gloves or extra stockings, as the case may be.

4. DIAGNOSIS. This is not always easy in non-paralytic cases, but in addition to clinical signs the virus may be detected in the faeces and tests for antibodies may be carried out on the blood.

5. PREVENTION. Poliomyelitis is a notifiable disease and during an epidemic a District Community Physician may close schools and swimming-baths in some districts. It is advisable to avoid crowded places and cinemas and, as already mentioned, procedures such as tonsillectomy and diphtheria immunization are postponed.

It must be remembered that every poliomyelitis patient carries the virus for 3 to 5 days in the upper respiratory tract before the onset of the acute stage and subsequently for 7 days. In all patients the virus is present in the faeces for about 14 days; in 50% it persists for 3 weeks and in 25% for 6 weeks.

The injection of immuno-globulin may give a temporary passive immunity for a few weeks, but this is rarely practicable on a large scale.

Vaccines give a more lasting active immunity and poliomyelitis is, therefore, essentially a preventable disease. Two types of vaccine are available:

(a) oral administration which is now usually employed, i.e. 3 drops of Sabin vaccine on a sugar lump every 4 weeks for 3 doses, with a booster dose at school entry and again at age of 15.

(b) by injection (2 with an interval of 3 weeks and a 3rd after 6 months).

In order to reduce the incidence of the disease it is important that a high percentage of the population should be immunized.

Meningitis

Surrounding the brain and spinal cord are membranes known as the dura mater, the arachnoid mater and the pia mater. The cerebrospinal fluid occupies the space between the arachnoid and pia mater.

Inflammation of these membranes, the meninges, may be produced by various organisms and the condition of meningitis is associated with changes in the cerebrospinal fluid.

Similar but less severe changes may be produced if irritation be caused by toxins circulating in the blood, without the presence of bacteria in the meninges. This condition and the associated symptoms is sometimes referred to as meningism. Meningeal irritation may occur in poliomyelitis.

The process of inflammation of the meninges is the same as that occurring in any other tissue of the body (see p. 9). The increased blood supply results in redness of the membranes, the accumulation of inflammatory cells, and a local outpouring of fluid. The cells pass into the cerebrospinal fluid which instead of being clear, becomes turbid. If the cells are very numerous it may become almost pure pus.

The following are the common varieties of meningitis:

1. Meningococcal meningitis (cerebrospinal fever).
2. Tuberculous meningitis.
3. Pneumococcal meningitis.
4. 'Septic' meningitis (usually due to the streptococcus) following (a) head injury, (b) disease of the middle ear and mastoiditis.
5. Virus meningitis.
6. Other organisms, which sometimes cause meningitis, include *Haemophilus influenzae, Esch. coli* and staphylococci.

Symptoms of meningitis (all types)

The symptoms of meningitis, which may occur at any age, develop rapidly in most types of the disease but tend to progress more slowly in tuberculous meningitis, which is now uncommon, than in other forms. They include:

(a) GENERAL SYMPTOMS. The onset is usually abrupt with pyrexia and increased pulse rate, general malaise with pains all over, furred tongue, vomiting, with rigors and convulsions in some cases.

Headache is often severe and continuous and may be either general, frontal or referred to the occipital region and down the back of the neck.

Irritation of the brain gives rise to restlessness and delirium, often associated with a shrill, unprovoked cry, known as the 'meningitic cry'.

The inflammatory process produces an increased formation and decreased reabsorption of the cerebrospinal fluid which causes a rise in the pressure within the skull. This increased intracranial pressure may be followed by progressive drowsiness, which develops into deep coma, with a slow pulse rate.

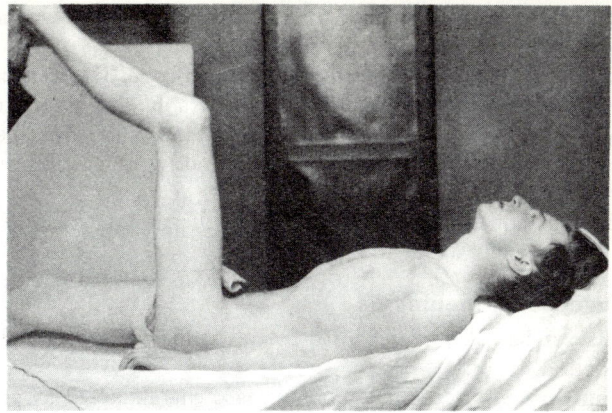

Fig. 80 Meningitis, showing head-retraction and tenseness of the ham-string muscles (Kernig's sign).

(*b*) SPECIAL SIGNS AND SYMPTOMS. Stiffness of the muscles at the back of the neck develops as a result of irritation of the spinal nerves. Any attempt to flex the head forward to bring the chin towards the sternum is resisted and may cause pain **(neck stiffness).** The next stage is the development of head-retraction in which the head is inclined backwards. In infants not only the neck but the whole back may be so arched and stiff that the infant can almost be made to rest on the back of the head and heels alone, a condition known as opisthotonos (see also p. 372).

Squints may occur and the pupils are often dilated. The patient resents interference and shows objection to noise and bright light (photophobia).

A very important sign of meningeal irritation is known as Kernig's sign. This consists of inability to extend the leg at the knee when the thigh is flexed to a right angle, and is due to tenseness of the hamstring muscles.

Complications and sequelae. These include broncho-pneumonia, retention of urine and more permanent conditions such as hydrocephalus, deafness, blindness and paralyses of various kinds.

Diagnosis. The diagnosis of meningitis is made on the history and symptoms combined with the presence of neck stiffness or head retraction and a positive Kernig's sign. The condition is confirmed by examination of the cerebrospinal fluid obtained by lumbar puncture. The fluid, instead of being crystal clear, is opalescent or turbid in appearance or may be purulent. It is most important to ascertain as soon as possible the actual organism present as this has a bearing on the antibiotic treatment of the case.

Prognosis. Meningitis is always a serious condition. The outlook in all types has, however, improved considerably since the introduction of chemotherapy and antibiotic drugs, and is largely dependent on the early treatment with the appropriate drug to which the infecting organism is sensitive.

Although sometimes necessary the intrathecal administration of drugs is usually avoided.

Meningococcal meningitis

The disease has also been known by the names Cerebrospinal Fever and Spotted Fever.

Definition. An acute infectious disease characterized by purulent inflammation of the membranes of the brain and spinal cord (meninges).

Cause. The condition is caused by an organism known as the meningococcus, and affects especially children and young adults.
Epidemics sometimes occur. Cases also appear from time to time, apart from an epidemic. Such cases are spoken of as sporadic.

The MODES OF SPREAD are by droplet infection and by the agency of carriers. The PATH OF INVASION is by means of the nasopharynx where the organisms first settle. They are conveyed from this site by the blood stream and lymphatics to the meninges where they produce inflammation. Pus forms, and is present in the cerebrospinal fluid.

The incubation period is 1 to 5 days.

Special symptoms of meningococcal meningitis

The general symptoms have already been described.

RASH. In some cases a rash develops, and it is for this reason that the disease has been called 'spotted fever'. The rash consists of small haemorrhages (purpuric spots) rather like flea-bites under the skin, and may be seen on the trunk and limbs.

The development of small vesicles on the lips (herpes), which is also seen in other maladies such as pneumonia, is common.

The condition may prove fatal or may improve rapidly with treatment. In fulminating cases bacteraemia may occur causing haemorrhage in the adrenal glands (Waterhouse–Friderichsen syndrome) in which acute circulatory failure occurs and which may respond to intravenous hydrocortisone.

Tuberculous meningitis

As has already been stated, this variety may be of more gradual onset than other types and tends to run a longer course. The signs and symptoms, however, are similar in character. There is often a period of ill-health for a few weeks before the meningeal symptoms arise.

There is usually a tuberculous focus elsewhere in the body, such as the lungs or lymph glands, so that the tubercle bacillus reaches the meninges via the bloodstream. It may also be a manifestation of miliary tuberculosis. Before the introduction of streptomycin, isoniazid, and PAS, cases were invariably fatal. Although 90% of early cases now recover some may relapse or be followed by permanent after effects, including mental changes and paralysis of various kinds.

'Septic' meningitis

This may be caused by any infection spreading from the skull to the meninges or may be part of a general septicaemia. The organisms usually found are the streptococcus or the staphylococcus. The common causes are:
1. Disease of the middle ear (otitis media) and mastoiditis.
2. Infection of the nasal sinuses.
3. Compound fractures of the skull, including fracture of the base.
4. Septicaemia associated with a boil, carbuncle or septic process elsewhere in the body.

The other types of meningitis are not very common and do not require separate description.

Special treatment of meningitis

Once the organism has been identified by bacteriological examination of the cerebrospinal fluid, an appropriate antibiotic, e.g. ampicillin, or sulphonamide to which it is sensitive is administered in full doses. It is usual to give one of them in anticipation without waiting for the bacteriological report and to change it later if the organism is shown to be insensitive.

Meningococcal meningitis. Combined therapy is administered with a sulphonamide, sulphadimidine or sulphadiazine, and penicillin intramuscularly *or* intravenously. Some strains of meningococci are resistant to sulphonamides.

Pneumococcal meningitis. Penicillin is given in doses of 1,000,000 units every 2 to 4 hours by intramuscular or intravenous injection. Intrathecal injections of penicillin (10,000 units) are sometimes necessary.

Streptococcal and staphylococcal meningitis. Massive doses of penicillin may be used as in pneumococcal meningitis. If the organism is penicillin insensitive one of the other antibiotics, e.g. cloxacillin, would be employed. Any septic focus would be dealt with by surgical means.

Influenzal meningitis. Chloramphenicol by intramuscular injection in full doses is the treatment of choice. Alternatively, ampicillin is given intramuscularly.

Tuberculous meningitis. The three most important drugs are streptomycin, isoniazid and ethambutol.

Streptomycin is given by intramuscular injection (20 mg per (1 lb) body weight), at first daily and later 2 or 3 times weekly for 3 to 4 months. Intrathecal injection is not usually necessary in early cases but, if employed, hydrocortisone may be required.

Isoniazid (10–15 mg per 500 g (1 lb) body weight daily), in 8-hourly doses for periods of a year or more.

PAS or thiacetazone may be required for some cases. Steroids, which lessen inflammatory reaction and so help to reduce the exudate causing complications such as hydrocephalus, may also be required for a period of about 3 weeks.

Virus meningitis. Most cases recover. There is no specific treatment which is, therefore, symptomatic.

General treatment of meningitis

Cases of meningococcal meningitis should be isolated. Other types of meningitis are not infectious in the ordinary sense of the word and special precautions are unnecessary once the diagnosis has been established. The patient is confined to bed in a quiet, darkened room. A cot-bed with padded sides may be necessary if restlessness is marked. In the acute stages a fluid diet is necessary, but the disease is an exhausting one and as much nourishment as possible should be administered, milk, eggs, beef tea and sugar being given freely. In stuporose cases swallowing is defective and nasal or oesophageal feeding must be commenced without delay.

The bowels are opened with aperients and careful watch is kept on the bladder since retention of urine with subsequent distension requiring catheterization is liable to occur. A fluid intake and output chart should be kept.

The mouth and eyes must be cleansed, and the back and pressure points attended to at regular intervals.

Special symptoms are treated as they arise. Headache may be relieved by an ice-bag or cold compresses to the head and drugs such as aspirin may be given. For restlessness chloral, paraldehyde or similar sedatives are required.

Diseases of the spinal cord

The spinal cord may be compressed by a tumour or abscess or damaged by disorders of the bone such as fractures, tuberculosis or secondary tumour. In some cases the pressure on the cord can be relieved by surgical means. Acute damage to the cord occurs in **myelitis** the cause of which is often unknown. Slower degeneration of the cord is found in certain types of syphilis and in multiple (disseminated) sclerosis, syringomyelia, motor neurone disease (amyotrophic lateral sclerosis, progressive muscular atrophy) and subacute combined degeneration of the cord. The last condition is due to deficiency of vitamin B_{12} (pernicious anaemia) and can be helped and even cured provided treatment is started early enough (p. 179).

Syringomyelia. This is a rare, slowly progressive condition the cause of which is not understood. Small cystic cavities develop in the centre of the cord, usually in the cervical region. These expand and gradually compress the adjacent anterior horn cells, motor and sensory nerve fibres. The symptoms include wasting of the small muscles of the hands and forearm muscles, with loss of sensibility to pain and temperature so that the patient may injure or burn his fingers without realizing that he has done so. In the later stages drainage of the cavities after laminectomy may be helpful.

Motor neurone disease (amyotrophic lateral sclerosis, progressive muscular atrophy). These constitute clinical variations of a slowly progressive, disabling and eventually fatal condition for which no cause or treatment is known. Either the anterior horn cells or the pyramidal tracts or both degenerate slowly. In progressive muscular atrophy the small muscles of the hands or feet are usually the first to be affected, producing a 'claw hand' or 'club foot'. The muscles of the forearm and shoulder or the peroneal muscles in the leg are involved later. With increasing weakness the patient takes to his bed.

When the motor nuclei in the medulla are involved which makes eating, swallowing and talking difficult the condition is called **progressive bulbar palsy.** In this condition nasal feeding may be necessary and there is a risk of fatal inhalation of food, drink or saliva.

Many disorders of the spinal cord progress to a state of **paraplegia** in which the legs are weak or totally paralysed, sensation in the legs and lower trunk is diminished or absent and control of the bladder and bowels is impaired or lost. The nursing care of such patients can be very exacting. The patient must be turned frequently and pressure points on the skin must be attended to with the greatest care. Where there is incontinence of urine the bladder is often catheterized to avoid soiling of the skin by urine. The catheter is usually of the indwelling variety. Sometimes it is possible to empty the bladder by manual compression above the symphysis pubis and the patient may even learn to do this himself. Loss of rectal control is usually accompanied by constipation which is relieved by an enema given twice a week.

Where the cause of the paraplegia is not progressive it is remarkable how much can be achieved by devoted nursing and careful physiotherapy. One of the most important aspects is to encourage the patient to regain hope for the future and cooperate to the fullest degree in making the best of his disabilities, and the nurse is often in a position where she is specially able to do this. Where the underlying disease, however, is progressive or the patient's psychological or physical state is poor, deterioration due to deepening bed sores or intractable urinary infection occurs and death is usually due to terminal bronchopneumonia, renal failure or general toxaemia.

Diseases of the nerves

The cranial and peripheral nerves are subject to a number of morbid conditions which interfere with their functions. Inflammatory or degenerative changes may take place producing the symptoms of **neuritis.** It has been seen, for example, that diphtheria toxin produces degenerative changes which cause paralysis. Similar results may follow the action of other bacterial toxins and drugs such as alcohol, arsenic and lead. Injury or pressure on nerves by tumours, tight splints or crutches may also cause degeneration. Innocent tumours of the nerves themselves (neuromas) are sometimes seen. Neuritis is also a complication of diabetes and sometimes occurs in association with carcinoma of the lung.

Aneurine (vitamin B_1) deficiency, though rare in this country, is a cause of peripheral neuritis and is possibly the basic factor in alcoholic neuritis.

The symptoms produced by such lesions will depend on the actual nerve affected and its distribution. Most peripheral nerves contain motor and sensory fibres combined with fibres which influence the blood supply and nutrition of the part (trophic fibres). Depending on whether one or all of these sets of fibres are affected the symptoms of neuritis may be classified as:

1. Motor symptoms, i.e. paralysis or weakness of muscles.
2. Sensory symptoms, i.e. loss of sensation (anaesthesia), tingling (paraesthesia) or actual pain.
3. Trophic changes, i.e. wasting of muscles, defective circulation, a tendency to bed or splint sores and atrophy of skin, which assumes a dry, glossy, appearance.

Polyneuritis. This term is used when many nerves in the body are affected at the same time. The condition is usually toxic in origin (e.g. diphtheria toxin, alcohol, arsenic or lead) but occasionally appears to be infective or allergic in character.

A particularly serious form resembles the bulbar type of polio-myelitis, and requires similar treatment, with postural drainage, pharyngeal suction, tube feeding and, possibly, tracheostomy. Steroids may be of value in the early stages.

Disorders of special nerves

Almost any nerve in the body may be affected by a pathological process, but only a few more common conditions require special mention.

Optic neuritis. Damage to the optic nerve may be due to toxic states or to pressure on the nerve within the skull. It is associated with defective vision but, if the damage be severe, degeneration of its fibres and permanent blindness may take place (optic atrophy).

When the retina is examined with an ophthalmoscope the entrance of the optic nerve is seen as a pale circular area having a sharp outline.

When the intracranial pressure is raised (e.g. in cerebral tumour), the margins of the disc become blurred (papilloedema).

Ophthalmoplegia. Affections of the third, fourth and sixth nerves, which supply the muscles of the eye, lead to paralysis of eye movements (**ophthalmoplegia**) and squints (**strabismus**). This is often associated with double vision (**diplopia**). Drooping of the eye-lid (**ptosis**) may also occur.

Trigeminal neuralgia. The fifth cranial or sensory nerve to the face is sometimes the site of attacks of excruciating pain radiating over the area of its distribution, mainly in the elderly. The origin of this condition, which is known as tic douloureux or trigeminal neuralgia, is not always clear, but the pain is often so severe that the patient may become suicidal. Many cases respond to treatment with carbamazepine ('Tegretol') 200 mg 6-hourly, others may be treated by injecting the Gasserian ganglion with alcohol or section of the sensory nerve root.

The seventh nerve. Paralysis of the seventh cranial nerve (the facial) results in **facial paralysis**. This may occur:

1. As a result of tumours of the parotid gland, inflammation of the middle ear and operations on the mastoid process.
2. In Bell's palsy.
3. In association with hemiplegia resulting from a cerebro-vascular accident, e.g. cerebral thrombosis.

Bell's palsy is probably due to a neuritis of the seventh nerve and is sometimes said to be due to exposure to a draught. Milder cases (e.g. 80%) clear up completely in a few weeks but in a few there is some residual paralysis.

A lesion of the seventh nerve results in a paralysis of the muscles of one side of the face, which becomes expressionless and looks as if it has been 'ironed out'. There is inability to close the eye properly and the angle of the mouth droops, so that the whole mouth appears to be pulled over to the normal side. Food debris tends to collect in the affected cheek which must, therefore, be carefully cleaned. It may be necessary to place a pad over the affected eye. Bell's palsy may be helped by local heat and physiotherapy and a covered wire splint may be fixed from the ear into the corner of the mouth in some cases. Intramuscular injections of ACTH or prednisolone by mouth, are helpful if given early enough.

In the facial paralysis associated with hemiplegia the eyelid movements usually escape and only the lower part of the face is affected.

The eighth nerve (Auditory). This is a sensory nerve which consists of two parts, (a) the true auditory nerve of hearing and (b) the vestibular nerve from the semicircular canals which is concerned with equilibrium, posture and balance. Lesions of the auditory fibres, therefore, produce deafness and noises in the ear (tinnitus), while those of the vestibular fibres cause giddiness (vertigo).

Motion sickness (sea-, car-, air-sickness) in which giddiness is associated with nausea and vomiting is due to disturbances in the semi-circular canals. It may be prevented and relieved by the use of drugs such as hyoscine, 'Avomine' and 'Marzine'. **N.B.**—Most of the modern drugs should be avoided in early pregnancy.

Menière's disease is characterized by recurrent, sudden attacks of vertigo and tinnitus often associated with nausea and vomiting. There is usually some degree of progressive deafness which is usually unilateral. The attack may cause the individual to stagger or he may fall to the ground. The cause of the condition has not been fully explained. There appears to be impairment of the microcirculation of the inner ear. Endolymph accumulates because it is not properly re-absorbed by the ischaemic endolymphatic sac. Pressure from the excessive volume of fluid (endolymphatic hydrops) causes the symptoms of Menières disease. Phenobarbitone, 'Stemetil', or diuretics may be helpful in reducing the frequency and severity of attacks but betahistine ('Serc'), a histamine-like compound appears

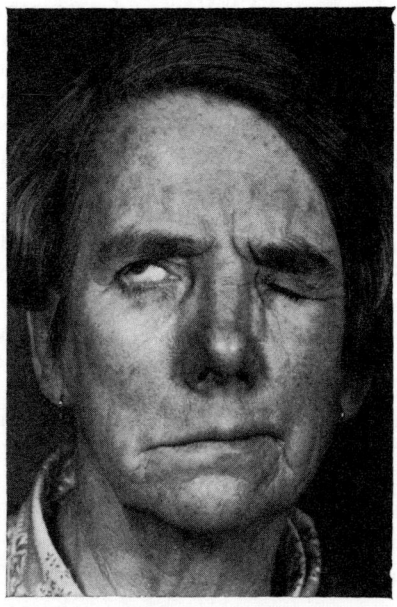

Fig. 81 Case of right-sided facial palsy. (From Mawson, 1967, *Diseases of the Ear*, Edward Arnold, London.)

to give the best results; the dose is 8 to 16 mg 3 times a day. Surgical measures may be required for the refractory cases.

Tinnitus or noises in the ear are described as hissing, ringing, buzzing etc. They may be constant or intermittent and with or without deafness. There are many causes including toxic drugs, salicylates, hypertension, otitis media etc.

Vertigo. In addition to motion sickness and Menière's disease, giddiness or the sensation of loss of equilibrium may result from many other conditions, e.g. disorders of the middle and inner ears, eye conditions such as glaucoma, toxic drugs including salicylates, alcohol, nicotine and streptomycin, variations in blood pressure (both hyper- and hypotension), anaemia and cerebral tumours.

Brachial neuritis is a term sometimes used for pain and paraesthesia felt in the arm. It is rarely a true neuritis but the symptoms are generally due to the protrusion of a cervical inter-vertebral disc, osteo-arthritis of the cervical spine or pressure on nerves of the brachial plexus by a cervical rib.

Carpal tunnel syndrome. Quite a number of cases of pain and paraesthesia in the arm and hand are due to compression of the median nerve in the ligamentous tunnel in the flexor surface of the wrist. There may be recurrent attacks. The condition is most common in the busy housewife who puts a considerable strain on her hands in the course of her work. The symptoms are often worse at night, causing loss of sleep. Conservative treatment consisting of rest and a night splint is often effective. Surgical decompression may be necessary, the restraining band (flexor retinaculum) being divided.

Sciatica. This is a symptomatic term given to describe pain felt in the distribution of the sciatic nerve, viz. in the buttock, back of the thigh and outer side and back of the leg.

CAUSES. (*a*) For a long time the main cause was considered to be an actual neuritis of the nerve; although this may be true in some cases it is a rare cause of the condition.

(*b*) In some cases the pain may be due to arthritis of the inter-vertebral or sacro-iliac joints. In others, a tumour of the vertebra may be present.

(*c*) By far the commonest cause is a prolapsed intervertebral disc.

Prolapsed intervertebral disc

The disc between each vertebra consists of a tough, round mass of fibro-cartilage having a softer centre, the *nucleus pulposus*. If the outer ring of fibro-cartilage is damaged by a back strain such as sudden bending or twisting or heavy lifting, the *nucleus pulposus* may protrude through or push in front of it some of the damaged fibres. This may occur suddenly or gradually. In the first instance the pain produced may be limited to the back. If, however, the protrusion is large, or in certain positions, it will tend to press on one or more of the nerve roots which form the sciatic nerve and cause pain of sciatic nerve distribution.

The disc most commonly affected is the fifth lumbar between the last lumbar vertebra and the sacrum. The fourth and third lumbar discs may also be affected. As previously mentioned, a similar lesion can occur in the cervical region but lesions elsewhere in the spinal column are rare.

Symptoms. The characteristic symptom is pain either immediately after the strain or injury or some days or weeks later. Although it may be limited to the small of the back, it usually extends to the buttock, thigh or leg, depending on which nerve root or roots are affected. This pain may be very severe and is made worse by bending, turning in bed, coughing and sneezing. Flexion of the thigh at the hip causes pain on the affected side. (This straight-leg raising is called Lasègue's sign and is elicited very much in the same way as Kernig's sign in meningitis.) Sometimes there is a little wasting of

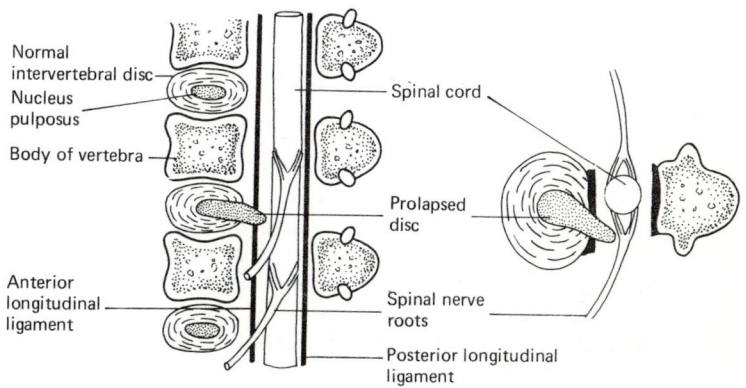

Fig. 82 Diagram illustrating prolapsed disc pressing on spinal nerve.

muscles and the knee or ankle reflexes may be lost. An x-ray of the spine may show some narrowing of the affected disc space.

Treatment. As a rule symptoms clear up gradually over a period of 6 weeks to 6 months, but may recur. In the acute stage, rest in bed on fracture boards is necessary. Occasionally, limitation of the movement of the lumbar spine by a plaster may be helpful. Later a surgical belt may be required.

Analgesic drugs such as aspirin, codeine, phenylbutazone and in very acute cases, even morphine are given for pain. Heat in the form of an electric pad, hot-water bottle or radiant heat may be helpful. Manipulation and traction of the spine is effective in some cases and may be followed by physiotherapy and exercises.

If there is no response to medical treatment it may occasionally be necessary to perform a laminectomy and remove the herniated portion of the disc.

Obstetric paralysis

Nerve injuries sometimes occur in infants at birth when labour has been difficult. The brachial plexus is most often affected producing paralysis of either

(*a*) the shoulder (Erb's palsy) in which the arm is rotated and the palm of the hand faces backwards and outwards (the waiter's tip position).

or (*b*) the forearm and hand (Klumpke's palsy) producing a 'claw hand'.

Syphilis of the nervous system (Neurosyphilis)

The treponeme of syphilis may cause organic disease of the nervous system in the following ways:

1. By direct action on the nervous tissue.

2. By causing syphilitic disease of the arteries which predisposes to conditions such as cerebral thrombosis.

Almost any part of the nervous system may be affected, thus cerebral syphilis, syphilitic myelitis and chronic syphilitic inflammation of the meninges (meningo-vascular syphilis) all occur. It is for this reason that the Wassermann reaction is usually performed on the blood and cerebrospinal fluid in neurological cases. In some instances the disease may be of congenital origin.

Two nervous diseases of syphilitic origin are of importance, viz. tabes dorsalis (locomotor ataxia) and general paralysis of the insane, although the efficient treatment of primary syphilis with antibiotics has considerably reduced their incidence. Changes in the cerebrospinal fluid are generally found in these conditions and the Wassermann reaction is positive.

Tabes dorsalis (Locomotor ataxia)

This disease may be defined as a degenerative condition of the posterior root ganglia caused by syphilis. It is most common in men between the ages of 30 and 50 and generally develops about 15 years after the primary infection with the treponeme has taken place. It is slowly progressive so that cases in various stages of the disease may be encountered and, therefore, it is conveniently described as having early, advanced and terminal symptoms.

Early symptoms. The most constant features in this stage are sharp shooting pains in the limbs which are called **'lightning pains'**, the absence of knee and ankle jerks and small pupils which fail to react to light (**Argyll-Robertson pupils**). Occasionally there is trouble with sight and difficulty in micturition.

Advanced symptoms. As the disease progresses other symptoms develop. Owing to secondary degeneration in the posterior columns

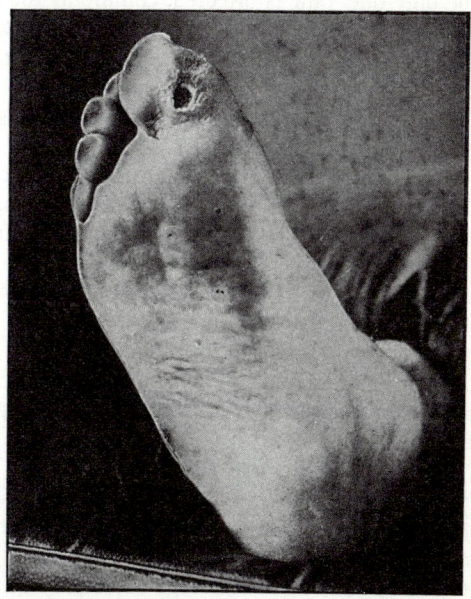

Fig. 83 Perforating ulcer of the foot in a case of tabes dorsalis.

of the spinal cord, which contain fibres relaying the sense of position to the brain, accurate control of muscular movements becomes impossible and the condition of **ataxia** occurs. This is usually confined to the lower limbs with the result that a typical 'ataxic gait' is produced. The patient is unable to feel exactly where his feet are in space and, in order to co-ordinate his movements as far as possible, he looks to the floor and obtains some assistance by means of vision. He tends to walk on a wide base, to raise his feet too high, to throw them too far forward and finally to bring them sharply to the ground.

Attacks of severe abdominal pain and vomiting, known as **gastric**

crises, may occur from time to time and are occasionally mistaken for perforation of a peptic ulcer.

Difficulty in micturition, with retention of urine and cystitis become more frequent and the bladder must be watched carefully for distension.

Changes in the nutrition of the tissues (trophic changes) are liable to take place, the common ones being deep ulcers on the foot in the neighbourhood of the toes (**perforating ulcers**) and changes in the joints. As a rule only one joint is affected, commonly the knee, hip or shoulder, and the lesion is characterized by painless swelling with destruction of the cartilage and ligaments so that deformities occur (**Charcot's joints**).

The visual trouble may progress to complete blindness associated with atrophy of the optic nerve.

Terminal symptoms. In the terminal stage, which may not appear until 10 to 15 years after the onset of symptoms, ataxia and muscular weakness are so marked that the patient is confined to bed; there is very little control over the bladder and rectum, and death may ensue from infection of the urinary tract or pneumonia.

Treatment. In the early stages attention is paid to the general health and, although the patient can usually continue his occupation, he should avoid undue mental strain and physical exertion. The diet must be nourishing in order to avoid serious loss of weight which is a common feature of the disease.

The usual anti-syphilitic remedies are employed and consist of a full course of penicillin. This will probably prevent any further progress of the disease so that recognition and treatment of the early stages is most important.

In the ataxia stage re-education exercises are often of value. Special symptoms are treated as they arise. Catheterization may be necessary for retention of urine. Various drugs such as aspirin and codeine may be used for pain. Morphine, pethidine or 'Tegretol' (carbamazepine) may be required for severe gastric crises.

The diagnosis is confirmed by a positive Wasserman reaction and other changes in the cerebrospinal fluid.

General paralysis of the insane

This condition is sometimes spoken of as GPI or referred to as **dementia paralytica,** but the name describes the terminal stages of the disease rather than those encountered in general medical work. The main pathological change taking place in the disease is degeneration of nerve cells in the cerebral cortex, and treponemes may be found in the brain so that the condition is really a chronic syphilitic encephalitis. Like tabes dorsalis the symptoms commence about 15 years after infection with syphilis and consist of progressive deterioration of the mental and physical powers. With the modern treatment of syphilis, this is now a rare condition.

The early symptoms include mental changes, such as forgetfulness, outbursts of temper, inattention to business and gross extravagance in an individual whose conduct has hitherto been normal. Excessive cheerfulness (euphoria) is common and delusions, especially those of grandeur in which the patient imagines himself to be fabulously wealthy or to be some important, influential personage, are often present.

Later the speech becomes slurred, movements are tremulous, cheerfulness gives place to depression and convulsions may occur.

Muscular weakness is progressive and the patient finally becomes bedridden, incontinent and demented. With early and efficient treatment, however, the outlook is greatly improved.

Treatment. Many cases, even in the early stages, must be confined to a mental home. Treatment consists of administering a full course of procaine penicillin (e.g. 1·2 million units a day for 20 days).

Cerebral tumour

Tumour formation may affect any part of the brain or spinal cord, the new growths being either innocent (meningioma), which arises in the meninges and presses on the brain from without: or malignant (glioma), which invade the surrounding brain tissue. Not infrequently secondary deposits of cancer arising in other organs of the body occur (e.g. lung, stomach).

The symptoms produced depend on two factors:

1. The pressure of the tumour within the skull, causing the general effects of increased intracranial pressure, which include mental changes, drowsiness, headache, vomiting, slowness of the pulse and sometimes fits. Papilloedema (p. 389) is an important sign.

2. The local effects of the tumour on the nerve centres of that part of the brain in which it is situated. It is evident that these symptoms will be very variable and depend entirely upon its position. Paralysis of cranial nerves, or various other motor and sensory changes may occur. If the cerebellum is affected the symptoms of a cerebellar lesion will be present. Attempts may be made to remove the tumour by operation.

X-ray of the skull, ventriculography, angiography, electro-encephalography, radio-active isotope and ultra-sonic tests are important methods of investigation.

A procedure sometimes adopted in order to lower the intracranial pressure is to give up to 500 ml of 50% sucrose intravenously, or 170 ml (6 fl oz) of 25% magnesium sulphate solution per rectum, the intake of fluid by mouth being restricted at the same time. This has the effect of withdrawing fluid from the brain into the blood. The volume of the brain is consequently diminished so that the intracranial pressure falls temporarily. This may enable an operation to be performed with greater safety. Intravenous urea may also be used.

Cerebral abscess

An abscess may be formed in the brain and is generally secondary either to (1) disease of the middle ear in which there is a direct spread of the infection to the temporal lobe or cerebellum, (2) frontal sinusitis spreading to frontal lobe, or (3) to suppurative conditions of the lungs such as bronchiectasis or lung abscess when the organisms reach the brain via the bloodstream. The symptoms produced are similar to those caused by cerebral tumour and are due

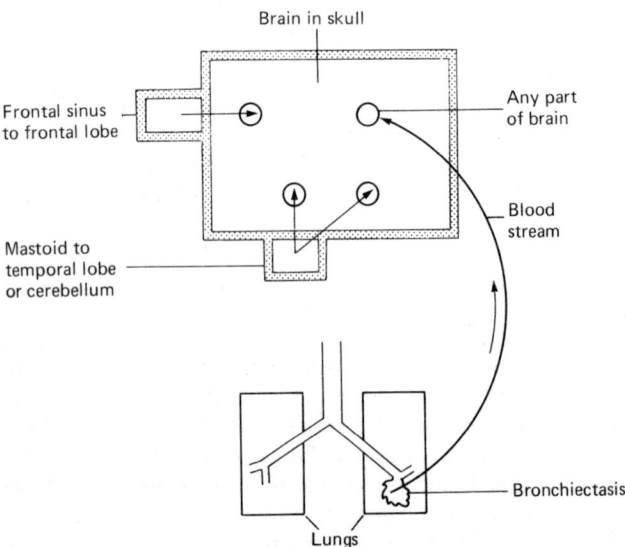

Fig. 84 Diagram illustrating common sites and origins of brain abscess.

both to raised intracranial pressure and to the local effects of the abscess.

The treatment is surgical, but penicillin or other antibiotic drugs are given first.

Apoplexy (Cerebrovascular accidents)

This acute cerebral catastrophe or stroke may be due to:

1. *Haemorrhage* from a cerebral artery.
2. *Thrombosis* of a cerebral artery.
3. An *embolus* such as a clot of blood from the left atrium in mitral stenosis, a clot dislodged from the wall of the heart after coronary artery thrombosis or a vegetation from a valve in bacterial endocarditis, becoming lodged in a cerebral artery.

Cerebral haemorrhage and thrombosis are incidents in the progress of atheroma of the cerebral vessels and are often associated with hypertension.

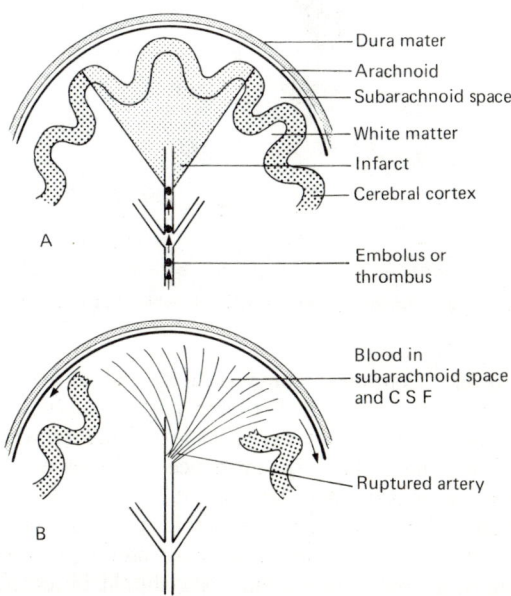

Fig. 85 Diagram illustrating: A. Production of a cerebral infarct by embolism or thrombosis. B. Destruction of brain tissue by haemorrhage.
N.B.—Infarcts and haemorrhage may also occur in the interior of the brain.

It must also be remembered that atheroma followed by thrombosis may affect arteries outside, but supplying, the brain including the internal carotid, vertebral and basilar arteries. Occlusion of any of these vessels will also produce cerebral symptoms.

The effects of these lesions will depend upon their size and the actual portion of the brain which is deprived of its blood supply. The symptoms may be sudden or gradual in onset and vary from coma with complete paralysis of one side of the body (hemiplegia) to transient weakness of a limb or temporary loss of speech (aphasia).

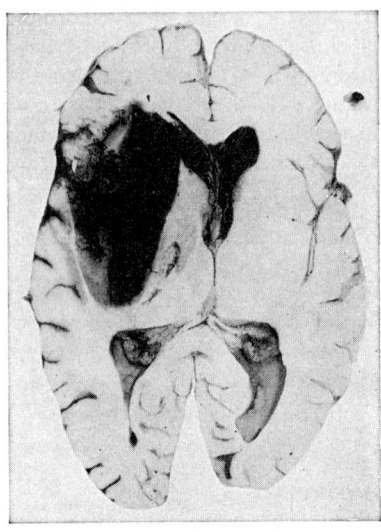

Fig. 86 Large recent haemorrhage on the left side which has ruptured into the lateral ventricle.

In the severe examples, coma is deep and is accompanied by stertorous breathing which, in the later stages, may develop into the Cheyne-Stokes variety. The latter cases are often fatal while in others partial recovery takes place. Incontinence of faeces and urine often occur. Retention of urine may be present.

Treatment. Since apoplexy is liable to occur in individuals affected by arterial disease (arteriosclerosis and high blood pressure), patients suffering from these conditions should be careful to lead a moderate life, avoiding indiscretions in diet and alcohol consumption and physical or mental strain. After the onset of the stroke the patient must be placed at rest in bed and kept as quiet as possible.

It is sometimes advisable to leave him in the room where the seizure occurred until the initial shock has passed off, a mattress or couch being arranged for him to lie on. Subsequently, he may be removed to bed when adequate assistance is at hand. The head and shoulders should be slightly raised and care taken that the neck is not bent and is free from any pressure which might impede the return of venous blood from the brain. In unconscious patients the head and shoulders should be turned to one side in order to prevent the tongue from falling back and obstructing respiration. Special care is always necessary to see that unconscious or paralysed patients are not burnt by hot-water bottles.

Liquid nourishment is given, if necessary by a nasal tube when swallowing is difficult. Neither aperients nor stimulants should be administered unless ordered, but the bowels may be opened with enemata. The bladder must be watched very carefully for retention of urine, and catheterization at regular intervals may be required. Lumbar puncture is sometimes performed for diagnostic purposes.

Paralysed patients are very liable to develop bed-sores, so that great care must be taken of the skin of the back and nursing on an air or 'ripple' bed is advisable. The patient should be moved from side to side at intervals of 2 to 4 hours and kept in position by pillows in order to avoid congestion of the lungs. Paralysed limbs should be put through a full range of movement several times daily. A bed cradle should be used to take the weight of bedclothes from paralysed limbs.

Patients should be got out of bed and physiotherapy commenced as soon as practicable. Occupational therapy may often be undertaken later in suitable cases.

Some cases of internal carotid artery thrombosis may be treated surgically.

Subarachnoid haemorrhage (Intracranial aneurysm)

Sometimes, as a result of a congenital weakness in its walls, one of the arteries forming the Circle of Willis at the base of the brain develops a small aneurysm. This is liable to rupture at any age and give rise to leakage of blood into the subarachnoid space which can be found in the cerebrospinal fluid on lumbar puncture. Various symptoms may be caused such as sudden unconsciousness, signs of meningeal irritation which may resemble meningitis (i.e. neck stiffness and a positive Kernig's sign), vomiting, squints and severe headache.

Although the condition may prove fatal, many cases recover, but subsequent attacks are liable to occur, often within a few weeks. The management consists of diagnostic lumbar puncture which may be repeated in some cases, and the administration of sedatives. The patient is kept in bed for 6 weeks. The patient who recovers should be advised to avoid all sudden exertion.

In some cases, after a cerebral arteriogram has been taken to demonstrate the site of the lesion, an operation may be performed (e.g. clips are placed on the artery on both sides of the aneurysm, or ligatures may be applied). Alternatively the pressure of blood in the aneurysm may be reduced by ligation of the internal carotid artery in the neck.

Multiple sclerosis (Disseminated sclerosis)

This is a chronic, incurable and relatively common disease of the central nervous system the cause of which is unknown.

Areas of degeneration and sclerosis appear at intervals in various parts of the brain and spinal cord, thereby producing fresh symptoms. Many months or even years may elapse between each episode, the first of which usually occurs in a young adult.

While it is unnecessary to describe in detail all the symptoms which may appear, sooner or later some typical features become prominent.

1. Intention tremor. This shaking movement of the limbs is not apparent at rest but becomes obvious when the patient makes a deliberate attempt to perform an act such as picking up a pin.

2. Nystagmus. This consists of oscillating movements of the eyes from side to side when an attempt is made to fix the gaze on an object placed to one side of the patient.

3. Scanning speech. The speech becomes slow and deliberate, equal emphasis being placed on each syllable. This is a type of dysarthria sometimes called staccato speech.

4. Spastic paralysis. The legs are often affected, becoming weak and stiff with ataxia in walking. At first they are extended (**paraplegia in extension**) but as the disease progresses **flexor spasms** occur and ultimately the legs remain flexed (**paraplegia in flexion**).

In addition, numbness in the limbs, mental changes, double vision (diplopia) and sometimes blindness may all occur. As the disease progresses the sphincters are affected, resulting in incontinence.

Although the disease tends to be progressive, remissions, in which there is a temporary or prolonged improvement, may occur. In the later stages the patient may become helpless, bedridden and incontinent; bedsores may develop and death ensues from exhaustion, urinary infection or some other intercurrent disease such as pneumonia, often as long as fifteen or more years after the onset of symptoms.

No curative treatment is available, but in the early stages the general health must be maintained by good food, fresh air and moderate exercise. Physiotherapy and occupational therapy are useful. Corticotrophin (ACTH) or tetracosactrin ('Synacthen-Depot') may be tried in order to control acute episodes but do not prevent relapses. Victims of this disease have low serum levels of essential fatty acids and dietary supplements of unsaturated fats (e.g. corn oil) may diminish the frequency of relapses.

Multiple sclerosis 'Clubs' exist in which sufferers get together and often devise mechanical appliances which aid them in overcoming some of their disabilities. These clubs are usually branches of the Multiple Sclerosis Society, which helps sufferers in any way it can and finances research into the disease.

Paralysis agitans

Paralysis agitans or **Parkinsonism** is a condition which is not uncommon in old age. It is due to degenerative changes in the brain and tends to be slowly progressive.

The face becomes mask-like and emotionless, and there is a peculiar shuffling gait associated with tremor of the hands. This consists of a rhythmic movement of the thumbs over the first fingers which resembles pill or cigarette rolling.

Drugs including 'Artane', 'Lysivane', and 'Kemadrin' are used in order to reduce the muscular rigidity in Parkinsonism.

Neurosurgical procedures designed to destroy a small area in the thalamus are of value in some cases, particularly to abolish tremor. Levodopa may help dramatically in this condition, particularly in relieving akinesia (poverty of movement) and 'loosening up' the patient, who is consequently better able to fasten buttons, use eating utensils and turn over in bed. About 70% of patients with Parkinson's disease improve with levodopa therapy. The dose is gradually increased until optimal results are achieved (usually at a dose level of 3 to 6 g daily). Gastrointestinal bleeding is a rare side effect and the drug is contra-indicated in patients with a history of peptic ulceration. Other side effects of the drug are involuntary movements, mental disturbances (including hallucinations) and transient postural hypotension.

Disorders of the mind

Disorders of the mind are so common that the study of them constitutes the special branch of psychological medicine. They vary from quite minor emotional disturbances to the extreme of complete breakdown of the mind, personality and standard of behaviour.

Contact with such cases is not unusual in general medical work. This is a broad classification of the more common disorders.

1. Functional disorders or neuroses

These are relatively minor deviations from normal psychological health or unresolved mental conflicts which in themselves do not render individuals incapable of conducting their own affairs or cause them to be socially unmanageable. Although it is not always possible to ascertain any definite cause there is often some external factor which contributes to or precipitates their onset such as a severe emotional or domestic disturbance, insecurity, fear or worry. There may be some associated physical disorder or endocrine disturbance such as thyrotoxicosis present. The neuroses include:

1. Hysteria.
2. Anxiety states and depression.
3. Obsessional and compulsive neuroses.
4. Addiction to drugs, alcohol and (possibly) tobacco.

2. The psychoses and insanity

A psychosis may be primary or idiopathic, that is to say no known cause can be stated. On the other hand, many cases are secondary to organic disease such as GPI (p. 396), head injury, cerebral tumour, apoplexy or various toxic states.

The manifestations include mania, melancholia and schizophrenia, all of which involve lack of insight and of personal appreciation of the mental abnormality.

3. Mental defectives

All grades of severity may be observed from a backward and retarded child to an imbecile completely incapable of ordinary social life. Some cases are due to mongolism and some to cretinism. The latter can be treated satisfactorily.

4. Moral defectives (Psychopaths)

5. Psychosomatic disorders

This term is derived from the words 'psyche' referring to the mind and 'soma' referring to the body.

It has been seen that some mental disorders are caused by organic disease. By contrast, it is considered that some physical disorders are produced or influenced by emotional factors, abnormal stresses and nervous impulses. There is little doubt that conditions such as peptic ulcer, ulcerative colitis, asthma and some cases of eczema, for example, are adversely influenced by such stresses but it does not follow that this offers a full explanation of the causes of these conditions.

Functional disorders of the nervous system (Neuroses)

Hysteria

This condition is seen more frequently in women than in men. It is a disordered action of the mind unaccounted for by organic disease. There is, in fact, a loss of balance between will-power and emotion without disturbance of intellect, resulting in departure from the normal outlook and behaviour.

It has its origin in some conflict or confusion of emotions, or failure to cope with the environment and problems of life which surround the individual. Instead of exercising will-power to overcome the difficulties, an outlet is found in the manifestations of hysteria.

The desire to be a centre of interest and for sympathy is prominent and, to obtain this, illness is often imitated. This is not necessarily a deliberate act of the conscious mind but is due to the workings of the subconscious mind, the patient being unaware that the disorder of a function is due to a disturbed mental process and not a physical disease.

The symptoms of hysteria tend to mimic those of organic troubles and it is often difficult to ascertain the true nature of the condition.

1. Fits. Hysterical fits sometimes occur and must be distinguished from epilepsy. The patient falls to the ground and appears to be unconscious. She throws herself about wildly, resisting attempts to restrain her but neither hurting herself nor biting her tongue. Urine is not passed and 'consciousness' is recovered, usually with some display of emotion such as laughing or crying. Hysterical fits never occur in the absence of an audience nor during sleep, and their onset is often determined by emotional disturbances such as quarrels, disappointment in love, excitement or grief (see also p. 359).

2. *Disorders of sensation*. The patient may complain of a sensation of constriction in the throat ('like a ball of wind'); this is called the *globus hystericus*. Partial or complete loss of sensation in any part, especially the limbs, sometimes occurs. Its description as 'glove and stocking anaesthesia' indicates the common distribution. In order to attract attention the patient sometimes inflicts upon herself wounds or causes inflammation of the skin (*dermatitis artefacta*) particularly in insensitive areas. Hysterical deafness, blindness and loss of speech also occur.

3. *Disorders of movement, etc*. Hysterical paralysis is another manifestation of the condition and may be associated with contractures of the joints. On the other hand, an abnormal posture or gait may be assumed. In cases of malingering which may mimic hysteria a rise in temperature may be faked.

Treatment. It is essential for the medical attendant or nurse to gain the confidence of the patient and, at the same time, to avoid sympathizing with her infirmities. It is wrong, however, to give her the impression that she is thought to be malingering and that there is nothing wrong with her. Firmness and tact without harshness or unkindness must be employed. Foolish displays of emotion require reproof while any improvement should be followed up by encouragement. Severe cases of hysteria should be removed from home surroundings and the sympathetic attention of relatives and friends. Fresh air, nourishing food and absence of worry are necessary. In addition psychotherapy, suggestion, and electrical treatment are valuable.

Splashing cold water on the face is generally an effective method of dealing with an hysterical fit.

Anxiety state and depression

These are functional disorders and occur in the absence of organic disease of the nervous system, although factors such as prolonged mental strain, accidents or injuries and severe debilitating illness are common predisposing causes and may be related to the activities of the sub-conscious mind.

The main symptoms are loss of power in concentration, general muscular weakness and lack of energy. There is often loss of weight and a poor appetite together with headache, palpitation and insomnia. The patient tends to worry over trifles and to be very anxious about his health, taking special notice of unimportant symptoms and the slightest sensation of bodily discomfort. Certain fears (or phobias) may be appearent such as fear of being in an enclosed space (claustrophobia), fear of being in a crowd, fear of open spaces (agoraphobia).

The conviction that the abnormal sensations are due to organic disease is called **hypochondria.**

Depression may be mild or severe and constitutes a feeling of misery or sadness with a general feeling of lack of 'well-being'. There are two main types:

(a) Exogenous (reactive), that is depending on external circumstances such as bereavement or frustration.

(b) Endogenous, or arising from within.

Either type may lead to suicidal attempts particularly if the patient is agitated as well as being depressed.

Treatment. Attempts are made to discover and treat the cause by good history-taking, sympathetic listening, group therapy, etc. Psychoanalysis has contributed much to psychiatric thought but has not found its way into the NHS as a routine treatment because of the sheer impossibility of giving such large numbers of patients individually the time required. Fortunately, other less time-consuming methods of treatment are effective. There has been a move towards 'physical' treatment of mental disorders and this is not unreasonable when one considers the biochemical disturbances found in these patients. Physical treatments include drug therapy and electroconvulsive therapy (ECT), which is used in severe depression. Drugs used to counteract anxiety including amylobarbitone 50 mg tds, chlordiazepoxide ('Librium') 10 mg tds ('Valium') 2, 5 or 10 mg tds, and the phenothiazines, e.g. chlorpromazine ('Largactil') 25 to 50 mg tds. These drugs are called tranquillizers or ataractics.

Drugs used to treat depression (antidepressants) are of two types: the **tricyclic antidepressants** (e.g. imipramine and amitriptyline) and the **monoamine oxidase (MAO) inhibitors.** Patients taking MAO inhibitors should avoid cheese, Bovril, Marmite and certain wines since serious effects, even cerebral haemorrhage, may follow their ingestion. For the same reason amphetamines and ephedrine should be avoided. Other drugs are potentiated by MAO inhibitors and should be used with caution in reduced dosages, or not at all. Such drugs are morphine, pethidine, antihypertensive drugs and the tricyclic antidepressants. The following drugs are all MAO inhibitors: phenelzine ('Nardil'), isocarboxazid ('Marplan'), iproniazid ('Marsilid'), nialamide ('Niamid') and tranylcypromine ('Parnate').

Mental disorders

For practical purposes insanity may be defined as a disorder of the mind, manifesting itself in conduct or ideas which render the patient incapable of managing his own affairs or which are a grave source of annoyance or danger to the community. In these circumstances the law makes provision, under the Mental Health Act, for the confinement of the individual in a mental hospital if necessary, but many borderline cases occur, and these are often treated as voluntary patients in mental hospitals.

The causation of mental derangement is a wide subject. In some instances there is a hereditary mental taint, in others epilepsy, alcoholism and drug-taking play a part. General stress of life, especially at critical physiological periods such as puberty, the climacteric (menopause) and pregnancy, or ill-health associated with bodily disease, toxaemia, etc., are all factors which may be present. In addition, it has been seen that mental changes occur in organic diseases of the brain such as cerebral arteriosclerosis, cerebral tumour and general paralysis of the insane.

While it is not proposed to discuss the various types of insanity some of the symptoms which may occur will be mentioned.

1. Mania. The patient is excited, restless and talkative. In severe cases he may be violent and dangerous. Food may be refused and habits become dirty.

2. Melancholia. This is more common than mania. General depression and apathy are the main features. In addition, refusal of food, lack of personal attention, and suicidal tendencies may be present.

3. Dementia. This means progressive loss of intellectual power, memory and social instincts, the general behaviour becoming simple and childish. It tends to occur in elderly patients with cerebral arteriosclerosis. Possibly remediable causes such as vitamin B_{12} deficiency and myxoedema should, however, be searched for.

4. Confusion. The patient appears completely confused (disorientated) as to where he is, why he is there and what he is supposed to be doing. Consciousness is clouded, distinguishing confusion from dementia in which the patient remains alert.

5. Hallucinations. These are common symptoms of many forms of insanity. A hallucination is a false perception of the senses— the patient sees, smells or hears something which does not exist.

Insane acts may be provoked by the voices which the individual hears, prompting or compelling him to carry them out.

6. Delusions are false beliefs or judgements which are untrue and not amenable to reason. The patient believes himself to be the Deity, royalty or some different personage. He imagines he is being persecuted or poisoned, etc. (paranoid delusions).

7. Schizophrenia, or 'split mind', is a term incapable of exact definition, but a common feature of all cases is their detachment from the realities of the world around them. The patient lives in a 'world of his own phantasy' which results in disorders of thought, emotion and behaviour, i.e. a splintering of the personality without necessarily any loss of intelligence or physical health. Remissions and relapses often occur. Schizophrenia is treated with chlorpromazine ('Largactil') or other phenothiazines often in large doses.

8. Moral insanity. These symptoms include the performance of various anti-social acts such as stealing (kleptomania), setting fire to property (incendiarism), uncontrolled drinking bouts (dipsomania), various sexual crimes, homicide and suicide.

Mental deficiency. Varying degrees of lack of mental development may occur, from an idiot whose intellectual faculties are so poor that he is unable to acquire any power of looking after himself to an imbecile who, although he can carry out simple rules of conduct, is unable to earn a living; and a feeble-minded person, whose willpower and mental development is inadequate for independent existence without some supervision.

Mongolism (Down's syndrome). This is a special form of mental

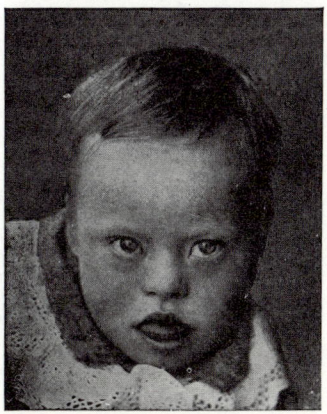

Fig. 87 A Mongol.

deficiency which is quite commonly seen. The physical appearances are characteristic. The child has a small head with the slanting, slit-like eyes of an Oriental. The face is red, the nose small and flattened at the bridge. The mouth is small but the lips tend to be thick and the tongue large. The hands are flat, broad and have short fingers. The little finger is incurved. The transverse palmar crease is single. As a rule, mongols are good-natured, affectionate and fond of music.

The condition is congenital and is associated with chromosomal abnormalities. The incidence of the condition is greatest in infants born to mothers over the age of 35.

Cretinism. This is a form of dwarfism and mental deficiency associated with lack of secretion of the thyroid gland in infancy (see p. 458).

Autism. This has been defined as 'a clinical state, transient or persistent, characterized by a failure to develop or sustain normal relationships with human beings and associated with an exceptional degree of self involvement'. It is a behaviour disorder caused by delayed or arrested maturation of the brain. A lack of normal baby speech usually brings autism to notice during the second year of life. A difficulty in communication is also shown by the fact that the child neither makes nor appreciates gestures.

An autistic child does not smile spontaneously, lacks interest in other children and is often quiet and passive.

Special schooling may help the child to become practically normal by the age of six or seven years.

9 Auto-immune Disease and Connective Tissue Diseases

There are a number diseases, some relatively common and others rare, the causes of which have not been fully explained. Among the well-known conditions are rheumatic fever, acute nephritis and rheumatoid arthritis.

Less well-known connective tissue diseases are systemic lupus erythematosus (SLE), polyarteritis nodosa, dermatomyositis, progressive systemic sclerosis (scleroderma) and Wegener's granulomatosis.

The general principles of immunity to infection and the production of gamma-globulin antibodies to the toxins of bacteria have been known for a long time, namely that the toxic antigens stimulate the individual to produce antibodies which do not cause any abnormal reaction in his own tissues.

Under certain circumstances it would appear that damage to the tissues of some individuals by bacteria, viruses, drugs or other toxic substances may cause the liberation of an antigen to which certain tissues of the individual become sensitive. The antigen–antibody reaction in these tissues or organs causes pathological changes which give rise to the symptoms of another disease which is often more serious than the initial infective condition.

Any organ so affected might be called a **target organ**. For example, in rheumatic fever the original streptococcal infection in the tonsils causes tissue reactions in the joints and often in the heart which can, therefore, be regarded as the target organs in this disease. In the same way the kidneys are the target organs in nephritis.

In some auto-immune diseases the antibodies are directed against particular target organs and are said to be **organ specific**. This is the case in acute nephritis, in pernicious anaemia (anti-gastric antibodies) and in Hashimoto's disease (anti-thyroid antibodies). In other conditions such as disseminated lupus erythematosus the antibodies are non-organ specific and damage cells throughout the body so that the disease involves many organs.

The idea can be carried further to explain other conditions such as some cases of meningeal irritation complicating infectious diseases in which no bacteria or viruses have been found in the brain or cerebrospinal fluid. Likewise, the orchitis of mumps in which the virus has not been demonstrated in the testis. In ulcerative colitis there are changes in the mucous membrane of the colon not associated with any particular infection.

Although all the facts are not known it is possible that all these conditions are in some way due to the sensitivity of the target organ to an antibody produced by the lymphocytes and plasma cells of the individual themselves and can be classified as examples of auto-immune disease.

The fundamental abnormality in auto-immune disease is the failure of the immune mechanism to distinguish between foreign proteins and 'self', allowing the antibodies which it has produced against the former, for reasons unknown, to attack its own tissues.

It is interesting to note that many of these diseases respond, at least temporarily, to the administration of steroids which damp down local inflammatory reactions.

Rheumatoid arthritis and some rarer conditions such as dis-seminated or systemic lupus erythematosus (SLE) and periarteritis nodosa have one feature in common, namely the degeneration of collagen with histological changes in the various connective tissues of the body. Collagen is a substance found in bone, cartilage and the cells which make fibrous tissue (**fibroblasts**). It can be broken down by chemical means into gelatin, polysaccharides and other sub-stances. These diseases are, therefore, sometimes referred to as 'collagen diseases' but are more accurately known as connective tissue diseases. As previously mentioned a common factor is the temporary response to steroids.

It is not possible at the present time to say more than that infection, allergy, heredity and endocrine factors may all play a part in the cause of rheumatic disease. It seems that the changes in the connective tissue produce an antigen which stimulates the reticulo-endothelial system to produce an antibody which brings about further degenerative changes.

Systemic lupus erythematosus (SLE). This disease may affect almost every organ in the body. Common features include skin lesions, sometimes with a crusting erythema of 'butterfly' distribu-tion over the nose and cheeks, joint pains, pleurisy, anaemia, leucopenia, thrombocytopenia, an increase in the serum gamma-globulin, albuminuria and raised ESR. Sometimes typical LE cells are found in the blood. The serum of patients with SLE contains a variety of abnormal antibodies which react with the patient's own cells and are therefore known as auto-antibodies (Greek: autos = self). One of them, which reacts with constituents of cell nuclei, is the *antinuclear factor* (ANF). It is this auto-antibody which induces the formation of *LE cells*. These are neutrophils, each with a large globular inclusion body composed of phagocytosed nuclear material from other leucocytes. Spontaneous remissions of symptoms may occur and rest and simple analgesics may suffice, but most patients require corticosteroid therapy. Cytotoxic drugs (e.g. 6-mercaptopurine and cyclophosphamide) may be used in resistant cases. Antimalarial drugs (chloroquine or hydroxychloroquine) may improve the affected skin and joints but do not control the disease. They may be used in combination with steroids if the latter alone do not adequately control skin and joint manifestations.

Periarteritis nodosa. In this disease there is inflammation of many arteries and the alternative name of polyarteritis nodosa is often used. The term 'nodosa' refers to the little nodules (aneurysms) which develop on the vessels in some cases. The disease is more common in males than in females and tends to start in young adulthood. The manifestations of the disease depend upon which organs are principally involved. Thus there may be, for instance, evidence of hypertension, nephritis, peripheral neuritis, blindness in one eye, asthma or cardiomyopathy. Sometimes the disease presents as a pyrexia of unknown origin. An eosinophil leucocytosis and an increased blood sedimentation rate support the diagnosis, but complete confirmation is only obtained by biopsy, usually of a muscle. Treatment is with steroids, for example prednisolone.

10 Diseases Affecting Joints, Bones and Muscles

I. JOINTS, ETC.

The term arthritis is used to describe changes in the joints which may be either inflammatory or degenerative in character. If only one joint is affected the condition is referred to as monarticular arthritis; if several joints are involved it is called polyarticular arthritis or polyarthritis (Greek: *poly* = many).

A joint consists of the ends of the articulating bones which are covered with cartilage. It is surrounded and kept in position by a capsule and special ligaments which are lined by synovial membrane.

Any or all of these structures may be involved in a disease process, depending upon the type of arthritis present.

The more common types of arthritis include:

1. Infective.
2. Rheumatic fever.
3. Rheumatoid arthritis.
4. Gout.
5. Degenerative, e.g. osteo-arthritis.
6. Traumatic.
7. Neurogenic, i.e. associated with neurological disorders such as Charcot's joints in tabes dorsalis (p. 396).

Rheumatoid arthritis

This disease is more common in women and often has its onset between the ages of 20 and 50 years. The cause of the condition is not fully understood but its progress is not materially affected by climate or diet. The blood of most patients contains an abnormal type of globulin (rheumatoid factor) which may possibly act as an antibody towards the patient's connective tissues. In other words, it is a type of auto-immune disease but the auto-immune disturbance may be secondary. The primary cause may be infective e.g. viral.

It is characterized by painful swelling of the small joints of the fingers which develop a typical spindle-shaped or fusiform appearance. Subcutaneous nodules similar to those seen in rheumatic fever may occur. In course of time other joints such as the wrists, ankles, elbows and knees become involved. It is therefore a polyarthritis which tends to be symmetrical in distribution.

The onset is sometimes acute, with fever, malaise and sweating. In other cases the onset is more gradual and its course is unpredictable, but eventually a chronic state may supervene and last for many

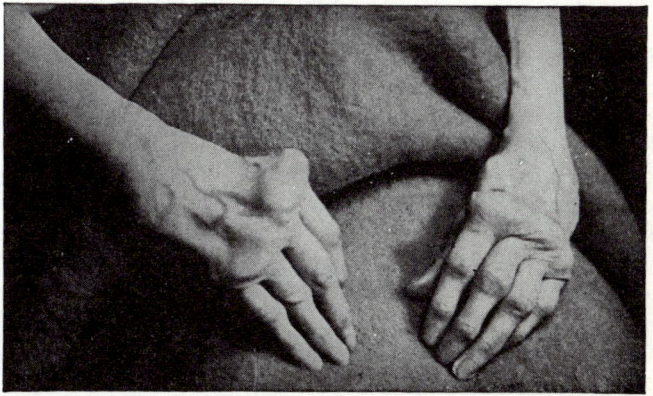

Fig. 88 Rheumatoid arthritis in a woman, showing deformity of wrists and fingers.

years, often leaving the patient severely crippled with deformed, stiff joints and wasted muscles. During the acute stages of the disease the blood sedimentation rate (ESR) is raised and the Latex test is positive. There is often loss of weight and anaemia.

This condition differs from rheumatic fever in several ways. The joint pains are not so efficiently controlled by salicylates, although aspirin may give considerable relief; permanent damage to the joint structure often follows; the smaller joints of the hands and feet are liable to be affected first; the inflammation does not tend to wander from one joint to another, and endocarditis does not usually occur.

Treatment. The aims of the treatment are:
1. To improve the general health of the patient.
2. To relieve the symptoms, e.g. pain.

3. To arrest the progress of the disease.
4. To preserve or restore the functions of the damaged joints and to prevent deformities.

Improvement or even cure may be obtained in many cases, but response to treatment is often slow and requires great patience both from the sufferer and his attendants.

GENERAL MEASURES. Attention to the general health is most important and the patient should preferably be placed in favourable hygienic surroundings including fresh air and sunshine in a warm dry climate. A generous diet with added vitamins, especially vitamin C, is given and any septic foci are removed if they are found. Anaemia, which is common, is treated with iron, or by blood transfusion if necessary. In some cases this anaemia may be due to chronic gastro-intestinal bleeding caused by aspirin.

Bed rest is important in the acute stages, but care must be taken to counteract the possible ill-effects of prolonged immobility. In other words, deformities must not be permitted to develop as a result of defects of posture. The patient should be placed on a firm mattress supported by fracture boards if necessary. When sitting up he should have a firm back-rest with a minimum number of pillows so that the back is kept straight rather than curved. He should be allowed to lie flat with one pillow at night. The weight of bedclothes should be removed from the feet by a cradle. The feet should be maintained at a right angle by sandbags or some form of foot-rest. No pillows should be placed behind the knees, which should be kept as straight as possible.

Massage and simple daily exercises, with full movements of those joints which are not too painful, is important.

TREATMENT OF JOINTS. Affected joints may be kept at rest in the proper position during the acute stages by the application of light splints or plaster. Night splints for wrists and knees are of special importance in some cases. Later, remedial exercises and physiotherapy are given to increase joint movement, and may be supplemented by appropriate occupational therapy. Orthopaedic measures may be necessary, e.g. excision of synovial membrane; finally, replacement with an artificial joint (arthrodesis).

RELIEF OF PAIN. Rest and splinting helps a great deal, but often analgesic drugs such as *aspirin*, which are very valuable in this condition, or codeine are needed and a hypnotic may be required at night. Other anti-rheumatic drugs are ibuprofen ('Brufen'), ketoprofen ('Orudis'), naproxen ('Naprosyn') and benorylate ('Benoral'). The application of methyl salicylate liniment, or kaolin poultices to

TABLE COMPARING DISEASES OF JOINTS

	Rheumatic fever	Rheumatoid Arthritis	Osteo-Arthritis	Gout
Age	Children and young adults.	25 and over.	Middle and old age.	Middle and old age.
Sex	Either.	Chiefly women.	Either.	Chiefly men.
Cause	Unknown. Auto-immune reaction to streptococci?	Unknown.	Trauma, old age, degenerative changes.	Uric acid in blood and tissues, due to disordered purine metabolism.
Joints	Usually large joints, subsiding in one and commencing in another.	Multiple, including small joints of hands and feet.	Usually one large joint, e.g. hip, knee,	Several, e.g. great toe, knee, elbow,
Pyrexia	At onset.	In acute stages.	Nil.	During acute attack.
Permanent Deformity	Nil.	Spindle-shaped joints. Often gross deformity.	Often slight.	Deformity mainly from 'chalky' deposits.
Heart	Often affected.	Infrequently affected.	Not affected.	Often arterio-sclerosis.
Treatment	Salicylates. Steroids. Rest in bed.	Local heat, etc. Physiotherapy. Gold. Steroids. Phenylbutazone. Indomethacin. Anti-malarials. Analgesics.	Analgesics, physiotherapy. + Orthopaedic measures.	Colchicine. Probenecid. Phenylbutazone. Steroids. Allopurinol. Local applications. Diet.

the joints may be appreciated and radiant heat or infra-red rays or paraffin-wax baths may be used. **Hydrocortisone** may be injected into the joints.

Phenylbutazone ('Butazolidin') is a drug which is often used. It has both an analgesic and anti-inflammatory action. Sometimes this drug produces toxic symptoms such as rashes, gastro-intestinal upset and occasionally is very dangerous because it can, quite suddenly, cause agranulocytosis, which may prove fatal, especially if a dose of 400 mg daily is exceeded. Anticoagulant drugs should not be given at the same time. The average dose is 100–300 mg daily.

Indomethacin ('Indocid'), which should be avoided in peptic ulcer and pregnancy, also has an analgesic and anti-inflammatory action. Side effects sometimes occur.

Gold, e.g. 'Myocrisin', is given by intramuscular injection and may be valuable in early cases. (Dose = 50 to 100 mg weekly until a total of up to 1 g has been given. The course may be repeated after an interval of some months.)

Steroids. These drugs have a remarkable effect in rheumatoid arthritis and may give very great symptomatic relief and increased joint movement within a few hours of administration. In rheumatoid arthritis, the joint cells are destroyed by enzymes liberated from minute intracellular bodies called lysosomes. One of the effects of steroids is to reduce the permeability of the membranes enclosing these bodies so that enzymes leak out less easily. Unfortunately, however, their use may be attended by serious side-effects and, if they are discontinued, the condition usually relapses rapidly. The psychological effect of giving them up is, therefore, very bad for the patient. The best method of using them has not yet been decided, but perhaps it is wise, in selected cases, to use small doses (e.g. prednisolone, less than 10 mg daily) sufficient to give some relief which will allow joint movement and physiotherapy to be carried out over a long period rather than to attempt to obtain a more complete remission of symptoms of a temporary character. Intra-articular injections of hydrocortisone may give considerable temporary relief.

Anti-malarial Drugs, e.g. 'Plaquenil' (hydroxychloroquine), if given in doses of 400 mg daily for 2 to 3 months may be helpful in some cases. These drugs may, however, cause permanent eye damage.

Some cases of chronic rheumatoid arthritis appear to benefit from spa treatment where, in addition to the use of the particular waters and baths, routine treatment can also be given.

When the acute symptoms have subsided encouragement and occupational therapy are of great importance.

Adaptation of the simple objects used in everyday life such as shoe horns with long handles, small rakes to draw light objects towards them, modified furniture, door-handles, etc., may help to make life much easier for patients crippled by this disease.

Suitable cases may be sent to a rehabilitation centre where specially designed apparatus may enable them to learn a productive trade. Simple handbooks on the disease are available for patients.

Still's disease

A disease, similar to rheumatoid arthritis occurring in children, in which polyarthritis with pyrexia is associated with enlargement of the lymph glands and spleen, is called Still's Disease. Steroids may be used in treatment.

Ankylosing spondylitis (spondylitis deformans)

This is a chronic arthritic condition affecting the joints of the spinal column and involving the sacro-iliac joints, producing what is called a 'poker back' or 'bamboo spine'. Its cause is unknown and probably differs from rheumatoid arthritis. It is more common in men. Physiotherapy, salicylates, phenylbutazone, indomethacin and steroids (which are not very effective) may be used in treatment. Spinal osteotomy may help patients with gross spinal deformity.

Osteo-Arthritis

This is a chronic condition which is distinguished by degenerative changes affecting primarily the articular cartilage and adjacent bone which can usually be seen on x-ray. Sometimes only one joint is affected, and it is usually a large one such as the hip, knee or shoulder joint.

It may follow some injury, but tends to occur in older subjects (40–60 years). There is no obvious inflammation present, but the joint becomes deformed and fluid may accumulate within the capsule. Creaking and grating may be heard or felt when it is moved, while pain is variable and tends to be worse in wet weather and at night.

Treatment similar to that described for rheumatoid arthritis is employed. For example, physiotherapy, aspirin, phenylbutazone and indomethacin. Oral steroids are not indicated. Shortwave diathermy is helpful and infra-red rays with exercises for wasted muscles are important. Walking-caliper splints may be used when the knee or hip joints are affected and in some cases operative measures may be necessary, e.g. in osteo-arthritis of the hip joint the diseased head of the femur may be removed and replaced by one made of plastic or stainless steel.

Other types of arthritis

Special types of acute arthritis occur if a joint becomes infected by pus-producing organisms, such as staphylococci, streptococci and pneumococci. These cases usually require operative treatment combined with antibiotics.

Tuberculous arthritis also occurs.

Gonococcal arthritis is a complication of gonorrhoea (p. 495).

The neurogenic type of arthritis associated with tabes dorsalis or diabetic neuropathy and known as a Charcot's joint is referred to on p. 396.

II. BONES

Bones may be affected by injury (fracture), inflammation (osteitis and osteomyelitis) and tumours both innocent and malignant. The treatment of these conditions is surgical.

Deformities of the skeleton occur in rickets (p. 433) and in various forms of dwarfism.

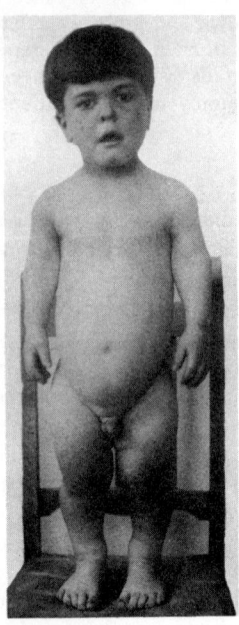

Fig. 89 Achondroplasia in a boy aged eight.

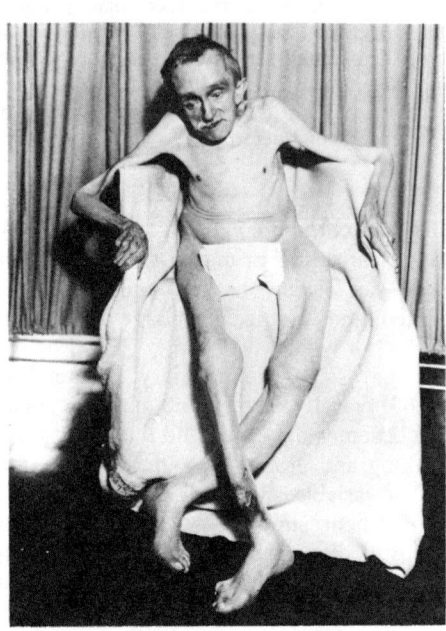

Fig. 90 Paget's disease.

Achondroplasia is a skeletal defect associated with dwarfism, the appearances of which are characteristic. Examples of the condition are often seen in public and in circuses.

The trunk is normal in length; the head appears large although the face is relatively small and has a 'pug-nose' appearance. The diminished stature is due to shortness of the long bones, especially the femora. The humerus is also affected so that the tips of the fingers only reach the iliac crests instead of over halfway down the thighs.

Paget's disease (Osteitis deformans). This is a chronic disease of bone, occurring in the latter half of life, the cause of which is unknown. The skull becomes enlarged and the tibiae thickened and bowed forwards. Other bones may also be affected. Bone pain may be severe. **Calcitonin** ('Calcitare'), obtained from porcine thyroid tissue, inhibits the excessive resorption of bone and may slow down the progression of the disease or arrest it. There are preparations for subcutaneous or intramuscular and for intravenous use. Transient nausea occurs as a side-effect in a few cases.

III. DISEASES AFFECTING THE MUSCLES

The muscles may be subject to congenital defects, important muscles failing to develop.

Inflammation of muscles is called myositis and may be associated with inflammation of the connective tissue (fibrositis, p. 422).

Wasting or **atrophy of muscles** is a common condition which the nurse can frequently observe for herself. It may be general or local in distribution and is due to a number of causes.

1. It is often part of a general wasting of the whole body due to chronic conditions such as cancer, tuberculosis, malnutrition or a prolonged illness, e.g. typhoid fever.

2. Disuse atrophy occurs if a part is kept at rest for a long period such as a limb retained in a splint or plaster. Physiotherapy is of value in preventing this condition.

3. Local muscular wasting may also be due to disease affecting the nerve supply and consequently the nutrition of the affected part. Examples of atrophy of this type have been referred to in connection with peripheral neuritis and poliomyelitis. Other lesions of the nerves or spinal cord have a similar effect.

4. Progressive muscular atrophy (Motor neurone disease) see p. 387.

There is a rare group of muscle diseases known as the **myopathies** and **muscular dystrophies**, e.g. pseudo-hypertrophic muscular dystrophy which only affects males. The latter conditions are often familial. There is degeneration of the muscle fibres which may be replaced by fat and connective tissue with consequent loss of power. No special treatment is known.

Myasthenia gravis is a rare condition of obscure origin (probably an auto-immune disease) in which the muscles become rapidly exhausted by voluntary movement but recover after a period of rest. A typical example occurs when the muscles of the eyelids are affected. The lids gradually droop until the eyes become closed. After a while the patient is able to open the eyes and the procedure is repeated. Double vision (diplopia) may occur. The jaw muscles may also be affected and mastication becomes gradually slower and less effective until a period of rest enables the patient to recommence eating. Neostigmine ('Prostigmine'), pyridostigmine ('Mestinon') and ambenonium chloride ('Mytelase') are used in treatment. Surgical removal of the thymus gland (which is an immunological organ) during the 7-year 'active' stage may have a very favourable effect, reducing or sometimes abolishing the need for drugs. A tumour, benign (thymoma) or malignant (thymic carcinoma), may occasionally be present and, paradoxically, surgery is then less likely to have a favourable effect.

'Fibrositis' (non-articular rheumatism)

This rather vague term is sometimes used to describe painful and tender areas in muscles and the fibrous tissue of the body, especially fascia, the sheaths of muscles and their ligamentous attachments. The causes of the condition are presumed to include exposure to damp and cold and possibly the presence of septic foci. It may be associated with minor trauma.

The symptoms are tenderness and pain, particularly on movement of the muscles in the affected area. It is for this reason that the condition is sometimes referred to as myalgia. Common examples of the condition are '**lumbago**' where the muscles and fascia of the back are affected, stiff neck (trapezius muscle), and pain in the chest caused by affection of the intercostal muscles and their attachments (intercostal myalgia).

The treatment consists of local applications of radiant heat or infra-red rays and massage. Aspirin and similar analgesic drugs, e.g. Tab. Codeine Co. ('Veganin'), help to relieve the pain. The injection of hydrocortisone or a local anaesthetic into painful spots is also effective.

There is probably no actual inflammation of the fibrous tissue and the nodules sometimes felt are due to localized spasm of muscle fibres.

11 Disorders of Metabolism and Deficiency Diseases

The normal metabolism of most of the important substances required and used by the healthy human body are discussed in the subject of Physiology. They include:

Carbohydrates, fats and proteins.

Mineral salts, including those of sodium, potassium, calcium, iron, chlorine, iodine, etc.

Vitamins and hormones.

Water.

Abnormalities and defects may occur in:

The intake,

The absorption,

The utilization,

of any of these substances. In some instances the gastro-intestinal tract may be at fault, in others the liver function and the secretion of bile may be defective.

While it is not possible to deal with all these abnormalities in this section of the book, reference to most of them is dealt with in connection with the major disorders which they cause.

Carbohydrates

(*a*) The main disorder of carbohydrate metabolism occurs when there is deficiency of insulin which is secreted by the islets of Langerhans in the pancreas. This results in diabetes (p. 439).

(*b*) Defects may occur in the storage of glycogen in the liver.

(*c*) Disturbance may occur in disorders of the pituitary and thyroid glands.

Fats

(*a*) Fat metabolism is closely linked with carbohydrate metabolism and, in the absence of insulin and the proper breakdown of glucose in the tissues, the complete combustion of fats is interrupted at the fatty acid stage so that diacetic acid (aceto-acetic) and acetone accumulate in the blood. These substances are then excreted in the urine (ketosis or acidosis, p. 441).

(b) This also happens in starvation and with excessive vomiting, especially in children (p. 212).

(c) Fats are not properly digested and absorbed when:

(i) The secretion of pancreatic juice is defective and the enzyme lipase is absent.

(ii) Bile salts are absent, as in some cases of jaundice.

In these cases excess of fat is found in the faeces which are pale, bulky, frothy and often offensive. Stools of this character are seen in sprue and coeliac disease, conditions in which fat absorption is defective (p. 244).

Proteins

Proteins taken in the diet are not stored as such but, after being broken down into amino acids, are used for the repair and growth of tissues. One of the end products of protein metabolism is the nitrogen-containing substance urea which is excreted in the urine. In cases of acute nephritis and other disorders of kidney function urea accumulates in the blood (p. 338).

Protein deficiency may be acute in such conditions as severe haemorrhage, extensive burns etc. Chronic shortage may result from inadequate intake or absorption. It is characteristic of **kwashiorkor**, a deficiency disease of children in underprivileged parts of the world. The clinical picture of kwashiorkor is of a wasted, anaemic child with dry skin, dependent oedema and a large fatty liver. If protein-deprivation continues the child dies.

Mineral salts. Sodium and potassium. Chlorides.

Sodium metabolism is closely linked with that of potassium and the most important salt concerned is the chloride. The various salts present in the tissues and body fluids are sometimes known as **electrolytes**. Sodium chloride or common salt is a very important constituent of the body fluids from which follows the frequent use of saline solutions in clinical medicine and surgery.

Generally speaking, in health a steady balance between the amounts of sodium and potassium is maintained in the body fluids and if, in pathological states, the sodium falls the potassium rises, and vice versa. (This is seen in some cases of Addison's disease, a disorder of the suprarenal glands which play an important part in the metabolism of sodium and potassium.) (p. 462.)

Chlorine, being an element present in hydrochloric acid, may be lost from the body when hydrochloric acid is lost by excessive vomiting. Excessive perspiration may also induce chloride loss as sodium chloride is one of the constituents of the sweat.

Replacement of water alone in cases of excessive vomiting and sweating is not enough since water is not retained by the tissues in the absence of sufficient salt. It follows, therefore, that the treatment of these conditions involves the administration of saline solutions.

Salt retention, on the other hand, results in water retention, and the opposite condition of dehydration, namely oedema, will occur. Hence the importance of a low salt diet in heart failure and nephritis, conditions in which oedema may be a prominent symptom.

Potassium. In advanced chronic renal failure the level of potassium in the blood reaches high levels and in acute renal failure, especially anuria, the level may rise rapidly to dangerous and even fatal values. A raised blood potassium may occur when there is sodium deficiency as in Addison's disease. On the other hand in severe diabetic ketosis, repeated vomiting and profuse diarrhoea, particularly where no food is taken by mouth, much potassium may be lost from the body and the blood level falls. Potassium loss may be aggravated further if too much intravenous saline alone is given to correct the dehydration associated with these conditions. Diuretic drugs may also cause the loss of large amounts of potassium in the urine. Marked potassium deficiency causes cardiac weakness with changes in the electrocardiogram, mental sluggishness, tingling in the limbs, general muscular weakness and impaired gut motility which may progress to complete paralysis of the bowel (paralytic ileus). In this condition abdominal distension and vomiting of increasingly faeculent material lead to rapid deterioration of the patient's condition and ultimately his death if the potassium deficiency is not corrected.

Low blood potassium is also known as hypokalaemia.

Calcium, see also p. 459.

Water. The following is a summary of some of the important points concerning the physiology of water metabolism.

1. Water accounts for about 60% of the body weight of a lean male adult (about 45 litres; 8 gallons) and is the main constituent of all the tissues, including the blood plasma and lymph.

2. The body requires up to 3 litres (5 pints) in 24 hours.

3. The intake is mainly in fluids taken by mouth and regulated by thirst up to 2 litres (3 or 4 pints). The remainder is contained in foodstuffs.

4. Water is excreted   (i) by the kidneys as urine,
                       (ii) by the skin as sweat,
                       (iii) by the lungs as water vapour,
                       (iv) by the bowels in faeces.

Excessive sweating, diarrhoea and vomiting, haemorrhage and loss of fluid from extensive burns will all result in increased water loss which may be serious and lead to dehydration.

5. In health there is a normal water balance in the tissues which, provided there is an adequate intake, is maintained by the excretory function of the kidneys. When this is disturbed in illness it is usual to keep a fluid balance chart on which the intake and output of fluid is accurately recorded. On such a chart are stated:

Intake: (*a*) by mouth, nasal or gastric drip,
          (*b*) by intravenous, subcutaneous, rectal or intra-peritoneal routes.

Output: (*a*) by urine,
          (*b*) by vomit,
          (*c*) by bowels, including diarrhoea.
          (*d*) by excessive sweating or copious discharge which cannot be measured accurately.

N.B.—In many instances it may be helpful to test the urinary chlorides at regular intervals (p. 322).

6. It has been seen that water is distributed in:
   (i) the blood plasma (3 litres) ⎱ Extracellular fluid
   (ii) the tissue fluids (12 litres) ⎰   (15 litres).
   (iii) the cells   Intracellular fluid
                                         (30 litres).

The balance between the intracellular and extracellular fluids is maintained by their respective osmotic pressures. The osmotic pressure depends on the protein and salt content of these fluids. If the osmotic pressure of one of them rises it extracts water from the other until the pressures are equalized. Solutions which have the same osmotic pressure are said to be 'isotonic'. A stronger solution is called 'hypertonic' and a weaker one 'hypotonic'. In order words, if hypertonic and hypotonic solutions are separated by a cellular membrane the hypertonic solution will withdraw water from the hypotonic solution until a balance is reached and both are isotonic.

If, therefore, there is water deficiency in the body, the plasma and tissue fluids will become hypertonic and will withdraw water from the intracellular fluid, causing the cells to become dehydrated.

On the other hand, if there is an excess of salt in the body, water is retained in the tissues and is not excreted by the kidneys. This accumulation of fluid results in oedema.

Water deficiency; 'Dehydration'

Lack of water in the body may be due to:
  (*a*) Deficient intake of fluid.
  (*b*) Excessive loss of fluid (a more common pathological cause).
    (i) Excessive sweating in febrile illness.
    (ii) Working in excessive heat, e.g. tropical countries, miners, stokers.
    (iii) Overheating of unconscious patients.
    (iv) Severe diarrhoea and vomiting from any cause.
    (v) Severe haemorrhage and burns.
    (vi) Diabetes and diabetic coma.

Signs and symptoms include thirst, which is not always present, dry tongue, dry inelastic skin, sunken eyes, tachycardia, decreased urinary output and raised blood urea, leading eventually to acute renal failure.

In infants the anterior fontanelle is depressed.

Treatment. Supply water and salt by oral, intravenous, subcutaneous or rectal administration. Normal saline or electrolyte solution may be given. Depending on the severity of the case between 2 and 4 litres are required in 24 hours. It must be remembered, however, that an excess of water introduced into the circulation may lead to 'water intoxication' and pulmonary oedema, which may prove fatal.

Water retention; oedema

The accumulation of fluid in the tissues may be either general of local in distribution. Subcutaneous oedema is characterized by pitting on pressure which causes temporary local displacement of the fluid away from the site of the pressure.

General oedema. The factors which cause water to be retained in the tissues are:
    (i) Increase in the general venous pressure, which occurs in heart failure and constrictive pericarditis and which results in increased capillary pressure so tending to force fluid through the walls of the capillaries into the tissue spaces.
    (ii) Failure of the kidneys to excrete water and salt either because they are damaged by disease, e.g. nephritis; or because their blood supply and circulation are defective.

(iii) Salt retention.

(iv) Lowered osmotic pressure of the blood due to lowering of the blood proteins, e.g. loss of albumin in the urine over long periods, as in the nephrotic syndrome and impaired production of albumin in the liver in cirrhosis.

(v) Serious malnutrition and starvation.

Local oedema. (i) Increase in the pressure of blood in local veins. This increase in venous pressure results in an increase in capillary pressure so that fluid is forced to pass through the walls of the capillaries into the tissue spaces. This may occur:

(*a*) As part of an increase in the general venous pressure which occurs in congestive heart failure.

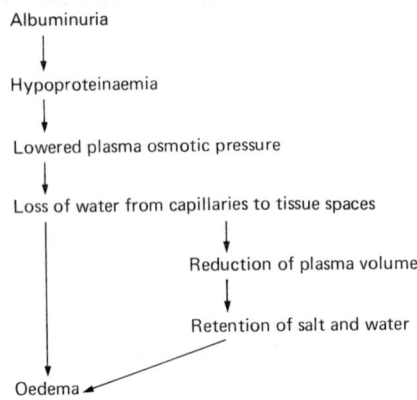

Fig. 91 Factors involved in renal oedema (Nephrotic Syndrome).

(*b*) Local pressure on a large vein by a tumour or constriction of any sort.

(*c*) Thrombosis of a large vein, e.g. femoral venous thrombosis which will cause oedema of the leg ('White leg').

(ii) Local damage to the capillary walls may cause similar leakage. Oedema fluid tends to collect:

(*a*) In the most dependent parts, mainly due to the effect of gravity and the fact that the venous and, therefore, the capillary pressure is also greatest in these parts.

(*b*) Where the tissues are loose and not closely attached to firm structures such as bone, e.g. the tissues around the eyes which become oedematous in nephritis.

(*c*) In large serous cavities such as the pleural cavities and the peritoneal cavity (ascites).

Treatment of general oedema

1. Restrict salt intake.

2. Increase urinary output by diuretics, e.g. chlorothiazide, frusemide ('Lasix'), 'Hygroton' etc. Spironolactone (a synthetic steroid) may be used especially in resistant cases.

3. Improve general circulation by administration of digitalis when the oedema is due to congestive heart failure, especially when there is atrial fibrillation.

4. Restrict fluid intake.

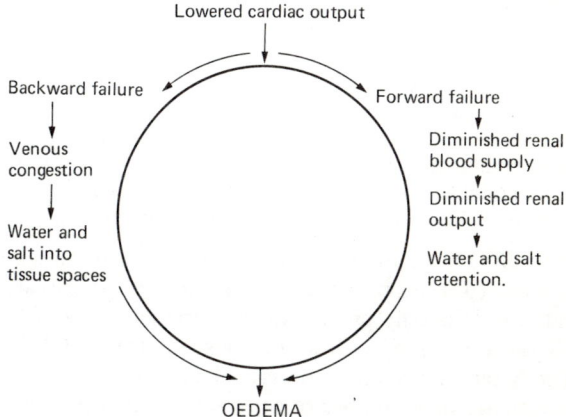

Lowered cardiac output

Backward failure

Forward failure

Venous congestion

Diminished renal blood supply

Diminished renal output

Water and salt into tissue spaces

Water and salt retention.

OEDEMA

Fig. 92 Some of the factors involved in cardiac oedema.

5. Remove fluid by tapping (paracentesis) when this is indicated.

6. Relieve venous obstruction when feasible.

N.B.—The local oedema due to inflammation is of a different character. It is an exudate of fluid into the tissues and one of Nature's methods of dealing with infection and diluting toxins.

Water intoxication. It is possible to overload the body with water. Mentally disturbed people may do this by drinking vast quantities of water. Water intoxication may also occur as a therapeutic misadventure during intravenous therapy or, in infants, during a period of tube feeding. The signs are apathy and epileptiform convulsions and the treatment is intravenous injection of hypertonic saline. Unless the condition is promptly recognized and treated, death may ensue.

Diseases due to vitamin deficiency

Vitamins are a class of substances of complex composition, existing in minute quantities in natural foods, which are necessary for normal nutrition and development.

In some instances the pure vitamin has been separated and its composition discovered.

The following is a brief account of the more important vitamins and the diseases associated with their deficiency:

Vitamin A. This fat-soluble vitamin is found in animal fats (e.g. milk, butter, cream, beef fat and cod-liver and halibut-liver oil). It is also present in eggs, raw carrots and green vegetables. It is not found in the vegetable fats (i.e. olive, linseed or coco-nut oil) and consequently is absent from margarine until it is specially vitaminized. It is closely related to the yellow pigment of carrots which is known as carotene. Deficiency in the diet is uncommon but results in **night-blindness** or difficulty experienced by some people in seeing in the dark. In some cases, eye troubles such as corneal ulcer, conjunctivitis and a condition known as **xerophthalmia** may develop. It is possible, but by no means certain, that resistance to infection, especially of the lungs and alimentary tract, may be lowered.

Vitamin B. This complex water-soluble vitamin is mainly found in yeast, seeds (pea, bean and lentil), in eggs, and in cereals such as wheat and rice. It is only present in the germ and husk of the cereals so that if these are removed, as in polished rice, a deficiency may occur. The vitamin originally described in this way has now been shown to consist of a number of separate substances each of which has a different action. The most important are:

ANEURINE (thiamine), *Vitamin B_1*. This vitamin is concerned in the metabolism of carbohydrates. Severe deficiency results in **beri-beri**, a disease affecting the heart (cardiomyopathy) and the nerves (peripheral neuropathy). This occurs mainly in the rice-eating populations of the East where the staple diet is polished rice. Aneurine is also used in many other conditions where minor degrees of deficiency are suspected. The dose varies from 25 to 100 mg daily by mouth or intramuscular injection.

RIBOFLAVINE (B_2). Deficiency of this vitamin is associated with soreness of the lips and tongue and the development of fissures at the angle of the mouth. The average dose is 6 to 12 mg daily.

NICOTINAMIDE (niacin). **Pellagra,** a disease causing intestinal upset, skin eruptions, nervous symptoms and mental changes is due to lack of this vitamin. This is also a tropical disease not seen in this country in its fully-developed form. Nicotinic acid is sometimes used as a vaso-dilator in a number of conditions, but its effect is uncertain. Doses vary from 50 to 250 mg daily.

CYANOCOBALAMIN, *Vitamin B_{12}*, is present in meat and other animal foods. It is used in the treatment of pernicious anaemia (pp. 177, 509).

FOLIC ACID is used in the treatment of tropical sprue, coeliac disease and certain types of macrocytic anaemia (p. 180).

Other substances in this group include pyridoxine, pantothenic acid and biotin, the importance of which is uncertain.

Broad spectrum antibiotics such as the tetracyclines may interfere with the absorption of vitamin B from the gut when given by mouth so that a suitable preparation is sometimes given at the same time.

Vitamin C (ascorbic acid, Anti-Scorbutic). This is found in fresh foodstuffs, especially fruits such as oranges, lemons, black currants, rose hips, tomatoes and green vegetables, and is therefore present in salads. It is rapidly destroyed by heat and is consequently lacking in tinned foods and boiled or dried milk.

Its absence from the diet results in the development of scurvy which is the main indication for its use (p. 433).

Ascorbic acid may also be a factor in the formation of haemoglobin and is sometimes given at the same time as iron in the treatment of anaemia.

It may be given in tablet form in therapeutic doses of 250 mg or more, daily in divided doses.

Vitamin D, Calciferol (Anti-rachitic). The distribution of this substance throughout Nature is similar to that of vitamin A and its chief sources of supply are milk, butter, margarine, sardines, cod-liver and halibut-liver oil, eggs, etc. (Normal daily requirement, 400–800 units.)

It is produced by the action of sunlight or ultra-violet rays upon a substance called 7-dehydrocholesterol which is present in the skin and may also be prepared artificially. It is only when this vitamin is present in adequate amounts that calcium and phosphorus are properly absorbed and utilized in the body in the processes of formation and growth of bones and teeth. Deficiency of vitamin D is responsible for rickets and for osteomalacia in adults.

Vitamin E, Tocopheryl acetate. This is found in wheat-germ, milk and green vegetables. In animals its absence has been found to cause sterility. Its action in the human being is not fully understood.

Vitamin K, (Menaphthone). This vitamin is present in green vegetables such as spinach, and egg yolk. It is also manufactured in the bowel by the action of bacteria but bile salts are necessary for its absorption. It is stored in the liver where it is essential for the production of prothrombin required in the process of blood clotting. Deficiency is most likely to occur in the premature or newborn infant whose bowel is sterile and results in 'haemorrhagic disease of the new born' in which melaena, epistaxis, etc. may occur. In this condition dosage should be limited to 1 mg daily. Overdosage may lead to blood destruction.

Prothrombin deficiency also occurs in some cases of jaundice, biliary fistula and gastro-intestinal disorders and can be detected by laboratory estimations. In these conditions dosage may be increased up to 5–15 mg daily.

Haemorrhagic symptoms may be caused by overdosage with anti-coagulant drugs (not heparin) which destroy prothrombin in the liver. In this instance a special chemical variety (K_1) is required and may be given either orally or intravenously. Blood transfusion may also be needed (p. 160).

'Vitamin deficiency.' The infrequent occurrence of deficiency diseases such as beri-beri, xerophthalmia and scurvy indicates that a complete absence of vitamins from the diet rarely exists in this country. On the other hand, a partial deficiency may be responsible for ill-health and lowering of resistance to infection which may be serious.

Cereals and carbohydrates form a large part of the diet, especially among the poor and elderly people, living on their own, on account of their relative cheapness and simplicity of preparation. They provide energy but are deficient in vitamins, while substances such as milk, butter, eggs and vegetables, having a high vitamin content, are relatively expensive, and take only a small place in the dietary of the elderly and poorer classes. Vitamins may be of real value in pregnancy, infancy, various diseases in which absorption may be defective and convalescence and care should be taken so that they are included in all special diets (e.g. some gastric diets), continued for long periods. The subject is one of importance in matters affecting the general health of the public, but there is no doubt that large quantities are taken unnecessarily by healthy people on the false assumption that they are 'tonics'.

On the other hand, excessive intake (hypervitaminosis) especially of A and D may cause serious undesirable effects.

Scurvy

The disease occurs in two forms:

(*a*) the adult, (*b*) the infantile.

In both varieties the condition is due to deficiency of **vitamin C.** The adult type is characterized by debility, anaemia, delay in the healing of any wound or ulcer which may be present, sponginess of the gums which bleed when touched and a tendency to haemorrhages, especially into the skin. It may occur in old people living alone and some travellers who do not obtain fresh fruit and vegetables.

Infantile scurvy, now uncommon, usually appears between the eighth and twelfth month in bottle-fed babies, especially those having only condensed milk or milk habitually subjected to prolonged boiling, which destroys vitamin C (ascorbic acid).

After a preliminary period in which fretfulness and refusal of food are present, the onset of acute symptoms is sudden. There is extreme tenderness of the limbs, the child screams when moved and swellings may develop over the lower end of the femur or upper part of the tibia. These are due to haemorrhages under the periostium of the bones. Occasionally haematuria may occur. If any teeth are present the surrounding gums are swollen, 'spongy' and bleed when touched. In the absence of teeth, the gums are normal.

Treatment. The essential point of both the prophylactic and active treatment of scurvy is the supply of an adequate amount of the anti-scorbutic vitamin C in the diet. This is most conveniently given to children in the form of orange juice or tomato juice. (Four teaspoonsful, sweetened with sugar, daily.) Adults may take the whole fruit, together with green salads, unboiled milk, etc. Tablets of ascorbic acid may be used in doses of 50 mg for prophylaxis or up to 500 mg for the treatment of the established condition, three times a day.

The general management of infantile cases is important. The child must be handled with great care. If it is necessary to move the child he should be carried on a pillow. The affected limbs should be wrapped in cotton-wool and may be steadied by light splints. The clothing must be such that it can be removed without lifting the infant and bedclothes should rest on a cradle.

Rickets

Rickets is a disorder of nutrition occurring in early childhood which results from a disturbance of calcium and phosphorus metabolism associated with deficiency of **vitamin D.**

It has been seen that vitamin D is present in milk, butter, eggs, etc., and that it may also be formed in the body by the action of sunlight upon the substance 7-dehydrocholesterol, which is present in the skin. It therefore follows that the condition may occur either as a result of deficient vitamin D in the diet or as a result of bad hygienic surroundings, with lack of sunlight and fresh air.

In the absence of vitamin D, the body is unable to absorb and utilize the calcium and phosphorus in the diet which leads especially

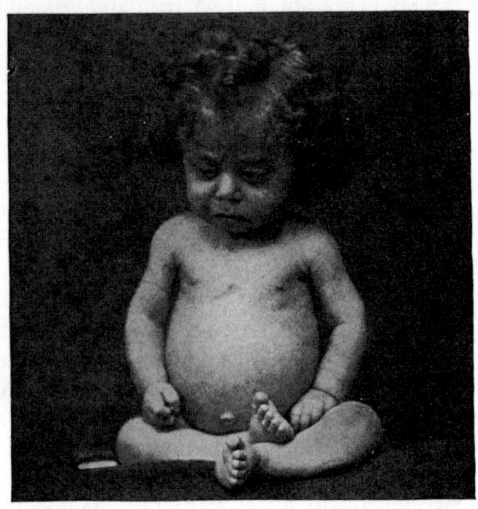

Fig. 93 Rickets, showing square head, 'pot-belly' and method of production of the curves in the tibiae.

to bony changes, for these substances are of great importance in the production of strong bones. In addition, other structures of the body are affected and this is shown by the common occurrence of bronchitis, gastro-intestinal upsets, loss of tone in the muscles, and nervous symptoms, e.g. convulsions and tetany (p. 461).

The characteristic features of the disease are:
1. General symptoms including gastro-intestinal, respiratory and nervous complications.
2. Bony deformities.
3. Delayed dentition.

1. General symptoms. The disease, now fortunately much less common may make its appearance between the ages of 4 months and 3 years in bottle-fed babies, living in bad conditions, especially among coloured immigrants. However, it is not common in tropical countries where there is adequate sunlight irrespective of a poor diet. It is most likely to occur in the spring, after the winter months when sunlight is scarce, the vitamin content of foods is at its lowest and infants tend to be kept indoors on account of the cold.

The earliest symptoms to attract attention are restlessness, irritability and sweating, especially about the head when the child is asleep, in a flabby infant who has been having a diet high in carbohydrate but low in fat. Loss of appetite, vomiting, diarrhoea, bronchitis and convulsions may also occur. As the disease progresses other symptoms may be observed, such as distension of the abdomen (pot-belly) and anaemia.

2. Bony deformities. Owing to the lack of lime salts (calcium phosphate), the bones become soft and easily bent, with the production of deformities, e.g.:

(a) THE LIMBS. The long bones become enlarged at the epiphyses and the shafts may be curved, a typical deformity being bowing of the femur and tibia resulting either in bow-leg or knock-knee. X-ray changes in the epiphyses occur early and are characteristic.

(b) THE HEAD. The skull assumes a box-shaped appearance with flattening of the top, and prominence of the frontal and parietal portions.

The fontanelle which normally closes at 18 months remains open. An early sign of rickets is the presence of localized areas of softening in the bones of the skull called craniotabes. When this is present these spots can be indented like a rubber ball, the bone rebounding into position when the finger is released.

(c) THE THORAX. The epiphyses at the junction of the ribs and the costal cartilages become enlarged, forming a row of small knobs down each side of the chest (the rickety rosary).

The so-called 'pigeon-chest' with a very prominent sternum may develop later together with spinal deformities (kyphosis and scoliosis).

(d) THE PELVIS. This may become narrowed or flattened, giving rise to difficult labour in later life in affected females.

3. Delayed dentition. In the normal infant 6 teeth are present by the 12th month and this number is usually doubled by the end of the 15th month.

In rickets there are often no teeth at the age of 1 year. When they do appear the enamel is soft and defective and they are subject to early decay.

Complications. A rickety child is liable to the development of bronchitis and gastro-intestinal disorders and, while rickets itself is not a fatal disease, when associated with these complications it becomes serious.

A definite increase in the irritability of the nervous system to which the name 'spasmophilia' has been given is also liable to occur in rickets. This includes symptoms of tetany (p. 461) and laryngismus stridulus (p. 268). In these conditions the blood calcium is usually low.

Treatment. This may be considered in three sections:

1. Prevention   ⎰ by diet, sunlight and vitamin
2. Treatment of the active disease ⎱   D.
3. The prevention and treatment of bony deformities (orthopaedic or operative measures).

(1) Prevention. The best safeguard against the development of rickets is breast-feeding for 6 months, but it must be remembered that the disease is liable to develop later in infants who are kept entirely on the breast after this period. When weaning has taken place an adequate amount of cow's milk must be given and the diet should contain fat in the form of butter or vitaminized margarine. An excess of starchy foods is to be avoided.

Infants who are entirely bottle fed should be given daily cream, cod-liver oil or a few drops of one of the vitamin D preparations (e.g. radiostoleum), in addition to orange or other fruit juice which supplies especially vitamin C.

During the second year of life a child should have 1 pint of milk a day together with the yolk of an egg which also contains vitamin D.

Although these dietetic measures are important the value of sunlight in the prevention of rickets cannot be over-emphasized. It has been seen that the disease is most prevalent during the winter and early spring and, in the rare instances in which rickets develops in breast-fed babies, it will be found that they have had very little outdoor life. It has been stressed that breast milk and fresh cow's milk contain vitamin D, but it must be clearly understood that the amount present is not high. Therefore, all infants should be placed out of doors for a period every day, whenever possible, with the hood of the perambulator down. Sunburn should be avoided, however.

Cod or halibut liver oil are satisfactory methods of giving vitamin D. A few drops may be added to the feeds during the first few weeks and gradually increased in the course of a fortnight to 2 ml, 30 minims, 3 times a day. Excessive doses may cause digestive disturbances, while older children sometimes prefer cod-liver oil and malt. Prolonged excessive dosage can be dangerous giving rise to 'infantile hypercalcaemia' with mental retardation and renal damage.

Prophylactic treatment should be given to:

(*a*) All artificially fed infants.

(*b*) Breast-fed infants who have little fresh air and sunshine.

(*c*) Premature infants.

(2) Treatment of the active disease. Careful management of the general health is necessary. The diet must be carefully standardized to contain, milk, eggs and meat, avoiding excess of starchy material. Fresh air is essential. The child should wear light but warm clothing and proper hours of sleep must be arranged.

Vitamin D is supplied either as cod or halibut liver oil or one of the proprietary preparations, or by exposing the skin to ultra-violet rays (direct or artificial sunlight) whereby it is formed from 7-dehydrocholesterol. The dose of vitamin D given is approximately twice that used in prophylaxis.

X-rays show that healing commences in about a fortnight and is complete in 1 to 4 months, depending on the severity of the case.

(3) The prevention and treatment of bony deformities. The bony deformities can to some extent be prevented by remembering that the bones are soft and that curvature will result if they are subject to a prolonged strain. In the early stages light splints projecting beyond the foot may be applied to the legs in order to prevent the child from standing. These are removed when healing takes place.

Physiotherapy is given to improve the nutrition and tone of the muscles. If permanent deformities such as bowed tibiae, knock-knee, etc., are present in later life they may be remedied by orthopaedic or operative measures.

Gout

Gout is a disorder of metabolism, the origin of which is not clear. It results in the accumulation in the blood of uric acid which is deposited in the form of salts (crystals of sodium urate) in and around the joints with the production of recurrent attacks of acute arthritis. Uric acid is derived partly from the nuclei of cells taken in the food (**exogenous**, from without) and partly from the nuclei of worn-out cells in the body (**endogenous**, from within).

It is most common in males of middle age, especially but not always those accustomed to good living, rich foods and alcohol. A family history of the condition is often obtained and the condition

may be brought on in patients taking chlorothiazide and similar
diuretics.

Acute gout. An acute attack is of sudden onset with severe pain,
swelling and redness of one or more joints. The pain may subside
after a few hours only to recur next day. The great toe is commonly
affected first but other joints including the ankles, knees, hands and

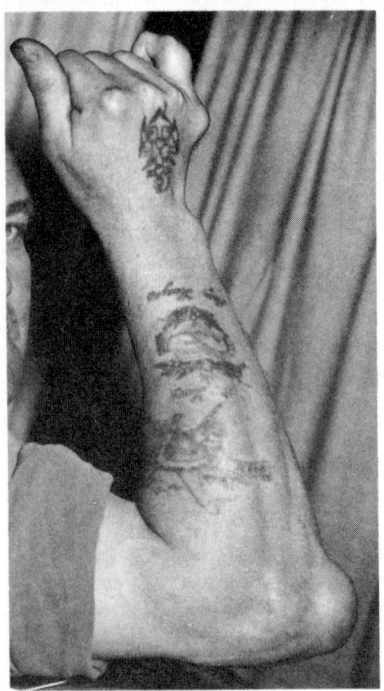

Fig. 94 Gout, showing deposits in meta-
carpal joints and olecranon bursa.

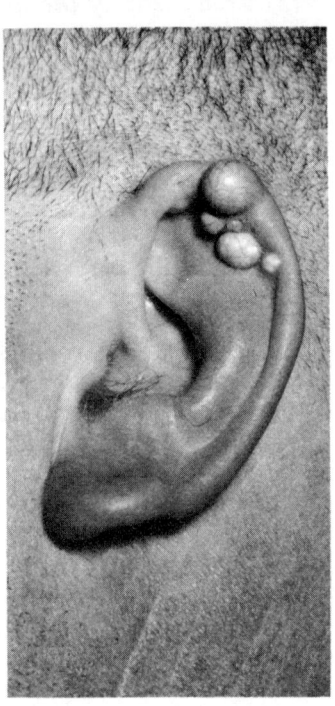

Fig. 95 Gout, showing tophi in
ear.

elbows may also be involved. The temperature is raised and there
is often marked irritability of temper. (The comic artist always
endows peppery colonels with an attack of gout!) An attack usually
subsides with treatment in the course of a few days.

Chronic gout. Chronic changes in the joints cause them to
become permanently deformed. Deposits of urates remain as 'chalky'
masses in the surrounding ligaments as well as in the articular
cartilages and bones.

Similar masses called **tophi** may be found in the cartilage of the ears. These are popularly called 'chalk stones' because when situated close to the surface of the skin, ulceration may occur with the extrusion of white material consisting of urates but looking like chalk.

Chronic gout may be complicated by arteriosclerosis affecting coronary, cerebral and renal vessels which may ultimately shorten the life of the patient.

Treatment. During the acute stages the painful joints may be wrapped in cotton-wool, supported on pillows and the weight of bedclothes carried by a cradle. Applications of lead lotion or spraying with ethyl chloride may afford some relief. A light diet with plentiful fluids is given and the bowels are kept open by saline aperients if necessary.

Colchicine, 0·5 mg every 1 or 2 hours until the pain is relieved or diarrhoea and vomiting supervene, was the traditional treatment in acute attacks but has been superseded by phenylbutazone, 600 mg daily for 2 or 3 days, then 300 mg daily.

Other drugs used in gout include:

(a) Acute gout.	(b) Chronic gout.
Phenylbutazone.	Sulphinpyrazone ('Anturan').
Indomethacin ('Indocid').	Probenecid.
Steroids.	Ethebenecid ('Urelim').
	Allopurinol ('Zyloric').

Salicylates and thiazide diuretics should not be given at the same time as sulphinpyrazone. Allopurinol administration may at first cause an increase in symptoms which may be covered by other drugs such as colchicine, phenylbutazone, indomethacin etc.

Between attacks and in chronic gout the diet should be strictly moderated and alcohol is usually avoided. Meat should only be taken once a day, but sweetbreads, liver, kidneys, duck and rich game are best avoided.

Diabetes mellitus

Diabetes is a disorder of carbohydrate metabolism due to relative or absolute deficiency of the internal secretion of the pancreas, insulin, and is associated with a rise in the sugar content of the blood and the appearance of sugar in the urine. It may, therefore, be regarded either as a disorder of metabolism or as a disorder of internal secretion.

Normally the islets of Langerhans in the pancreas secrete **insulin** into the bloodstream but they take no part in the formation of the pancreatic juice which is poured into the intestine and aids the process of digestion. Insulin is, therefore, an internal secretion or hormone. Much of the energy of the body is obtained by the burning up of sugar in the form of glucose (also called dextrose) derived from carbohydrates, but this can only take place in the muscles and tissues when an adequate amount of insulin is present. In the absence of sufficient insulin, sugar which the tissues cannot use accumulates in the blood (hyperglycaemia) and, when this reaches a certain level, it is excreted by the kidneys and appears in the urine (glycosuria).

Ketosis. The metabolism of carbohydrate is intimately connnected with that of fat. It is only when sugar is being burnt that an equivalent amount of fat can be fully broken down into carbon dioxide and water. If sugar is not being used by the tissues owing to lack of insulin, fats are broken down at an increased rate to provide energy. An intermediate product of fat katabolism, aceto-acetic acid, accumulates in the blood and appears in the urine together with acetone. These two substances are referred to as ketone bodies and their accumulation in the body as ketosis, acetonaemia or acidosis. In diabetes, ketosis may be severe, the toxic effects on the nervous system contributing to the state of diabetic coma. Milder degrees of ketosis also occur in starvation and cases of excessive vomiting (p. 320).

Cause. Although the mechanism by which glycosuria is produced is understood, little is known of the cause of the diabetes in most cases. Sometimes diabetes is due to chronic pancreatitis. Excessive secretion or administration of adrenal cortical hormones (Cushing's syndrome) or growth hormone (acromegaly) may cause a diabetic state.

All ages may be affected including children, but the commonest incidence is between 30 and 60 years. In younger patients the disease is often severe in type. Not infrequently hereditary factors may be present and the condition is particulary common among elderly Jews. In some individuals who appear to have a latent tendency to the condition it may be brought on by the use of some drugs such as steroids and thiazide diuretics.

In the maturity-onset diabetes of obese persons, insulin levels in the blood are actually raised above normal. However, the levels are insufficient for the increased requirements imposed by the obesity. The pancreatic islet cells pour out large quantities of insulin in response to the increased demand but, because of inherited or acquired defects, cannot sustain the high output.

Symptoms. The onset of the disease may be gradual or sudden, the patient complaining of thirst, a large appetite and increasing weakness. In some cases there is loss of weight, often marked in young subjects.

The glucose content of the blood is raised to such a high level that it also appears in the urine in large amounts. Glucose in the urine acts as a diuretic with the result that the amount of urine secreted in increased (polyuria). This is further increased by taking large quantities of fluid to relieve thirst.

Characteristics of the urine. The daily quantity is increased; it is pale in colour but has a high specific gravity (1025–1045) on account of the sugar which it contains. The presence of sugar may be detected by Benedict's test, the 'Clinitest' or with 'Clinistix' which the patient may be taught to use himself (p. 319).

When ketosis is present, acetone and aceto-acetic (diacetic acid) are demonstrated by Rothera's and the ferric chloride tests or the 'Acetest'. Albumin is occasionally present.

Complications. *1. Skin lesions.* Boils and carbuncles may occur. Itching of the skin (pruritus) due to monilia infection, especially about the vulva and anus, is common, and may be the first symptoms indicating the disease.

2. Arterial disease. Arteriosclerosis, hypertension and coronary thrombosis are liable to occur. In elderly patients (over 50) with arteriosclerosis, gangrene of the toes may develop, especially in the presence of corns or neglected toe-nails, hence the importance of care of the feet and suitable foot-wear in diabetes. Spreading gangrene sometimes necessitates amputation of the limb.

3. Renal disease with albuminuria (Kimmelstiel-Wilson syndrome).

4. Eye changes, these include cataract (opacity of the lens), and haemorrhages, exudates and microaneurysms in the retina (retinopathy) which may lead to blindness.

5. Neuropathy, especially in the lower limbs, producing tingling sensations, pain and loss of reflexes.

6. Diabetic coma. This is the most important complication and is connected with the accumulation of ketone bodies in the blood, but since the introduction of insulin treatment it has become less common. The onset is gradual and may be preceded by epigastric pain, headache, loss of appetite and obstinate constipation. Sometimes emotional disturbances occur. Increasing drowsiness develops and may proceed to deep coma. The pulse becomes weak and rapid and the temperature is subnormal. A common feature is the presence of marked dyspnoea with deep, sighing respirations described as 'air-hunger'.

Sugar and acetone are present in large amounts in the urine and the breath is found to have a sweet odour, resembling 'new-mown hay' and due to acetone. The presence of a positive ferric chloride test in the urine is always a danger sign in diabetes. Unless efficient treatment is instituted at once the condition may prove fatal.

Very rarely coma develops without the presence of urinary ketones in diabetic patients with severe dehydration, especially in the older age group. The treatment consists in giving insulin and large quantities of water as intravenous hypotonic saline.

Diagnosis. The diagnosis of diabetes is suggested by the history and the appearance of sugar in the urine but is often discovered on routine examination, especially if the test is carried out after a meal as sugar may be absent in an early morning specimen. The following investigations may also be performed.

1. Blood sugar. A sample of blood is taken, usually in the morning when the patient is fasting and sent to the laboratory for examination. The normal fasting blood-sugar is between 80 and 120 mg per 100 ml and the level should not rise above 180 mg per 100 ml after a carbohydrate meal.

2. Glucose tolerance test. Before any food has been taken in the morning, a specimen of blood is collected. The patient is then given 50 grams of glucose dissolved in 300 ml ($\frac{1}{2}$ pint) of water. Blood and urine are collected at intervals of half an hour for two and a half hours.

Treatment. Before the introduction of insulin by Banting in 1922 the treatment of diabetes consisted of reducing the amount of carbohydrate in the diet until the urine was free from sugar and, at the same time, adjusting the amount of fat so that ketosis did not occur. Periods of starvation were employed with the object of resting the pancreas and allowing the excess of sugar in the blood to be utilized by the tissues and excreted by the kidneys.

As a rule a standard diet is used, the calorie value of which depends on the weight and energy requirements of the patient, and consists of:

Carbohydrate	100 to 250 grams
Protein	60 to 90 grams
Fat	60 to 100 grams
Calories =	1200 to 2200

N.B.— 1 gram of carbohydrate supplies 4 calories
1 gram of protein supplies 4 calories
1 gram of fat supplies 9 calories

The average man requires the following number of calories which must be increased 10–20 per cent if muscular work is being performed. This is an average of 30 calories per kilogram (14 calories per pound) bodyweight.

8 stone	112 lbs	52 kg	1700 Calories
9 stone	126 lbs	60 kg	1900 Calories
10 stone	140 lbs	65 kg	2100 Calories
11 stone	154 lbs	70 kg	2200 Calories
12 stone	168 lbs	77 kg	2500 Calories

The quantities of the actual foodstuffs taken are calculated from diet tables in such a way that the total amounts of carbohydrate, protein and fat correspond with those permitted in the diet. By consulting diet tables (p. 554) the menu may be varied from day to day, but care must be taken to weigh out accurately each portion of food. The diet is so arranged that the greater part of the carbohydrate allowed each day is taken at the morning and evening meals.

The **Line Ration Scheme*** outlined by Lawrence is a scheme readily adaptable to all cases. Each line ration represents 155 calories and is divided into two portions as follows:

Black Portion	10 g carbohydrate
Red Portion	$7\frac{1}{2}$ g protein and 9 g fat

Any black portion may be combined with any red portion to make a ration and the number of rations a day divided, as necessary, between the different meals according to the time of insulin administration.

One Black Portion added to one Red Portion = one Line Ration.

CARBOHYDRATE FOODS (containing Sugar or Starch)
Black portions (10 g Carbohydrate)

	oz
Rice, Sago, tapioca (raw)	$\frac{2}{5}$
Biscuit, Toast or Breakfast Cereals; Flour, Oatmeal, Macaroni (all dry); Jam or Marmalade	$\frac{1}{2}$
Bread (all kinds)	$\frac{2}{3}$
Potato, Peas or Beans (dried or tinned); Banana or Grapes; Dried Apricots (stewed)	2
Parsnips, Ripe Greengages; Prunes (stewed)	3
Raw Apple, Pear, Cherries, Gooseberries, Plums, Damsons, Orange (skinned); Young Peas or Beetroot	4
Peach or Apricot or Black Currants (ripe); Greengages (stewed); Broad Beans	5
Strawberries; Stewed Pears, Damsons or Plums	6

* The 'Line Ration' diet scheme is published in card form by Messrs. H. K. Lewis & Co.

Milk (also contains 1 Red); Black Currants (stewed); Raspberries or Melon (ripe)	7
*Apples or Cherries (stewed); Carrots or Leeks	8
*Jerusalem Artichokes; Loganberries; Blackberries (stewed)	10
*Grapefruit (in skin); Tomatoes; Red Currants	12
*Onions, Turnips or Radishes	14

Negligible Starch Content in Average Helpings of:

Asparagus, Green Artichokes, French Beans, Brussels Sprouts, Cabbage, Cauliflower, Celery, Cranberries, Cress, Cucumber, Egg Plant, Endive, Stewing Gooseberries, Greens, Horseradish, Lemons, Lettuce, Marrow, Mushrooms, Radishes, Rhubard, Salsify, Scarlet Runners, Seakale, Spinach.

Red Portions (Proteins and Fat)
$7\frac{1}{2}$ g Protein and 9 g fat

One Egg
Bacon or Ham (both lean) 1 oz
Kidney $1\frac{1}{4}$ oz and Fat $\frac{1}{4}$ oz
Liver 1 oz and Fat $\frac{1}{4}$ oz
Tongue (tinned or fresh) 1 oz
Tripe or Sweetbreads $1\frac{1}{4}$ oz and Fat $\frac{1}{4}$ oz
Lean Beef or Veal 1 oz and Fat $\frac{1}{4}$ oz
Lean Lamb or Mutton 1 oz and Fat $\frac{1}{4}$ oz
Lean Pork 1 oz
Chicken or Pigeon 1 oz and Fat $\frac{1}{4}$ oz
Duck 1 oz
Pheasant, Grouse or Partridge $\frac{3}{4}$ oz and Fat $\frac{1}{4}$ oz
Rabbit or Hare $\frac{3}{4}$ oz and Fat $\frac{1}{4}$ oz
Crab or Lobster $1\frac{1}{4}$ oz and Fat $\frac{1}{4}$ oz
Herring 1 oz and Fat $\frac{1}{4}$ oz
Kipper 1 oz and Fat $\frac{1}{4}$ oz
Salmon 1 oz and Fat $\frac{1}{4}$ oz
Sardines 1 oz
White Fish (all kinds) $1\frac{1}{4}$ oz and Fat $\frac{1}{4}$ oz
Cheese $\frac{3}{4}$ oz
Milk 7 oz (also contains 1 Black).

Fats are Meat Fats, Suet, Dripping, Butter, Margarine, Lard, Olive Oil; Thick Cream in twice the amount stated for other fats

Extras of no food value: Tea, Coffee, Soda water, etc., ordinary condiments and flavouring.

Insulin. The discovery of insulin has enabled the majority of diabetics to lead a normal life and to enjoy an interesting even though restricted diet. In many cases the patient can learn to give his

Half portions of these are usually enough.

own injections, test his own urine, and often adjust his diet to his daily requirements. The risk of diabetic coma has been very greatly reduced, but the possibilities of insulin over-dosage must not be forgotten.

Four types of insulin are commonly employed:

1. Soluble insulin BP (Rapid acting).
   'Nuso' and 'Actrapid' insulins are similar in action but are preferable in special circumstances.
2. Protamine zinc insulin (PZI).
3. Globin insulin.   (Slow acting).
4. Insulin zinc suspension (IZS).
   'Rapitard' insulin is similar in action.

Each of these may be used alone but a dose of soluble insulin is usually needed in addition to the slow and long-acting protamine zinc or globin insulin.

Soluble insulin is rapidly absorbed and has its maximum effect in about 4 to 6 hours. At least 2 injections are necessary in each 24 hours. Increased frequency of injections (as compared with the long-acting insulins) may, however, be compensated by improved control of the diabetes.

Protamine zinc insulin acts more slowly. It has little action immediately after injection, but has its greatest effect in 16 to 18 hours.

Globin insulin comes between the other two with a maximum effect at 12 hours. It is used less frequently.

Insulin zinc suspension (lente) is a mixture of special types of short-acting (semilente or amorphous) and long-acting (ultralente or crystalline) insulins which is administered in a single morning dose and exerts its influence over the whole 24 hours in a manner similar to the mixture of soluble and protamine zinc insulin. Insulin zinc suspension must not be mixed with any of the other insulins and should not be used if the total dose is above 50 units or if the patient shows a marked tendency to develop ketosis.

The aim is to reduce the number of injections to 1 in 24 hours if possible, so that the dose and type of insulin must be carefully selected for each individual.

The various types of insulin are supplied in vials containing 20, 40 or 80 units per ml and it is most important for both the nurse and the patient to be quite sure which strength is being used. In the case of protamine zinc and globin insulin the bottle must be shaken gently so that the suspended matter is evenly diffused throughout the mixture before any is withdrawn.

Insulin keeps well if stored in a cool, dark place, but soluble insulin should not be used if it becomes cloudy. It may be administered with an ordinary hypodermic syringe or one specially graduated in units. This is kept in a metal case filled with spirit and may be rinsed in

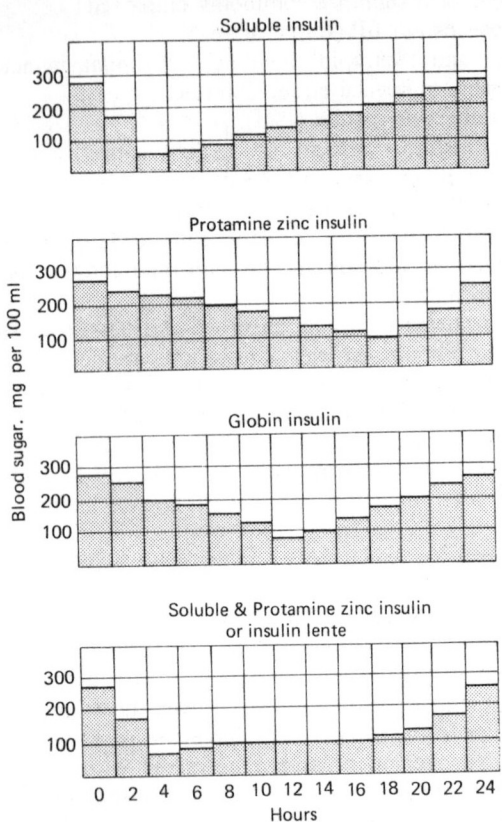

Fig. 96 The effect of a dose of the various types of insulin on the blood sugar of a diabetic patient.

boiled water before use. It is wise to keep one needle for piercing the rubber cap and a separate one for injecting the insulin as the rubber is apt to cause blunting. The top of the rubber cap having been cleansed with spirit the requisite amount of insulin is drawn into the syringe. A small amount of air injected into the bottle facilitates the removal of the liquid. The skin is cleaned with spirit or ether and the injection given subcutaneously. It may be made either into the arms or thighs, the latter being chosen is the patient is administering it himself. The thorax or abdominal wall may also be used, but care must be taken to select a different spot for successive injections.

Soluble insulin is given $\frac{1}{2}$ hour before a meal which must contain some carbohydrate food. The other types are given before breakfast.

While the process of standardization of insulin and diet is going on, the urine must be tested for sugar and acetone before each meal. When the regular dose of insulin has been determined daily tests should be carried out on the morning specimen.

The dose of insulin generally requires to be increased if the patient is suffering from any infection (e.g. a boil, severe cold, bronchitis, etc.).

It must be clearly understood that insulin is not a cure for the disease and, once being necessary, it is probable that the patient will have to continue taking it for the rest of his life, adjustments in the dosage being required from time to time.

Because of their delayed action protamine zinc, 'Lente' and globin insulin should not be used in diabetic coma.

Unless the dose is carefully adjusted, protamine zinc and globin insulin are liable to produce hypoglycaemia especially during the night.

Hypoglycaemia drugs (oral)

There are a number of substances, e.g. tolbutamide ('Rastinon') and chlorpropamide ('Diabinese') which when taken by mouth will lower the blood sugar and may sometimes be employed instead of insulin. Their main use is in middle-aged non-obese diabetics who show no tendency to ketosis and who do not require more than 40 units of insulin daily. Occasionally toxic symptoms occur and there is a tendency for tolerance to develop. The average dose of tolbutamide is 0·5 to 1·5 g in 2 or 3 doses daily, and chlorpropamide 100 to 500 mg once daily. Side effects such as vomiting, headache, intolerance of alcohol, blood platelet deficiency and rarely jaundice may occur. Glymidine ('Gondafon') acetohexamide ('Dimelor') and glibenclamide ('Euglucon') are similar in action and, like tolbutamide and chlorpropamide, are chemically related to the sulphonamides. They act by stimulating the release of insulin from the pancreas.

Phenformin ('Dibotin') and metformin ('Glucophage') are members of the diguanide group of drugs and act differently from the previously mentioned drugs. They augment the action of whatever insulin the patient has in his circulation. They may be used alone, in combination with the sulphonamide-like drugs, or with insulin.

Hypoglycaemia. This may occur if too much insulin or too little food is taken. The subject is of great importance to the nurse as she is often the first person to witness the symptoms of this condition which can easily be remedied if prompt measures are adopted.

When a dose of insulin is injected it covers the metabolism of a definite amount of carbohydrate and results in a lowering of the blood sugar.

Provided equivalent quantities of these substances are present, the blood sugar can be maintained within normal limits (e.g. 100 to 180 mg per ml of blood). If the amount of insulin is increased or that of the carbohydrate decreased the blood sugar will fall. When it reaches an abnormally low level (e.g. 50 mg per 100 ml), the symptoms of hypoglycaemia are produced.

The early symptoms are anxiety and irritability, double vision, sweating, pallor, coldness of the extremities and a sense of constriction about the waist. These are followed by faintness, collapse, drowsiness or complete loss of consciousness which, in severe cases, may pass into deep coma. Occasionally convulsions or delirium are seen.

These symptoms are liable to come on about 2 to 3 hours after an injection of soluble insulin or later if protamine zinc, lente or globin insulin has been used. Great care must be taken to warn patients of their occurrence. It is for this reason that patients taking insulin must have a sufficient amount of carbohydrate in their evening meal in order to prevent the development of hypoglycaemia coma during sleep. It may also occur if unaccustomed or excessive muscular exercise is undertaken.

The treatment of hypoglycaemia is to give sugar in order to restore the blood sugar to its normal level. If he is conscious he may take 2 lumps of sugar or a stick of barley sugar by mouth. When unconsciousness supervenes a solution of glucose may be given directly into the stomach by a nasal tube. In severe cases, glucose is injected intravenously (20–40 ml of 50% dextrose solution). 1 mg of glucagon may be given by intramuscular injection in an emergency because it liberates any glycogen remaining in the liver.

It is wise for all patients having insulin to carry a supply of sugar about with them and to take some directly they are aware of the onset of hypoglycaemic symptoms. In addition, all diabetics should carry a card with them indicating that they are taking insulin and therefore liable to hypoglycaemia.

DIAGNOSIS OF DIABETIC AND HYPOGLYCAEMIC COMA

	Diabetic Coma	Hypoglycaemic Coma
Onset	Gradual.	Often sudden except with PZI
History	Often of acute infection in a diabetic or no previous history of diabetes.	Recent insulin injection, or inadequate meal or excessive exercise after insulin.
Skin	Flushed, dry.	Pale, sweating.
Tongue	Dry and furred.	Moist.
Breath	Smell of acetone.	No acetone.
Respiration	Deep (air-hunger).	Shallow.
Pulse	Rapid, feeble.	Normal or bounding.
Eyeball tension	Low.	Normal or raised.
Urine	Sugar and acetone.	No sugar or acetone unless bladder has not been emptied for some hours.
Blood Sugar (or 'Dextrostix')	Raised [over 200].	Subnormal [20–50 mg]
Blood Pressure	Low.	Normal.
Abdominal pain	Common and often acute. Occasional vomiting.	Sometimes sense of constriction.

If there is any doubt as to whether the patient is suffering from diabetic coma with hyperglycaemia or insulin hypoglycaemia, a specimen of urine should be obtained by catheterization, if necessary. If no sugar or acetone is found the condition is certainly due to hypoglycaemia. If a large quantity of urine is withdrawn and contains sugar it is impossible to say that some of this was not secreted before the last injection of insulin so that a second specimen must be obtained after the bladder has been emptied.

Treatment of diabetic coma. Any diabetic whose urine gives a positive ferric chloride reaction (p. 320) is suffering from a severe degree of ketosis which, unless checked, may progress rapidly into coma, a serious condition which may prove fatal.

Ketosis and diabetic coma are likely to occur (*a*) in a severe diabetic who has not received treatment, (*b*) in one who has failed to continue with his correct dose of insulin, (*c*) in one who has a severe infection during the course of which the insulin dosage has not been increased.

Although with severe ketosis the patient is not unconscious, this state must be regarded as the **pre-coma** stage and treated on the same general lines as fully-developed coma, but the dosage of insulin given will be less and the other steps taken proportionately less drastic.

In diabetic coma there is a serious disturbance of metabolism and it is necessary to combat the following important abnormalities:

1. Raised blood sugar due to disordered carbohydrate metabolism.
2. Ketosis due to disordered fat metabolism.
3. Dehydration and water loss.
4. Loss of electrolytes, i.e. sodium, potassium, chlorine and phosphorus.

I. The disordered carbohydrate metabolism and raised blood sugar (often 500 to 1,000 mg per 100 ml) is treated by giving large doses of soluble insulin. Owing to the fact that there may be some resistance to insulin in the tissues this is at first given intravenously and later by intramuscular or subcutaneous injection, the dose being reduced gradually as the patient improves, e.g.:

1. 100 units of soluble insulin initially, one half being given intravenously and the other half intramuscularly.
2. Further doses of soluble insulin intramuscularly every 4 hours according to the results of blood sugar estimations.

The exact details of the administration of these doses are checked by obtaining and testing the urine before each is given, together with the estimation of the blood sugar at intervals.

II. The severe ketosis, dehydration and loss of electrolytes is dealt with by giving intravenous fluids. An intravenous drip is set up and a combination of the following fluids given, usually in this order:

1. Isotonic saline, to replace fluid and the sodium chloride deficiency.

2. A mixed electrolyte solution containing salts of sodium, potassium, etc.

3. 5% glucose in isotonic saline, to help to combat the ketosis, to prevent insulin over-dosage and to supply more fluid.

As much as 15 litres of fluid may be required over a period of 72 hours, but care must be taken not to overload the circulation by giving too much too rapidly.

Sometimes 5% sodium bicarbonate or $\frac{1}{6}$ molar sodium lactate is given intravenously with a view to combating ketosis.

The bowels may be opened with enemata.

When recovery from coma has occurred the diet is given by mouth and gradually increased until the necessary standard and its corresponding dose of insulin has been reached.

Summary. The main points for the nurse to remember about diabetes are:

1. It is a disorder of carbohydrate metabolism due usually to disease of the islets of Langerhans in the pancreas.

2. There is a rise in the blood sugar (hyperglycaemia), and sugar appears in the urine (glycosuria) because the tissues are unable to utilize sugar in the absence of insulin.

3. The disturbance of carbohydrate metabolism results in incomplete combustion of fats with the production of ketone bodies which appear in the urine and may accumulate in the blood leading to diabetic coma.

4. Over-dosage with insulin is followed by hypoglycaemia the symptoms of which must be recognized and distinguished from those of diabetic coma. The treatment of both must be understood.

5. Treatment is carried out by suitable dieting supplemented when necessary by the injection of insulin.

6. Oral anti-diabetic substances (e.g. tolbutamide, chlorpropamide, metformin) may be used in mild, middle-aged or elderly cases.

Obesity

A patient may be said to be suffering from obesity when he or she is substantially above the average weight for persons of the same race, sex, age and height. (In Britain 6% of men and 20% of women are said to be more than 20% over-weight.

The condition may be nutritional, that is due to over-eating, or it may be associated with endocrine or other metabolic factors, e.g. hypothyroidism and Cushing's syndrome. Many cases probably result from a combination of both but no one becomes overweight unless their calorie intake exceeds their energy requirements. However, some people undoubtedly put on weight more easily than others. (A fat mobilizing substance (FMS) is found in the urine of normal subjects which is absent from that of many obese patients, unless they are fed on diets consisting almost exclusively of fat.)

Where obesity is due primarily to gross over-eating, psychological and emotional factors may be responsible for the latter both in adults and children and may require investigation.

Obesity may have serious effects. For example, the life expectancy of a man of 45 who is 11 kg (25 pounds) overweight is reduced by 25%. Diabetes, hypertension, coronary artery disease and cerebrovascular disease are all more common in the obese. In addition, the overweight patient is more liable to suffer from gallstones, osteoarthritis and hiatus hernia.

The treatment of obesity, apart from any special underlying cause, is essentially a matter of strict and prolonged adherence to a low calorie diet. An initial period in hospital on a very low calorie diet or 'fluids only' may help in severe cases. Much publicised 'fad' diets tend to come and go with contemporary fashion but offer little advantage over the standard low calorie reducing diets outlined in hospital diet sheets. Appetite suppressing drugs such as 'Duraphet,' 'Preludin' and 'Ponderax' should only be used in the early stages of treatment under strict medical supervision as they often have side-effects and tend to become ineffective after a short time. Apart from 'Ponderax' they are potentially drugs of addiction. Generally speaking their use should be discouraged because many of them have a stimulating effect on the central nervous system and produce a feeling of euphoria.

12 Diseases of the Ductless Gland (Endocrine System)

The ductless glands or endocrine organs consist of those structures in the body which manufacture hormones and are known to pour their secretion directly into the bloodstream. The majority, such as the thyroid, have only internal secretions (hormones). The pancreas, on the other hand, produces an external secretion, the pancreatic juice, which passes to the duodenum via the pancreatic ducts; and an internal secretion, insulin, formed in the islets of Langerhans, which passes into the circulation. Hormones are chemical messengers. There are basically 3 types of hormone from the biochemical point of view: steroids (e.g. hydrocortisone), amines (e.g. thyroxine) and polypeptides (e.g. insulin).

The functions of ductless glands are in many cases intimately connected not only with each other, but also with the nervous system. They take an important part in controlling the processes of metabolism in the body and a balance exists between the activity of the individual glands, so that if the function of one is disordered an alteration in the general endocrine balance is to be expected.

In a broad sense, disordered function of a ductless gland may result in either an increase in the amount of its secretion or a decrease, and different symptoms will be produced in each case. A different clinical picture may appear if disease of a gland (e.g. pituitary or suprarenal) occurs in infancy or childhood.

The important glands having an internal secretion are: the thyroid, parathyroids, suprarenals, pituitary, thymus, sex glands (ovary and testes) and pancreas.

The thyroid gland

This consists of two lobes, one on each side of the trachea, joined by a narrow portion, the isthmus.

The gland secretes an iodine-containing substance, thyroxine (T4), which exerts an important influence on the metabolism of the body and on the nervous system. Most tissues are able to convert thyroxine to tri-iodothyronine (T3), which is probably the active hormone. Most thyrotoxic patients have raised serum T4 levels but up to 10% have normal T4 levels; these patients have raised serum T3 levels and are sometimes said to have 'T3 toxicosis'.

Persistent enlargement of the gland is called a **goitre**. This, however, is not necessarily associated with disturbance of its functions. In other words, a goitre may be either toxic or non-toxic. A large goitre may produce symptoms by causing pressure on the trachea.

Goitre

Temporary enlargement of the thyroid is often seen at the age of puberty in girls and may recur at each menstrual period.

Chronic enlargement of the gland is liable to occur in certain districts (e.g. Derbyshire and Switzerland) and is due to a lack of iodine in the local water supply and is sometimes called endemic goitre. The thyroid may increase enormously in size and produce pressure symptoms. In order to prevent the development of the condition, the use of 'iodized salt' instead of ordinary cooking salt has been recommended for use by the inhabitants of these goitre districts.

Benign tumours (adenomas) may be either toxic or non-toxic; malignant disease may also occur.

The conditions in which disturbances of thyroid secretion associated with metabolic disorders occur may be divided into two groups.
1. Hyperthyroidism or thyrotoxicosis, in which the activity of the gland is increased.
2. Hypothyroidism, in which it is diminished (i.e. myxoedema, cretinism).

1. Hyperthyroidism (Thyrotoxicosis)

This is also referred to as **Graves' Disease, Exophthalmic Goitre, Toxic Goitre,** and is characterized by moderate enlargement of the thyroid gland, protrusion of the eye-balls (exophthalmos), a rapid pulse (tachycardia) and general nervousness.

Cause. The cause of the condition is not fully known. It is more common in women than men and has its onset, often, between the ages of 15 and 30 years. Auto-immunity appears to play a part. In some cases the onset appears to date from a sudden fright, shock or grief.

It is possible that the condition is due to a long-acting thyroid stimulating gamma globulin produced by abnormal lymphocytes. In other words, this may be an auto-immune disease.

Symptoms. The main symptoms have already been mentioned and include moderate enlargement of the thyroid gland, exophthalmos, a rapid pulse and general nervousness. In addition there is a fine muscular tremor which can be demonstrated by asking the patient to hold out the hands with the fingers widely separated.

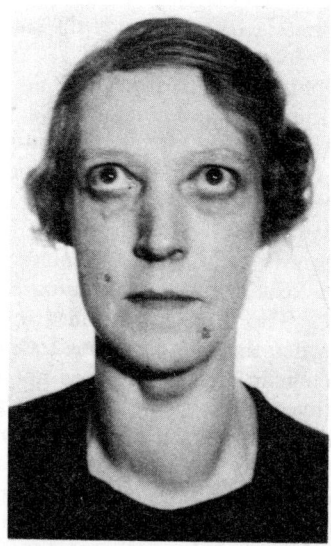

Fig. 97 Thyrotoxicosis (Graves' Disease).

Excessive sweating also occurs and the hands feel hot and often moist.

The general impression conveyed by the appearance of a patient in the advanced stages is one of fear or excitement.

Hyperthyroidism is associated with an increase in the body metabolism so that loss of weight is common.

Diarrhoea, glycosuria, and disturbance of menstrual function may be present.

The muscle of the heart is often affected and tachycardia may be followed by the development of atrial fibrillation and, later, heart failure.

The course and severity of the disease is variable. Some cases appear to recover completely, others are benefited by treatment but relapse later. Occasionally very acute symptoms occur (thyroid crisis).

Treatment. One of the following lines of treatment may be adopted:

1. Surgical.   2. Medical.   3. Radio-iodine.

The **surgical** treatment consists of removing a portion of the gland thereby diminishing the amount of thyroid secretion reaching the blood (partial thyroidectomy). A preoperative course of medical treatment is given first in order to avoid the risk of a postoperative thyrotoxic crisis.

The main points of **medical** treatment are the use of 'anti-thyroid' drugs together with physical and mental rest in the early stages.

In hot weather the amount of exercise permitted should be reduced to a minimum, for it will be found that heat tends to aggravate the symptoms while patients often improve during the winter months.

The most important 'anti-thyroid' drug used in the medical treatment of thyrotoxicosis is carbimazole ('Neomercazole'). The dose is carefully adjusted as toxic symptoms including rashes and agranulocytosis may develop. The drug is continued for some months but some cases relapse when the drug is stopped. One of its effects is to lower the basal metabolic rate, but it does not usually abolish the exophthalmos or thyroid enlargement. Other 'anti-thyroid' drugs include the derivatives of thiouracil which are more toxic. Potassium perchlorate is sometimes used but may cause fatal aplastic anaemia.

A shorter course of carbimazole may be given as a preoperative measure, but is usually discontinued two or three weeks before the operation, because, if the drug is continued, harmorrhage at the time of the operation is likely to be excessive. It is replaced by Lugol's iodine 0·3 ml (5 minims) twice or three times daily or potassium iodide, 60 mg tds. The anti-thyroid effect of iodine only lasts a short time (i.e. 2 to 5 weeks) and has no place in the long-term or routine treatment of thyrotoxicosis.

Atrial fibrillation, if present, is treated with digitalis and sometimes propranolol ('Inderal'). If it persists when the thyrotoxicosis has been controlled, DC cardioversion is usually indicated.

In hot weather, bedclothes must be reduced to a minimum and the judicious use of an electric fan will often render a seriously ill patient more comfortable. Alcohol and coffee should be avoided.

In all cases an accurate record of the pulse, especially the sleeping pulse, must be made and the weight recorded at regular intervals.

Estimations of the basal metabolism which is not very reliable, and the protein-bound iodine (PBI) in the serum may be carried out.

Radio-active iodine (^{131}I)

(i) A small dose of this substance may be used in the diagnosis of thyroid disease.

(ii) **Treatment.** A single calculated dose by mouth may be effective in curing thyrotoxicosis but as this might cause genetic changes it is not usually given to patients under the age of 40. In any case, response to treatment tends to be rather slow, and a long-term disadvantage is that many patients tend to develop myxoedema after some years. The fear that it might cause malignant changes is unfounded.

2. Hypothyroidism

Myxoedema. This condition exhibits symptoms which are the reverse of those occurring in hyperthyroidism, for the gland atrophies and its secretion is diminished. The severity of the disease depends upon the degree of atrophy present. The condition may also follow operative removal of the thyroid gland, excessive dosage of anti-thyroid drugs and radio-active iodine.

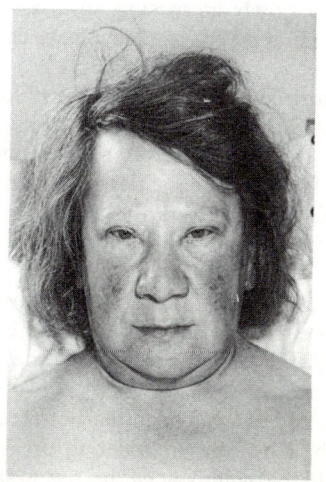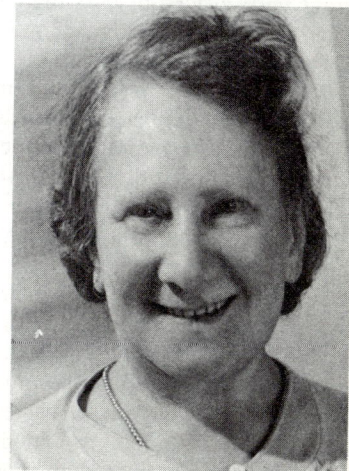

Fig. 98 Myxoedema before and after treatment.

The primary type of disease affects females much more commonly than males (7 : 1). The onset is very gradual and usually occurs about the age of 45.

In contrast with the appearance of extreme nervous stimulation seen in hyperthyroidism, the patient becomes mentally dull and complains of loss of memory while speech and movements are slow. The skin becomes dry and thickened and the eyelids are baggy, a condition which simulates oedema but does not pit on pressure. The hair is thin and the outer portions of the eyebrows are frequently lost. The weight increases and obesity may be marked.

The basal metabolic rate is low and there is a marked sensitivity to cold.

The blood cholesterol is high (i.e. over 220 mg per 100 ml).

In the radio-active iodine test the uptake is diminished.

The serum protein-bound iodine (PBI) content is reduced.

Constipation is usual and the temperature is subnormal.

Patients suffering from myxoedema, and other elderly patients, are liable to marked fall in temperature in very cold weather (hypothermia). However, such patients must not be actively rewarmed. They should be protected from further heat loss and placed in a room at a moderate temperature. Steroids may be very valuable in this stage. A special low-reading thermometer may be required in the management of this condition (p. 18).

The **treatment** of myxoedema consists in administering thyroxine starting with a dose of 0·05 mg daily slowly increasing up to about 0·3 mg daily, if necessary. If too much is given, headache, sweating and a rapid pulse will develop.

The improvement is generally marked, but the patient must continue to take thyroxine permanently.

Cretinism. Congenital deficiency of thyroid secretion sometimes occurs and results in dwarfism with failure of mental development. It is, therefore, a disease of infancy. Cretins may be the offspring of goitrous parents and are, therefore, more commonly seen in districts where goitre is frequent.

In untreated cases the body is broad and the limbs short. The nose is flat and the mouth and tongue large. Constipation is common and the child has a hoarse cry. Walking and talking are delayed and, in severe cases, the child may become an imbecile.

The condition may be suspected at birth but is often not recognized before the 2nd or 3rd month. However, in order to prevent irreparable damage treatment should be commenced in the first 6 weeks if possible.

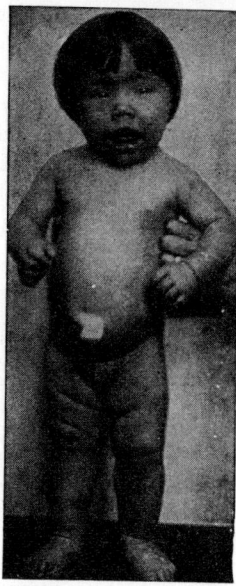

Fig. 99 A case of cretinism, aged 18 months. Note umbilical hernia.

If **treatment** with thyroxine, initially about 0·025 mg daily, is commenced early, growth and mental development may become normal. It must, however, be continued throughout life.

Calcitonin

The thyroid gland possesses a system of cells which are concerned with calcium metabolism. In response to a high serum concentration of calcium, the thyroid secretes **calcitonin,** which tends to reduce the calcium level.

The parathyroid glands

These are 4 small structures situated in the neck, behind the thyroid gland. Each is about the size of a pea and they secrete a substance, **parathormone,** which is concerned with **calcium metabolism.**

Disorder of their function may result either in decreased or increased activity.

It has been seen that calcium plays an important part in the formation of bones which owe their strength to the deposit of lime salts in their structure. It has also been mentioned that calcium metabolism is dependent upon an adequate supply of vitamin D, and that a deficiency of this vitamin results in rickets with its associated weakness of the bones.

In addition, calcium affects the excitability of the nervous and muscular tissues, so that if the amount of calcium circulating in the blood is decreased these tissues become more irritable.

It has been found that increased activity of the parathyroid glands is associated with an increased amount of calcium in the blood, and decreased activity with a diminished amount.

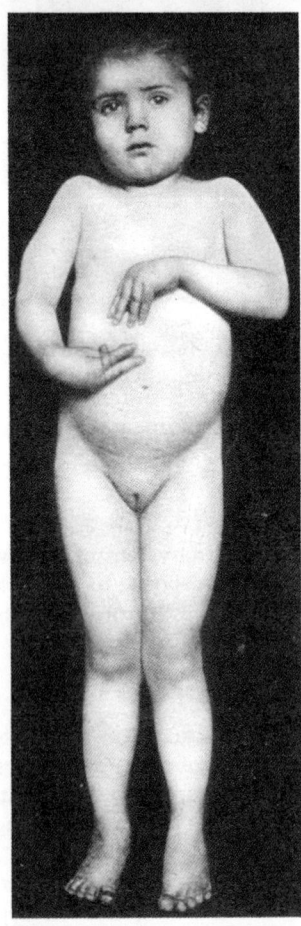

Fig. 100 Tetany, showing spasm of the hands.

(a) Decreased activity of the parathyroid gland. This state being associated with a low blood calcium and consequently in an increased irritability of the nervous and muscular tissues, results in a condition known as **tetany**. (This must not be confused with the disease tetanus or 'lock-jaw'.)

The symptoms of tetany are:

1. Muscular cramps affecting especially the hands and feet are sometimes called carpopedal spasm. The thumbs are held across the palms, the fingers drawn closely together and flexed at the meta-carpophalangeal joints. Flexion at the wrists and elbows may also be present. The toes are also drawn together with flexion and rotation inwards of the feet at the ankles.

2. Constriction of the limb with a tourniquet brings on or increases the spasm (Trousseau's sign).

3. Tapping over the facial nerve above the angle of the jaw causes contraction of the face muscles of that side (Chvostek's sign).

Tetany may occur in rickets, and reference has been made to the occurrence of 'Spasmophilia' (p. 436) in which there is increased excitability of the nervous system resulting from the low blood calcium. It is also seen in gastro-intestinal disorders such as pyloric stenosis, dilatation of the stomach, coeliac disease and prolonged vomiting. It may also be produced by overbreathing especially in patients with a nervous temperament. The parathyroid glands are sometimes damaged in the operation of thyroidectomy, causing tetany.

In addition to treating any obvious cause the administration of calcium, e.g. calcium gluconate, intravenously in emergency, and vitamin D will restore the blood calcium to normal and relieve the symptoms. A.T. 10 (Dihydrotachysterol) is sometimes used instead of vitamin D.

(b) Increased activity of the parathyroid glands. This may cause a rare disease known as generalized **osteitis fibrosa** in which a tumour (adenoma) of one or more of the glands is present.

The bones show cystic changes and the condition may be cured by removal of the parathyroid tumour.

The blood calcium is raised above 10 mg per 100 ml.

The adrenal (suprarenal) glands

These organs are situated immediately above the kidneys and consist of an outer layer or cortex and an inner layer or medulla each of which has a different function.

The adrenal cortex is closely concerned with the control of the metabolism of minerals, glucose and proteins. This control is exercised by means of hormones which are liberated from the adrenal cortex into the blood. Aldosterone is the hormone concerned with mineral metabolism. It causes sodium to be retained by the kidneys and potassium to be excreted. Glucose metabolism is controlled by hydrocortisone which has the opposite effect of insulin for it raises the level of blood glucose and encourages the deposition of fat. Hydrocortisone is vitally concerned in assisting the body to withstand 'stress' in the form of injury, infection, other inflammations, allergic responses and even certain malignant diseases. If secretion of hydrocortisone is seriously diminished or absent the body may react so feebly to 'stress' that it is overwhelmed and the patient unexpectedly dies. On the other hand hydrocortisone and synthetic 'corticosteroids' are used in a very great variety of conditions (see p. 522). The secretion of hydrocortisone is itself controlled by the anterior pituitary gland through another hormone called adreno-corticotrophic hormone (ACTH).

Protein metabolism is controlled by an androgenic hormone which promotes the building up of muscles and other tissues and which also tends to cause the development of male secondary sexual characteristics (facial hair, deep voice, etc.).

The adrenal medulla secretes noradrenaline and adrenaline. Noradrenaline raises the blood pressure. Adrenaline hastens the heart rate, increases the blood sugar and relaxes the spasm of the bronchial smooth muscles in asthma.

In the adult, over-secretion by the adrenal cortex, which may be due to a tumour of the gland, produces **Cushing's syndrome.** This may also occur as a result of over-stimulation of the adrenals by the pituitary. A similar syndrome is caused by prolonged treatment with steroids. Cushing's syndrome is characterized by obesity, abnormal growth of hair (hirsutes), hypertension and muscular weakness. An affected woman ceases to menstruate and may be troubled by facial hair and a deepening voice.

Addison's disease

(Adreno-cortical insufficiency)

This condition is characterized by increased brown pigmentation of the skin and mucous membranes, wasting, muscular weakness and a low blood pressure.

The blood sodium may be low and the blood potassium may be

raised. It is important, therefore, to check the blood electrolytes in this condition.

Although remissions may occur the disease tends to be progressive and, unless treated, ultimately proves fatal. Severe crises, associated with vomiting, diarrhoea and collapse, are liable to occur.

It is the commonest affection of the suprarenal glands and is due to their unexplained atrophy or sometimes to their destruction by tuberculosis. This disease is treated with cortisone. With this alone, sodium may not be adequately retained in the body. Fludrocortisone ('Florinef') 0·1 to 0·2 mg daily, will then also be required.

Phaeochromocytoma is a tumour of the medulla of the suprarenal gland characterized by attacks of high blood pressure. The diagnosis is confirmed by a fall in blood pressure following the intravenous injection of 'Rogitine'. It is also necessary to collect a 24-hour specimen of urine for catechol amines. The treatment is surgical.

The pituitary gland

This is situated within the skull in a small depression close to the base of the brain, known as the sella turcica.

It consists of 2 parts, the anterior lobe and the posterior lobe. The anterior lobe controls the secretion of the sex hormones by the ovary and testis, of milk by the lactating breast, of thyroxine by the thyroid gland and of hydrocortisone by the adrenal cortex. It also secretes growth hormone which profoundly affects growth in childhood and adolescence and which has an antagonistic action to insulin.

Tumours of the anterior lobe are not uncommon and the symptoms produced are of 2 types:

(*a*) Local: those of cerebral tumour giving rise to increased intracranial pressure by far the most important being the optic nerve causing various types of visual disturbance and eventual blindness, and pressure upon neighbouring structures (e.g. headache, vomiting).

(*b*) General or systemic: those associated with increased or decreased activity of the gland.

The function of the pituitary is closely connected with growth so that the symptoms of defective function depend on whether the onset of the disease occurs before or after normal growth has stopped.

Hyperpituitarism or over-secretion of the growth hormone before growth has normally ceased results in enormous overgrowth in the size of the skeleton (gigantism). When adults are affected the condition of **acromegaly** develops. Further growth of the long bones is not possible, but those of the skull, hands and feet are

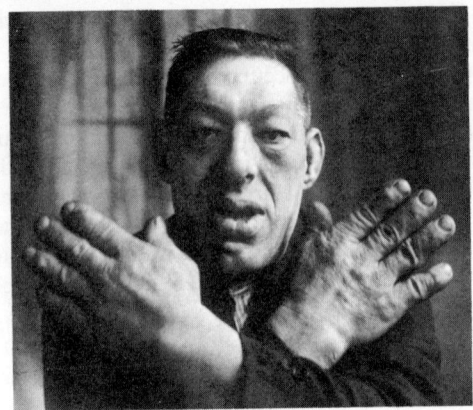

Fig. 101 Acromegaly, showing enlargement of the lower jaw and hands.

affected. The face increases in size, especially the lower jaw, the hands and feet enlarge. Curvature of the spine is generally present and the lips become thick and the skin coarse. Acromegaly is treated by

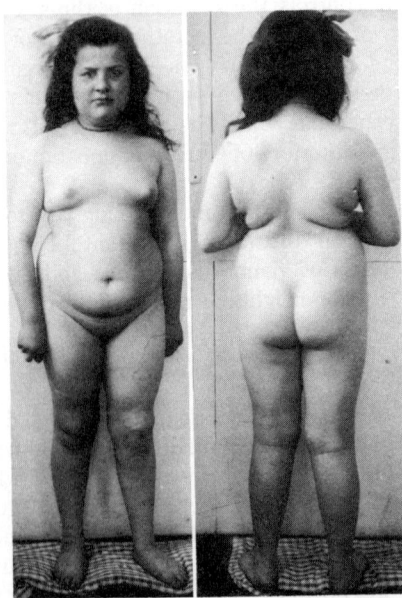

Fig. 102 Hypopituitarism, showing obesity and lack of pubic hair in a young girl.

x-ray therapy, radioactive implants into the pituitary gland or surgery (hypophysectomy).

Hypopituitarism or under-secretion. This may be associated with obesity and abnormalities of carbohydrate metabolism.

In adolescents sexual development may fail to occur, while in adults there is loss of sexual power.

Simmonds' disease is a rare condition due to destruction of the pituitary gland resulting either from harmorrhage into its substance, infarction or a tumour. There is marked wasting, loss of sexual function, loss of axillary and pubic hair, loss of energy, low blood pressure and slowing of the mental processes.

Diabetes insipidus. In some cases when the posterior lobe is diseased there is a deficiency of anti-diuretic hormone (ADH) and the quantity of urine excreted is greatly increased and of low specific gravity. Injections of pitressin tannate in oil (to prolong the effect of the drug) or nasal sprays of lysine-vasopressin (synthetic ADH) may be used in this condition and diuretics such as chlorothiazide are helpful in some cases.

TABLE SHOWING THE IMPORTANT RESULTS OF DISEASE OF THE DUCTLESS GLANDS

Gland	Name of Hormone	Hypersecretion		Hyposecretion	
		In Children	In Adults	In Children	In adults
Thyroid	Thyroxine	Thyrotoxicosis (exophthalmic goitre).		Cretinism.	Myxoedema.
Parathyroid	Parathormone.	Generalized osteitis fibrosa, with high blood calcium.		Tetany, with low blood calcium.	
Suprarenal (cortex)	Cortisone	Sexual precocity.	Obesity, increased hairiness. Cushing's syndrome.	Addison's disease.	
(medulla)	Adrenaline. Noradrenaline.	Hypertension (phaeochromo-cytoma)		—	
Pituitary (anterior lobe)	Growth hormone.	Gigantism.	Acromegaly.	Infantilism.	Simmonds' disease
(posterior lobe)	Vasopressin Oxytocin.	? Disorder of carbohydrate metabolism.		Diabetes insipidus.	

'**Pituitrin**' is an extract of the posterior lobe of the gland. When injected it raises the blood pressure and causes contraction of the muscular coats of the bladder, small intestine and uterus.

The thymus gland

This is situated in the thorax immediately behind the sternum. It is present during childhood but normally atrophies when puberty is reached. Its function is connected with the development of immunity and the formation of lymphocytes. Occasionally enlargement may be present or a tumour may develop in its substance, producing symptoms of pressure within the thorax.

The cases of unexpectedly sudden death under anaesthesia or as a result of shock which were formerly ascribed to 'status lymphaticus' are probably due to some reflex action on the heart through the vagus nerve and nothing to do with the thymus. (See also myasthenia gravis, p. 421.)

The sex glands

The ovaries and testes produce internal secretions which affect both the reproductive processes and general health.

The ovaries produce **oestrogens** and **progesterone** which prepare the uterus for pregnancy. The menopause results from the failure of the ovaries to continue their production of these hormones.

The testes secrete the hormone **testosterone** which is responsible for the development of the secondary sex characteristics—the external genitalia, facial hair and masculine voice.

13 Disorders of the Skin

The diseases affecting the skin are mainly of importance to the nurse on account of the frequency with which she has to carry out the treatment advised. In many instances, the rate of recovery is dependent upon the efficiency with which these duties are performed. However only a limited general account of common conditions can be included here.

The skin is made up of the epidermis and the dermis. The latter consists of fibrous tissue, blood vessels and nerves and contains the sebaceous glands, sweat glands and hair follicles.

A nail is a specialized portion of the epidermis growing from a root hidden under the fold of skin which partially covers the 'half moon' or lacuna situated at its base.

Types of skin lesion and their definitions

1. Abnormalities of sensation, e.g. itching (pruritus), and anaesthesia, hyperaesthesia or paraesthesia which are generally of nervous origin (p. 373).

Pruritus may be either general or local and instinctively causes scratching. It is common in many disorders of the skin and also occurs in general conditions, such as diabetes, leukaemia, Hodgkin's disease, obstructive jaundice and drug allergy. Local applications which may be helpful include calamine lotion, menthol and camphor lotions and steroid preparations. Oral drugs include the antihistamines, 'Dilosyn', 'Periactin' and cholestyramine (in obstructive jaundice).

2. Erythema. A diffuse area of redness associated with dilatation of the capillaries which disappears on pressure. It is seen in sunburn, erysipelas, scarlet fever, drug rashes, etc.

3. Macules. Small round spots which are not raised above the surface of the skin and are usually red or copper coloured, e.g. measles, rubella, secondary syphilis.

4. Papules. Small, solid elevations of the skin or pimples. Papules occur in the first stages of the small-pox eruption, secondary syphilitic lesions of the skin, etc. Papules of the larger size are sometimes called **nodules,** e.g. erythema nodosum.

5. Vesicles. Small elevated blisters containing clear fluid, e.g. chicken-pox, and the second stage of the small-pox eruption.

6. Bullae. Large blisters or blebs 1·25 cm ($\frac{1}{2}$ inch) or more in diameter; e.g. pemphigus.

7. Pustules. Vesicles containing purulent fluid which when they erupt produce crusts or scabs: e.g. the third stage of small-pox eruption.

8. Scales. Small dried portions of dead epidermis seen, for example, in psoriasis.

9. Crusts. Masses caused by the drying of serous or purulent exudates on the skin, also called scabs, e.g. in impetigo.

10. Wheals. Rounded or elongated elevations of a temporary nature associated with the outpouring of fluid into the skin. This transient oedema compresses the blood vessels in the area and produces a white elevation, which generally itches. The condition is seen in urticaria (nettle rash).

11. Excoriations. Scratches or abrasions of the superficial layers of the epidermis.

12. An ulcer. Loss of tissue involving the whole thickness of the epidermis.

13. Petechiae. Small red or purple patches due to haemorrhages into the skin. They do not fade on pressure, e.g. purpura.

14. Ecchymoses. Extensive extravasations of blood into the skin, e.g. large bruises, scurvy.

15. Disorders of pigmentation. Changes in the colour of the skin are encountered in various diseases, a number of which have been mentioned, e.g. the yellow discoloration in jaundice: the pale lemon tint of pernicious anaemia: the brown pigmentation of Addison's disease. Pigmentation may also occur in scars following ulcers, e.g. varicose ulcers, or burns, and in areas of skin which have been subject to inflammation. It is seen after the prolonged internal use of drugs such as arsenic or silver salts. A mottled discoloration of the skin on the front of the shins is often seen in persons addicted to sitting close to a fire and is called 'erythema ab igne'.

Occasionally a diminution in the pigment in the skin occurs and appears as irregular white patches scattered over the surface of the body (vitiligo). Complete absence of pigment from the skin, the hair and the iris is called albinism.

16. Disorders of the structure of the skin. These may be congenital deformities such as naevi, a naevus being a tumour formed by dilated blood vessels. Others include hairy or pigmented moles, warts (verrucae), and the locally malignant tumour known as a rodent ulcer (epithelioma).

Types of diseases which may affect the skin

The commoner affections of the skin may be divided into those which have their origin from causes arising outside the body (exogenous), and those arising from within the body (endogenous).

The **exogenous** causes include:

1. Traumatic conditions such as burns, scalds, the application of strong acids or alkalis. These are dealt with in surgical works.

2. Eruptions due to external irritation (dermatitis), e.g. (*a*) constant friction; (*b*) various cosmetic preparations (lipstick, nail varnish, deodorants, etc.) in certain individuals who are allergic to them; (*c*) chemical agents such as the metal nickel, fur dye, hair dye and those used in certain occupations, e.g. French polishers, surgeons and nurses (from the use of streptomycin, phenol, lysol or other antiseptic lotions, the local application of antibiotic and antihistamine ointments, also household detergents and soap-powders); (*d*) powerful rays, e.g. sunlight, ultra-violet, x-rays or radium.

3. Inflammatory conditions resulting from bacterial invasion of the skin, e.g. acne, boils, carbuncles, erysipelas, impetigo, lupus vulgaris (a lesion of the skin caused by tubercle bacilli).

4. Parasitic infections of the skin, e.g. ringworm, pediculosis, and scabies.

The **endogenous** causes include:

1. Eruptions due to the toxins or organisms causing the acute infectious diseases such as scarlet fever, measles, rubella, smallpox, chicken-pox and herpes.

2. Unknown toxins possibly of alimentary origin causing conditions like urticaria.

3. Eruptions due to certain foods in sensitive individuals (allergic type), see p. 15.

4. Drug eruptions caused, for example, by penicillin, codeine, iodides, bromides, barbiturates, salicylates, gold or serum.

5. Skin lesions associated with disorders of the circulation, e.g. varicose eczema and ulcers (see p. 156), chilblains, Raynaud's disease.

6. Tumours and cancer of the skin, e.g. basal-cell carcinoma (rodent ulcer).

It must be remembered that certain individuals have very sensitive skins or appear to be especially susceptible to eruptions, so that, in these cases, both exogenous and endogenous factors may operate in the production of a skin lesion.

There is no doubt also that in some cases anxiety states and psychological disturbances (psychosomatic causes) may be factors in the onset of certain skin conditions including eczema. These are sometimes classified as neurodermatoses.

INFECTIONS OF THE SKIN

Boils and carbuncles

A **boil** or **furuncle** is deep-seated inflammation commencing in a hair follicle or sebaceous gland and caused by the staphylococcus aureus. Any part of the body may be affected, but the neck, axillae and buttocks are the most common sites. Boils are especially liable to occur in diabetes so that the urine should always be examined for sugar. In other cases, the patient may be in a poor state of health and recurrent crops may occur. A boil starts as a tender, indurated mass deep in the skin which increases in size and is surrounded by oedema. It forms a painful red swelling about 1·0–2·5 cm ($\frac{1}{2}$ to 1 inch) in diameter. Later, a small pustule which eventually bursts appears at the centre. Finally, a slough separates from its interior and is discharged.

Once a boil has formed there is little that can be done to hasten its resolution. Hot poultices tend to damage the surrounding skin and spread the infection. 'Fucidin' ointment may be applied. Swabbing around and over the lesion with surgical spirit is probably as good as anything. When the boil discharges, plain dressings are usually adequate but magnesium sulphate paste may help if the boil is large.

Boils tend to be multiple (furunculosis), a new one starting as another one heals. The aim must be to break this chain of auto-infection. The staphylococcus resides particularly in certain carrier sites—the nose (anterior nares), the perineum and the backs of the hands. It may be attacked at these sites by an antiseptic nasal cream (e.g. 'Naseptin'), applied twice or thrice daily, and daily chlorhexidine ('Hibitane') baths. Vaccines of staphylococcus aureus are sometimes used in recurrent cases but their effectiveness is unproven.

Boils must not be squeezed because this process causes a breakdown of the barrier of defence put up by the tissues against the infection which consequently spreads to the surrounding healthy parts and increases the size of the lesion. This is especially important in boils on the face or lips for manipulation may cause the infection to spread by the veins to the blood sinuses in the skull and produce the very dangerous condition known as **cavernous sinus thrombosis.**

A **carbuncle** is a larger, deeper lesion than a boil and involves, also, the subcutaneous tissue. At the commencement it has the appearance of an ordinary boil, but the inflammation spreads rapidly and produces a red, painful, indurated area of swelling which may attain several inches in diameter, and eventually discharge through several openings on its surface. Fever is often present and sugar may be found in the urine which should, therefore, always be tested. The patient is generally in a debilitated state of health which requires attention during the after-treatment. With the administration of an antibiotic to which the organism is sensitive, surgical measures such as extensive incision or complete excision of the whole area which is afterwards packed with magnesium sulphate paste and allowed to heal by granulation are rarely necessary.

In **acne** greasy plugs accumulate in the ducts of the sebaceous glands, particularly those of the face, shoulders and back. These are known as comedones or 'black heads' and their formation is probably due to an organism called the acne bacillus. There are various grades of severity. In severe cases, infection by staphylococci occurs and results in local inflammation with the production of pustules. The condition is commonly seen in both sexes between the ages of 15 and 30 years. It is essentially a disorder of puberty and is associated with a hormone (androgen) imbalance which affects the sebaceous glands. (**N.B.**—It is never seen in eunuchs but can be induced by androgen therapy.) Excessive consumption of carbohydrate is said to be a contributary cause. While generally regarded as a trivial malady it should not be neglected, as it may become extensive, leaving permanent scarring and disfigurement of the face and considerable psychological trauma.

The **treatment** consists of frequent washing with soap and hot water and frequent shampooing. Heavy make-up should be discouraged. Hexachlorophane, 'Cidal' soap or 'Cetavlon' may also be used. Comedones, if not inflamed, may be removed by a special extractor, or by pressure with the fingers protected by a handkerchief. When suppuration is present they should not be squeezed.

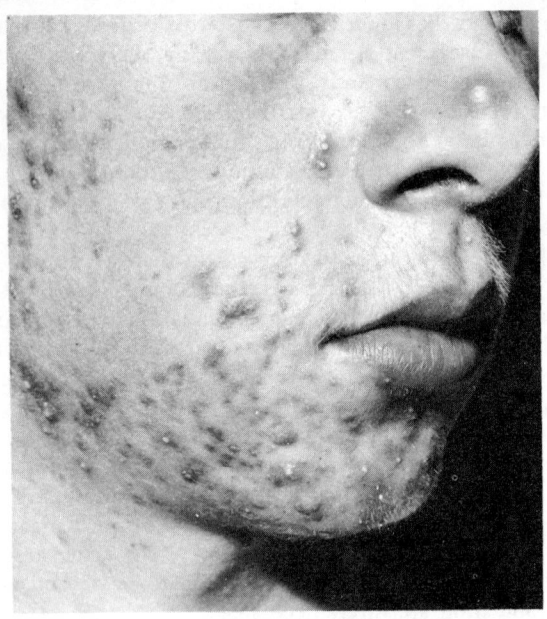

Fig. 103 Acne Vulgaris. (From Sneddon & Church, 1968, *Nursing Skin Disease*. Edward
Arnold, London.)

Calamine or sulphur lotion may be applied, but greasy ointments
are best avoided. However, the non-greasy ointment, 'Eskamel',
containing resorcinol, may be helpful. In severe cases, x-ray treatment is occasionally given. Others improve with ultra-violet rays.
Pustules may be broken with a pointed match-stick which has been
dipped in tincture of iodine. Stilboestrol is sometimes given and
severe cases may respond to tetracycline or doxycycline. The condition sometimes improves when the patient is taking oral contraceptives or is pregnant.

Acne rosacea

This condition is most likely to be seen in women after the age of 30.
General flushing of the face and the development of red papules are
characteristic. Various local applications may be helpful. Deep cystic
lesions may be treated by injecting the cysts with corticosteroids or
occasionally by incision and drainage. Pits and scars may sometimes be
eradicated or blended into healthy skin by **dermabrasion.**

Erysipelas

This is a now rare acute diffuse inflammation of the skin accompanied by toxaemia and fever and caused by a streptococcus. The organism gains entrance to the skin through an abrasion which may be minute and escape detection. The area feels hot, tense and painful. It becomes red, slightly raised and has a definite margin, which can be seen and felt. Frequently vesicles containing clear or turbid fluid develop on its surface. There may be considerable local oedema which, if the face is involved, causes swelling and closure of the eyelids. The condition being mildly contagious, contact with surgical patients and puerperal women should be avoided until the inflammatory process has subsided.

The main form of **treatment** is the administration of penicillin or other antibiotics. Various applications to the inflamed area, such as a saturated solution of magnesium sulphate, may relieve discomfort. The eyes may require treatment with lavage, followed by penicillin, sulphacetamide or chloramphenicol drops.

Impetigo contagiosa

This common condition caused by streptococci or staphylococci is seen chiefly in children and tends to affect exposed parts such as the face, scalp and hands. It is contagious and spreads not only from one person to another but also, by scratching or rubbing, the patient is liable to infect other parts of his own body. Patients with impetigo should, therefore, be segregated as much as possible with special care of washing and eating materials.

Small red spots appear and rapidly develop into vesicles and pustules which rupture and become covered with yellowish crusts. The neighbouring lymph glands are enlarged, and may suppurate. Impetigo is often superimposed upon the lesions of pediculosis or scabies which become infected as a result of scratching.

The **treatment** consists of removing the crusts in one of the following ways: (*a*) bathing in warm water or antiseptic lotion, (*b*) warm olive oil compresses, (*c*) starch poultices.

If the lesions are situated on the head the surrounding hair must be cut while, in severe cases, permission should be obtained to shave the whole scalp.

Neomycin and gramicidin ointment ('Graneodin') may be applied. Hydrocortisone may be incorporated in similar ointments. Sulphathiazole ointment and penicillin cream have been used, but they are liable to produce dermatitis and should be avoided. In children, who will not refrain from scratching, splinting of the arms may be necessary. Cloxacillin may be given orally.

If only scanty lesions are present, it is often sufficient to apply a small dressing of Elastoplast after removal of the crusts. When this is taken off after a few days, the skin will be found to have healed.

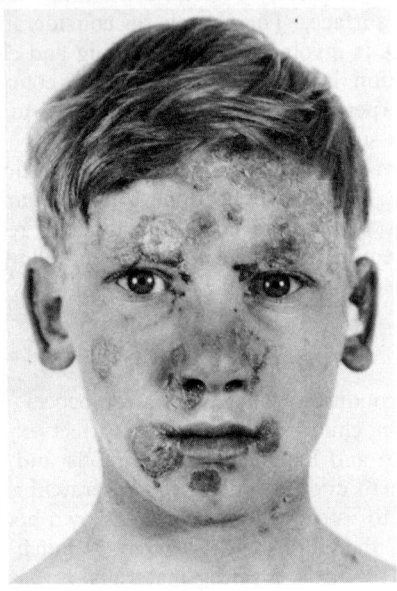

Fig. 104 Impetigo. (From Sneddon & Church, 1968, *Nursing Skin Disease*. Edward Arnold, London.)

'Cracked ears' are an allied condition, fissures appearing in the skin at the junction of the ear with the scalp, often as a result of inefficient drying. Strapping the ear forward, after an application of silver nitrate stick, is generally effective.

Sycosis (barber's rash). This is a similar condition seen in adults which affects the beard area and is spread by shaving. It is, however, usually staphylococcal in origin and may become chronic and resistant to treatment. Framycetin ('Framygen'), framycetin and gramicidin ('Soframycin') or clioquinol ('Vioform') ointments may be applied.

Parasitic infections of the skin

The common parasitic infections of the skin include:

(i) *Tinea* or ringworm, due to a fungus which is, therefore, a vegetable parasite. This may affect the scalp, beard, body or nails.

(ii) *Pediculosis* or lice, of which there are three varieties: (a) Pediculus capitis (of the head); (b) Pediculus corporis (of the body); (c) Pediculus pubis (of the pubic hair).

(iii) *Scabies* due to an insect (acarus or *Sarcoptes scabiei*).

Tinea or ringworm

This is due to a fungus. The form affecting the scalp is called tinea capitis (tonsurans) and commences with the formation of a small, circular, scaly patch in which the hair becomes thinner, individual hairs become brittle and break off close to the scalp, the stumps being visible with a magnifying glass. Rarely, suppuration occurs and the condition is then called a kerion. As a rule only children under the age of 12 are infected.

Diagnosis. Scrapings and hairs from a suspected lesion examined under a microscope will demonstrate the presence of the fungus. Another method is to examine the suspected area through a special Wood's Glass in a dark room under ultra-violet light. By this means selected rays only are seen and these have the power of illuminating hairs infected with ringworm.

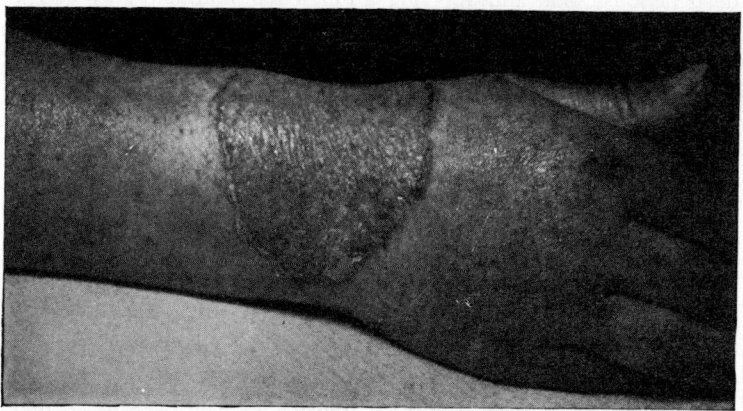

Fig. 105 Ringworm on the skin.

Ringworm of the skin is called tinea circinata because it produces circular patches with scaly margins.

Fungus infections of the finger- and toe-nails also occur and are slow to respond to treatment.

Treatment. Formerly ringworm of the scalp was only cured by removal of the hairs (epilation) from the infected areas. This was done by means of x-rays or by the application of special lotions followed by fungicide ointments. The modern treatment is to give the special fungicidal antibiotic, griseofulvin, 250 mg 4 times daily for several weeks.

This is also needed for ringworm of the finger-nails but a long course of up to 6 months is necessary. It is even longer if toe-nails are affected. (**N.B.**—Barbiturates should not be taken at the same time.)

These conditions are contagious, and great care must be taken that other individuals do not come in contact with the brush and comb, clothing, and toilet materials of infected patients.

In ringworm of the scalp, the head should be covered with a linen cap and all articles of clothing and bedding must finally be sterilized or destroyed.

Infected children should not be permitted to attend school or to mix with other children until cured.

Tinea pedis, also known as 'athlete's foot', is a common fungus infection which involves especially the skin between the toes, which becomes sodden with perspiration, sore and cracked.

The treatment consists of washing the affected parts, removing dead or loose skin and applying a fungicidal ointment, such as zinc undecenoate, Whitfield's ointment, tolnaftate cream ('Tinaderm'), 'Tineafax' or 'Mycil', night and morning. Foot baths containing a solution of potassium permanganate are useful.

It is also wise to dust the feet, socks and footwear with a similar powder for some weeks after, since the fungus may persist in them.

Pediculosis

Three different species of pediculi attack the human body, the head louse, the body louse and the pubic or crab louse.

The louse is an insect having six legs and is 1·5 to 3 millimetres in length.

Pediculosis of the head. Pediculi can be seen crawling about the head. They breed rapidly, and the females fix their eggs to the hairs by means of a cement. These can be seen as small white oval bodies

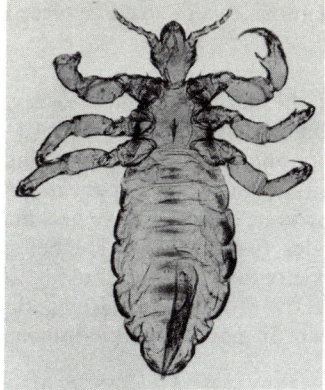

Fig. 106 Pediculus corporis × 10

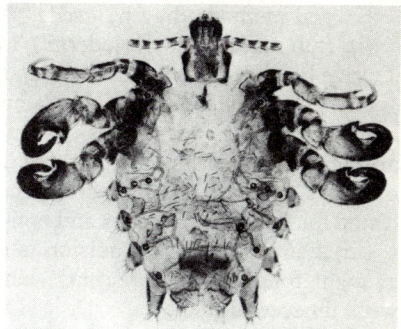

Fig. 107 Pediculus pubis × 10.

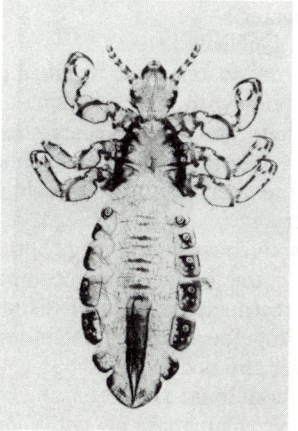

Fig. 108 Pediculus capitis × 10.

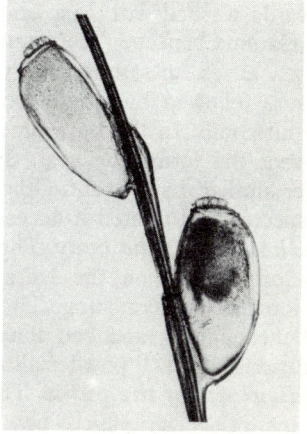

Fig. 109 Nits (eggs) of Pediculus capitis on hairs (magnified).

attached at intervals along each hair and are known as **nits**. The bite of the insect often causes itching which leads to scratching and subsequent infection of the skin with other organisms. The resulting lesion is an impetigo of the scalp. This is a common cause of enlarged glands in the neck which may suppurate and form cervical abscesses.

The aim of treatment is not only to kill the lice but also to destroy and remove the nits. When attending to this part of the toilet the nurse should wear an overall and a mackintosh cover should be placed round the patient's neck.

Several methods may be used:

(i) Rub malathion ('Prioderm') into the scalp and allow to dry. Twelve hours later, wash the hair and comb it whilst wet.

(ii) DDT (Dicophane) hair emulsion may be employed. This kills lice but does not always destroy nits so that 2 or 3 applications at intervals of 7 days are advisable. However, some lice have become resistant to DDT and other insecticides (e.g. carbaryl) are being tested for their effectiveness and non-toxicity for the human host.

(iii) Benzyl benzoate emulsion is effective if rubbed into the scalp at night followed by a morning shampoo. It may be repeated in one week if necessary.

(iv) Paraffin oil (Kerosene), 1 teaspoonful rubbed into the whole scalp may be used provided there is no naked light in the vicinity. The head should then be wrapped in a wet towel for 2 hours and afterwards washed with soap and water.

(v) Gamma benzene ('Lorexane', 'Quellada').

In all cases, nits must afterwards be removed by shampooing the hair, followed by careful combing with a special fine-toothed metal nit-comb. In the meantime, hats and hair brushes should be sterilized, the former by heat, the latter by immersion in hot lysol (2%) or similar disinfectant. Other members of the household should be inspected and treated if necessary.

Pediculosis of the body. The body louse lays its eggs both in the underclothing and on the hairs of the body. The accompanying irritation causes scratching. The treatment consists of disinfection of all the clothing and bed linen, together with baths followed by applications of DDT powder all over the body.

Pediculosis of the pubis. The crab louse is shorter and broader than the other varieties. The pubic hair may be cut short and applications of DDT or an ointment such as betanaphthol, or phenol lotion (1 in 40) on lint may be made.

Insect bites and stings

Those commonly affecting man are caused by the common flea (*Pulex irritans*), the bed bug, gnats, bees and wasps. The irritation may be due either to an acid or alkaline poison and may be relieved, viz. ant, hornet, wasp: by vinegar or lemon juice; bee: weak ammonia or bicarbonate of soda. Ointments containing one of the antihistamine drugs may be helpful. If reactions are severe one of these drugs may be given orally or even intravenously. Intravenous hydro-cortisone or subcutaneous adrenaline may also be used. Occasionally individuals become hypersensitive to bee and wasp stings and the allergic shock reaction can prove fatal. Sublingual isoprenaline tablets could be carried by individuals known to be sensitive.

Scabies

This condition is due to an insect called *sarcoptes scabei*. The female burrows in the horny layers of the skin where she deposits her eggs.

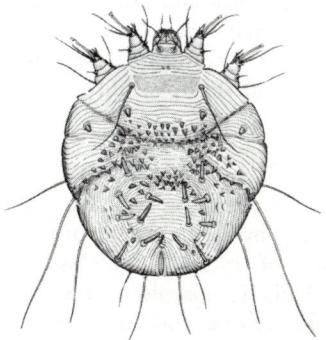

Fig. 110 Sarcoptes scabiei (female) ×20. The female burrows under the skin to lay her eggs, the burrows thus formed being typical and black with the faeces of the insect; they are most frequently found on the wrist. The male roams about over the body or clothes and is rarely captured.

These hatch in the course of several days and fresh lesions may be produced. The commonest sites for scabies to commence are between the fingers, on the front of the wrists and in the genital region, but any area of the body may be affected.

The burrows may be seen as small black lines at the end of which a vesicle or papule is sometimes present. Irritation, especially at night when the patient is warm in bed, followed by scratching and secondary infection with the production of impetigo, is common and may obscure the original lesion.

The routine of treatment must be carried out in detail and it is often necessary to apply it to all members of a family at the same time.

The preparations used are:

(a) Gamma benzene cream ('Lorexane', 'Quellada') may also be used in the treatment of pediculosis.

(b) Sulphur ointment (10%) is effective but less pleasant.

(c) Benzyl benzoate.

  (i) A hot bath is given and the body scrubbed with soap and a nail brush.

 (ii) Benzyl benzoate emulsion (25%) is applied all over the body from the neck downwards and allowed to dry.

(iii) Clothing is not changed for 48 hours.

 (iv) Another bath is taken and followed by a complete change of clothing and bed linen. The used clothes should be left unworn for 2 weeks and linen boiled or laundered.

It should be remembered that itching may persist for some days after the infection has been eradicated. Reactions may be caused by any of the medicaments in sensitive individuals.

Herpes

Herpes Simplex. Herpes is a recurrent inflammatory condition of the skin characterized by the formation of small vesicles in clusters, surrounded by an area of erythema. The lesion is commonly situated on the lips (herpes labialis) nostrils or external genital organs. It is often associated with febrile conditions such as a common cold (coryza) or lobar pneumonia and is also known as herpes febrilis. A virus is responsible for the condition, which is usually annoying rather than serious. The infection can, however, be very severe in patients with eczema and in those receiving immunosuppressive therapy.

Occasionally the herpes simplex virus causes severe stomatitis, vulvo-vaginitis or even meningo-encephalitis.

One strain of the virus (Type 2) may cause neonatal herpes, the infection being acquired by the baby from the mother's genital tract during delivery. Neonatal herpes may be mild or fatal; it may cause severe abnormalities of the eyes or central nervous system.

There is good evidence that Type 2 herpes virus is important in the causation of carcinoma of the cervix. Drying applications are used, 0·25% silver nitrate solution or 'Metanium'.

Herpes Zoster or **shingles** requires separate description. It is due to virus (of the neurotropic type), which produces inflammatory changes in the ganglia situated on the posterior (sensory) roots of the spinal nerves and other ganglia, e.g. the geniculate ganglion in which vesicles may appear on the external ear, together with some deafness and possibly facial paralysis.

The actual skin lesions are similar to those of simple herpes, but they are situated in the area of distribution of a sensory nerve. Thus, they commonly occur along the line of the intercostal spaces on the thorax or obliquely across the abdomen. In other instances a branch of the fifth cranial nerve may be affected, so that lesions appear on part of one side of the forehead (herpes ophthalmica). The attack is usually preceded by pain along the course of the corresponding nerve.

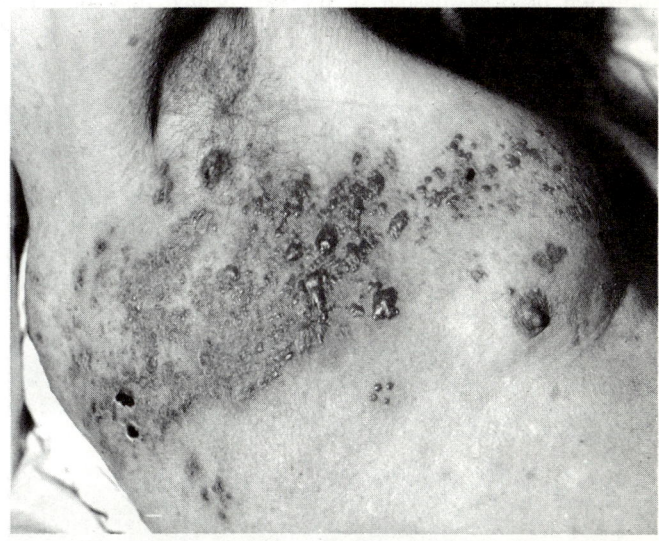

Fig. 111 Herpes Zoster.

This neuralgia may be severe and persist long after the skin lesion has subsided. Post-herpetic neuralgia is difficult to treat. A course of x-rays to the affected nerve roots is sometimes helpful. Before resorting to this, however, the effect of carbamazepine, chlorpromazine and an electric vibrator of the 'Pifco' type should be tried. In severe cases, local gangrene of the skin may take place leaving permanent scars.

A connection exists between herpes zoster and chicken-pox; cases of one condition sometimes being followed by the development of the other in a susceptible individual, after an incubation period of about three weeks. It is, therefore, advisable to separate persons suffering from herpes zoster from those who have not had chicken-pox.

Large-doses of vitamin B_{12} are sometimes given, but its action is uncertain. The lesion is painted with 5% idoxuridine solution, an antiviral agent. Alternatively it is dressed with zinc oxide powder or painted with collodion and analgesics are given as necessary.

Dermatitis (eczema)

These terms are used to describe superficial, non-contagious inflammation or breaking-out of the skin which may be due to a number of causes. Strictly speaking, the term dermatitis should be reserved for skin rashes caused by external irritants.

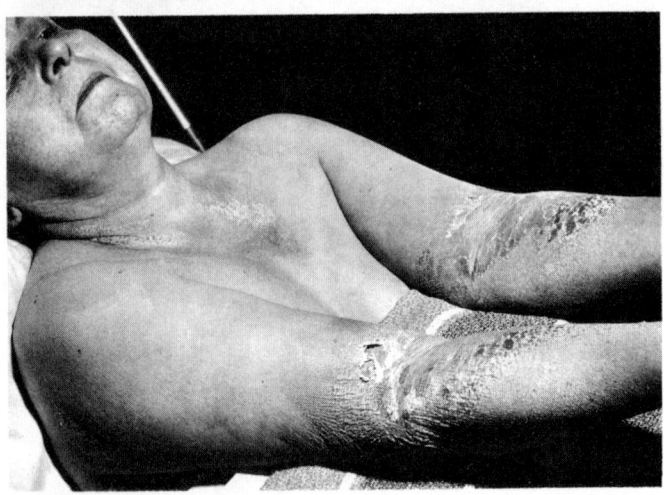

Fig. 112 Dermatitis of neck and cubital fossae due to dye in a frock.

The condition may be acute or chronic in character, and accompanied by various types of skin lesion, such as erythema, vesicles, pustules, scales or crusts. It may be either dry in type or associated with the exudation of serous fluid (weeping eczema).

The more obvious causes due to external irritants (exogenous causes) such as chemical and industrial agents, certain plants—e.g. primula, ivy—hair and fur dyes, cosmetics, household detergents, and powerful rays, have been mentioned. A common example of **contact dermatitis** is that caused by sensitivity to nickel, used on suspenders, ear clips etc. Industrial causes include rubber and oil.

In addition, obscure toxic states, psychological disturbances and increased sensitiveness of the skin may be responsible (endogenous causes).

Any part of the body may be affected, but when only folds of the skin, e.g. the groins, axillae, under the breasts, are involved the condition is called **Intertrigo.**

N.B.—Intertrigo is a fungus infection (Candida) causing an eruption in areas subject to friction. Treatment involves keeping the affected areas dry, using powder and applying an ointment or paint such as benzoic acid with salicylic acid or crystal violet paint.

The subjects most liable to eczema are those possessing a greasy skin. This condition, in which the sebaceous glands are over-active, is called **seborrhoea.**

Infantile eczema is a special type affecting babies and is sometimes associated with an excessive carbohydrate diet. In most instances, however, it is regarded as an allergic condition. It may be necessary to substitute goat's milk for cow's milk.

Treatment. Whenever possible the cause is removed and patch testing of the skin may be required to determine sensitivity. In the acute stages, ointments are avoided, and various lotions such as normal saline, calamine, or lead are applied. If there is much local sepsis, perchloride of mercury (1/4000) or flavine may be used. When acute inflammation has subsided, oily preparations, e.g. calamine liniment, are of greater value.

In the chronic stages, various ointments are employed, e.g. Hydrocortisone ointment, zinc paste (Pasta Zinci Co., known also as Lassar's Paste), calamine cream or coal-tar preparations. These should be spread on gauze or lint and bandaged gently on to the affected part. Dressings are changed twice daily, care being taken that the underlying skin is not injured when they are removed. Soap and water are avoided and the skin is cleansed with saline or olive oil. Attention is given to the general health, septic foci and the bowels, and a special diet may be ordered. A sedative drug is often required at night to promote sleep and to prevent irritation and scratching. Either a barbiturate or nitrazipam may be used. Anti-histamine drugs by mouth are sometimes helpful, but their local application may itself provoke dermatitis and should be avoided.

Notes on preparations used in disorders of the skin

Ointments are generally speaking greasier than **creams** which usually consist of oil in water emulsions. The choice is a matter for the individual patient to decide which happens to suit him.

Pastes are thicker preparations and contain a powder such as zinc oxide or starch. They help to form a protective covering for the skin. They are more porous than ointments and help to prevent scratching.

Lotions may be watery or oily (e.g. calamine). Some are antiseptic (e.g. eusol); others anti-parasite (e.g. gamma benzene) or anti-pruritic (e.g. hydrocortisone which may also be applied as an ointment or cream).

Powders. Simple dusting powders are of value in areas subject to friction, e.g. intertrigo in the groins and under the breasts.

Dressings. Special dressings include tulle gras and occlusive polythene preparations or gloves for the hands which are specially useful for covering steroid preparations.

In emergency clean linen, e.g. handkerchiefs, sheets, moistened with saline or treated with calamine lotion, if indicated, makes useful temporary dressings.

Other skin conditions

There are a number of skin conditions of doubtful aetiology, some of which may be the manifestation of obscure toxic or allergic processes. These include urticaria (nettle rash), pemphigus, psoriasis and erythema nodosum.

Urticaria

This allergic condition is characterized by the appearance of wheals which are localized areas of oedema. These are usually transitory in duration and are accompanied by severe itching. Urticaria commonly results from food poisoning or from the ingestion of strawberries, shell-fish, eggs, pork, milk or drugs such as penicillin, barbiturates or aspirin in individuals susceptible to any of these substances. It may also occur after the injection of serum (serum rash, p. 16).

The treatment consists in searching for and avoiding or removing the cause. Local applications to allay irritation, such as calamine, hydrocortisone, coal-tar or lead lotion, are useful. Injections of adrenaline or ephedrine are sometimes ordered. Antihistamine drugs, such as 'Benadryl', 'Anthisan' or 'Piriton', may be given by mouth or applied locally as an ointment but with the latter there is a considerable risk of producing sensitivity. In resistant cases steroids may be given orally.

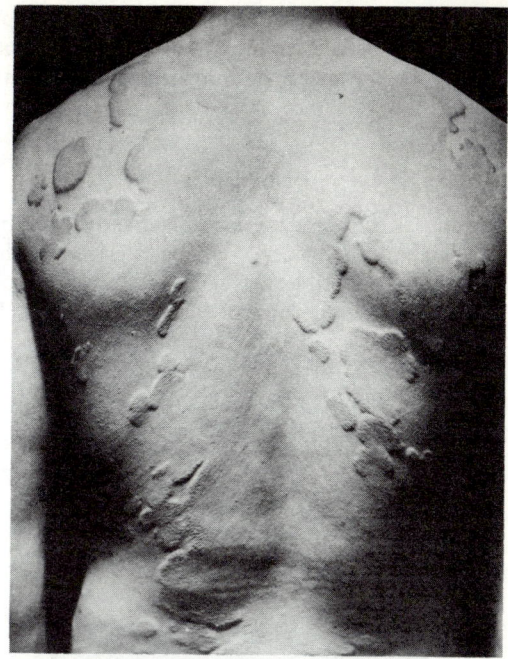

Fig. 113 Urticaria. (From Sneddon & Church, 1968, *Nursing Skin Disease*. Edward Arnold, London.)

Pemphigus

This is a rare skin condition characterized by the occurrence of crops of large blisters (bullae). It may be acute or chronic in type, and affects both adults and infants. Steroids may be used in the treatment of the adult form.

It is important to remember that two types occur in the new born:

(*a*) Simple *pemphigus neonatorum*, in an otherwise healthy, well-nourished infant affecting any part of the body. This condition is caused by a staphylococcus and is allied to impetigo. It is very contagious and cases should therefore be carefully isolated from other infants.

(*b*) *Syphilitic pemphigus*, occurring in congenital syphilis. The baby is wasted, and a copper-coloured macular eruption may also be present. The lesions are commonest on the soles and palms, and the Wassermann reaction is positive in the blood of the infant and the mother.

The local treatment of pemphigus consists in rupturing the bullae with a sterile needle and applying neomycin lotion. Antibiotic drugs may be given. Syphilitic cases require antisyphilitic treatment.

Psoriasis

This is a common affection of the skin of unknown origin, although there may be a familial incidence. It is characterized by the presence of red patches covered by silvery-grey scales in various parts of the body, with little or no disturbance of the general health. It is sometimes associated with a period of rheumatoid arthritis and sometimes produces its own peculiar arthritis (psoriatic anthropathy) affecting the terminal joints of the fingers.

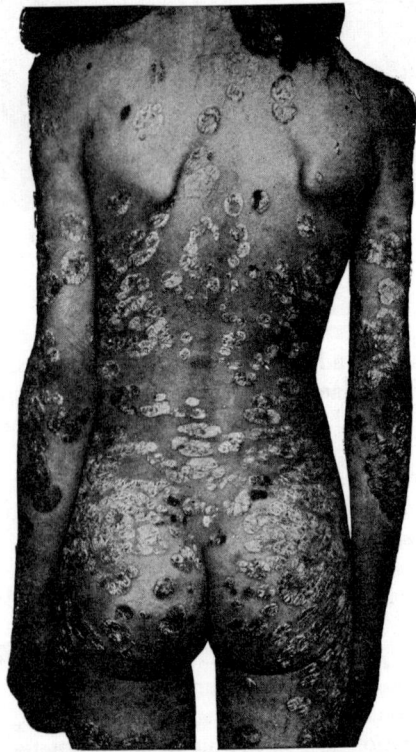

Fig. 114 Generalized Psoriasis.

Any parts may be affected, but lesions are common over the back of the elbows and front of the knees. The nails may also be involved. The condition is a chronic one and improvement may be followed by seasonal relapses (especially in the spring and autumn).

There are no special curative measures. Coal-tar preparations, steroids and ultra-violet light may be employed. Chrysarobin or dithranol ointment or paste are sometimes used as local applications. These have the disadvantage that linen is permanently stained, so that old materials should be utilized while the course of the treatment is being carried out. Methotrexate, a cytotoxic drug, is occasionally used for severe cases. It is given in tablet form. It may cause liver damage.

Pityriasis. This term means scaliness and is used to describe various skin lesions of unknown origin, e.g. pityriasis rosea and pityriasis rubra pilaris.

Erythema nodosum

This condition is an allergic cutaneous manifestation due to susceptibility to circulating toxins. In some cases toxins produced by the tubercle bacillus are responsible: in some, sarcoidosis, streptococcal infection and drug reactions are known causes.

The lesions consist of oval swellings on the extensor aspects of both limbs, more commonly the shins than elsewhere, varying in diameter from 1·25–5 cm ($\frac{1}{2}$ to 2 inches). They involve the skin and subcutaneous tissue and are well described as erythematous nodules, their colour at first being red but later changing to purple like a bruise. They are very tender and are often accompanied by pyrexia, malaise and joint pains.

The treatment consists of rest in bed with elevation of the affected parts, to which lead lotion is applied.

X-rays of the chest are taken in order to exclude pulmonary tuberculosis and sarcoidosis. A Mantoux test may be carried out and the blood sedimentation rate is observed. This is usually raised in the acute stages.

Erythema multiforme. The cause is often unknown but it may be due to drug sensitivity in some cases, e.g. sulphonamides. Scattered, usually symmetrical lesions of erythema surrounded by concentric rings (target type) which sometimes develop vesicles in the centre appear. A severe type is known as Stevens-Johnson syndrome. Mucous membranes and the conjunctiva may be affected. Steroids and anti histamines may be helpful in treatment.

Skin lesions associated with local circulatory disorders

These include varicose eczema and ulcers (p. 156), chilblains and Raynaud's Disease.

A **chilblain** or **erythema pernio** is a local exudation of fluid from the blood vessels following a spasmodic contraction of the small arterioles and capillaries in response to the stimulus of cold, especially in those whose peripheral circulation is sluggish. The lesions are ill-defined purple or reddish, irritating swellings which occur chiefly on the fingers and toes in cold weather. In severe cases fissures or ulcers may develop.

In treatment, attention to the general health and diet is necessary. Ultra-violet light may help to prevent their recurrence in susceptible individuals. Calcium salts and vitamins may be given by mouth. The local treatment by rubbing in ichthammol or iodine ointment after immersing the affected areas in equal parts of hot water and hydrogen peroxide for ten minutes may be helpful. In cold weather patients should be careful to keep the extremities warm, with loose woollen gloves and stockings.

Frost bite is a more severe form of cold injury.

Raynaud's Disease. Strictly speaking, this is a local disorder of the circulation rather than a skin disease, and occurs as a result of defective blood supply to the extremities. The diminished blood supply is probably due to alteration in the nervous control of the vessels which pass into spasm.

The lesions are usually symmetrical and affect the toes and fingers: in rare cases the ears and tip of the nose may be involved.

The disease, which is usually seen in women, is characterized by recurring attacks of pain in the affected parts which at first become cold, numb and white in colour. Later, engorgement of the veins and capillaries develops and the part assumes a hyperaemic appearance.

In severe cases, this may eventually be followed by gangrene involving either a small portion or the whole of a finger or toe.

Vasodilator drugs, e.g. 'Hexopal', tolazoline ('Priscol'). Dibenyline ('Ronicol'), may be given. Sympathectomy may be performed.

Affections of the sweat glands

The sweat glands are under the control of the sympathetic nervous system and also the heat regulating centre. The response to the latter is essentially physiological. The former may be associated with emotional conditions which are controlled by the frontal cortex and may affect the hands, feet and axillae in particular, and which may be a social handicap.

Excessive sweating is called **hyperidrosis**. In addition to emotional reactions it may occur in febrile illnesses, on exertion and in patients suffering from thyrotoxicosis and tuberculosis. It is also characteristic of malaria.

Sometimes the secretion accumulates in the openings of the ducts and these are then visible as minute glistening points on the skin. They may also appear under adhesive strapping, in obesity and in conditions of moist heat. They are known as sudamina.

Miliaria or prickly heat is a somewhat similar condition more common in hot countries. It is due to overactivity of the sweat glands associated with some blockage of the ducts so that the secretion passes into the skin rather than onto the surface. The lesions appear as numerous pale reddish papules especially at sites of clothing friction.

In axillary hyperidrosis local applications of aluminium salts which may be used in proprietary preparations, are useful. In very severe cases local excision of the axillary skin may be effective.

When decomposition of the sweat and sebaceous material as a result of bacterial action is added to hyperidrosis, an offensive odour is produced and the condition called **bromidrosis**. This may be associated with tinea pedis ('athlete's foot'), p. 476.

If the feet are affected, frequent washing followed by powder and changing the shoes and stockings twice daily are necessary.

Affections of the hair

Infection of the hair with ringworm has been mentioned.

Baldness (**alopecia**) is a common condition. General loss of hair is usually due to advancing age. The occurrence of localized patches is called alopecia areata. Some cytotoxic drugs may cause alopecia.

Affections of the nails

Alteration in the texture of the nails, with irregular transverse ridging, occurs when their nutrition is defective and may often be seen after a serious acute illness.

The nail takes about 4 months to grow 1·25 cm ($\frac{1}{2}$ inch) so that the approximate date of an illness which has produced a transverse groove across the nail can be estimated.

Spoon-shaped nails (koilonychia), in which the centre is depressed, are often observed in achlorhydric hypochromic anaemia (p. 181). Excessive curving of the nails is associated with the clubbed fingers seen in chronic pulmonary conditions and congenital heart disease (pp. 137, 309).

Hypertrophy of one or more nails, with the production of a claw or horn-like formation, is seen usually in old people. The big toe is commonly affected and the condition is known as **onychogryphosis.** The nail is discoloured, ridged, and often twisted. The treatment consists of softening the nail in hot water to which soda may be added. It can then be pared down and later filed. If the nail is very loose it may be removed and the nail-bed protected with zinc ointment spread on linen.

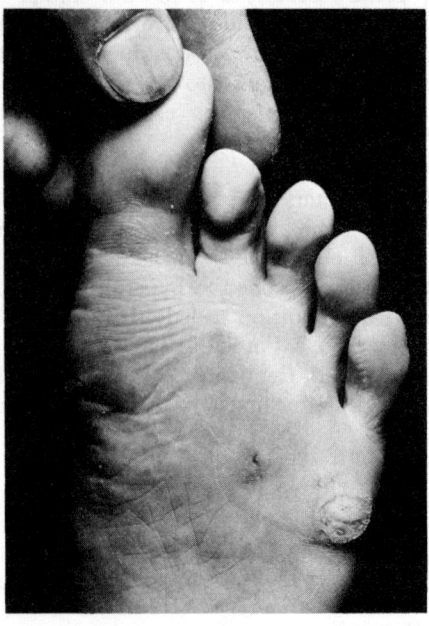

Fig. 115 Plantar warts. (From Snedden and Church, 1968, *Nursing Skin Disease*, Edward Arnold, London.)

The nail-beds may be involved in inflammation (onychia) or affected by ringworm and psoriasis.

A **Corn** (clavus) consists of thickening of the superficial layers of the epidermis produced by undue pressure or rubbing of its surface. Corns can be very painful and may sometimes become infected. They can be prevented by the use of properly fitting shoes and may be remedied by shaving off the thickened portions or by application of a corn paint or plaster containing salicylic acid. The attention of a chiropodist is usually advisable.

Warts (verrucae) are superficial tumours which may be single or multiple, which are usually seen on the fingers, hands or soles of the feet (plantar warts) mainly in children and young adults and are due to a local virus infection. Small lesions may be removed by the application of caustics, such as silver nitrate, phenol, trichloracetic acid or strong nitric acid. The surrounding healthy skin should be protected with petroleum jelly before these remedies are applied. 'Salactol'—a paint containing salicylic acid and lactic acid may be applied to all types of wart. X-ray treatment may cause local scarring and is usually avoided. Large warts can be scraped out with a sharp spoon under local anaesthesia. Applications containing podophyllin in linseed oil which are left in position for a week may be effective. The electric cautery or CO_2 snow may also be used. Some people claim to be able to remove warts by charms and hypnosis may be successful.

Bed sores (decubitus ulcers). Bed sores are gangrenous ulcers due to death of the tissues and result from continuous pressure, often associated with dirt and moisture which occur with incontinence.

They are especially liable to develop when the vitality is lowered by long and exhausting illnesses such as typhoid fever and by old age; also when there is interference with the nutrition of the part as a result of disease of the nervous system (trophic changes, p. 389). They are commonly seen on the sacrum, buttocks and heels. Their prevention and treatment is fully described in textbooks on nursing. A flotation bed ('water-bed') may help to heal pressure sores.

14 Venereal Disease

Venereal disease is propagated mainly by sexual intercourse. Three varieties, syphilis, gonorrhoea and non-specific urethritis, commonly occur. With the introduction of chemotherapy and antibiotics the immediate decrease in the incidence of these diseases and the effectiveness of their treatment gave hope that they would cease to be a major problem. Unfortunately, however, for a number of reasons there has been a considerable increase in all types in recent years. Among the causes for this have been increased promiscuity, greater travel facilities, homosexuality and the fact that the responsible organisms tend to acquire some resistance to treatment and need maximum doses of the available drugs. The following is a brief account of their more important features.

Syphilis

Syphilis may be defined as a contagious (sometimes congenital) disease caused by the Treponema pallidum (spirochaeta pallida). It may be acquired:

(*a*) By sexual connection.

(*b*) Occasionally by accidental infection, e.g. in medical practice, or through the use of infected articles.

The incubation period between exposure to infection and the appearance of the primary lesion is 2 to 6 weeks. The disease is described in 3 stages.

(i) The Primary stage. The initial lesion consists of a painless, hard, red papule developing at the site of inoculation which later ruptures and forms an ulcer. This is called a **chancre**. In the male this is usually on the penis. In the female it may be either on the vulva or the cervix. In the latter case it may be symptomless. The neighbouring lymph glands become enlarged.

(ii) The secondary stage. If the primary stage is missed or

untreated, this period indicates general infection of the body and commences about 6 weeks after the onset of the disease, and is prolonged for about 2 years. During this time any of the following symptoms may appear:

(*a*) Skin rashes consisting of copper-coloured macules or papules.

(*b*) Sore throat with small, 'snail track' ulcers on the tonsils.

(*c*) Condylomata or moist warty papules situated around the genitals and anus.

(*d*) Enlarged lymphatic glands in the neck, axilla, etc., which feel shotty but are painless.

(*e*) Loss of hair (alopecia).

(*f*) Anaemia.

Syphilis is especially contagious during the primary and secondary stages.

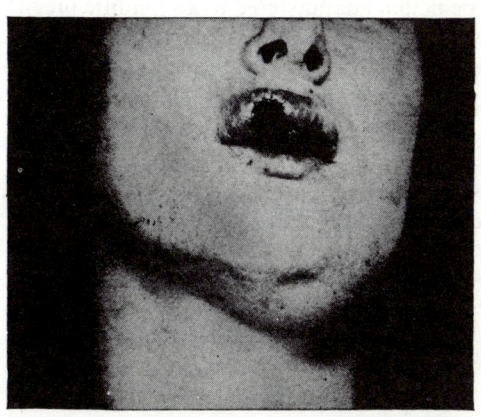

Fig. 116 Lip chancre and enlarged gland.

(iii) The tertiary stage. The lesions characteristic of the tertiary stage usually appear within 2 to 15 years from the onset of infection.

A typical pathological process occurring is the production of specialized granulation tissue called a gumma (see p. 25).

Syphilitic lesions may attack almost any tissue or system of the body; among the common parts affected are:

(*a*) The skin and mucous membranes, i.e. ulcers on the legs, palate, face or tongue.

(*b*) The cardiovascular system, e.g. disease of the aortic valves, of the walls of blood vessels leading to aneurysm.

(*c*) The bones and periosteum, causing osteitis and periostitis.

(*d*) Affections of the central nervous system (**neurosyphilis**), in which either the nervous tissues themselves may be involved, as in tabes dorsalis and general paralysis of the insane, or the meninges or blood vessels (see p. 394).

Congenital syphilis is inherited from the mother who may herself have been infected by the father. An untreated syphilitic mother will often give a history of repeated abortions followed later by a stillbirth and finally by a living infant which develops evidence of congenital syphilis.

N.B.—All antenatal patients and infants for adoption should have blood tests for syphilis.

The manifestations of congenital syphilis, which is now rare, may occur early in infancy, often within a few weeks of birth, or later in childhood.

However, penicillin administered to a syphilitic pregnant woman is effective in preventing congenital syphilis whether it is given early or late in pregnancy.

The early manifestations include:

(*a*) General wasting.

(*b*) Skin eruptions, e.g. pemphigus and macular rashes.

(*c*) Snuffles, which is a condition of syphilitic rhinitis, with nasal discharge often followed by destruction of the nasal bones leading to a depressed bridge of the nose.

(*d*) Enlargement of the liver and spleen.

(*e*) Inflammation of bones and their epiphyses.

The late symptoms are:

(*a*) Affections of the eyes, such as inflammation of the cornea in which permanent opacities ultimately develop (keratitis), and optic atrophy.

(*b*) Eighth nerve deafness.

(*c*) Various affections of the bones and joints.

(*d*) Hutchinson's teeth. These consist of peculiar peg-shaped and notched incisor teeth which tend to be widely separated from each other.

(*e*) Nervous symptoms, including juvenile tabes dorsalis and general paralysis of the insane.

Diagnosis. The diagnosis of syphilis is made on the clinical findings and, in the case of the primary lesion, on the discovery of the treponeme in scrapings from the chancre. In addition, the Wassermann, Kahn, treponemal immobilisation (TPI) and fluorescent antibody (FTA) tests are frequently made in the laboratory on the blood and cerebrospinal fluid.

Treatment. The treatment of syphilis is now less prolonged than formerly but may consist of several courses spread out over a considerable period until the Wassermann Reaction becomes negative.

A 10-day course of penicillin injections, e.g. single daily injections of 1·2 mega units of procaine penicillin or procaine penicillin in oily solution (PAM) 3 times weekly may be given. For patients who are

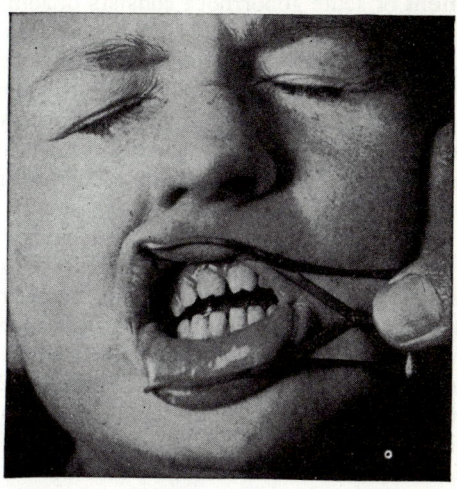

Fig. 117 Hutchinson's Teeth, showing characteristic notching and peg-shaped appearance of upper incisors.

sensitive to penicillin, erythromycin, cephaloridine or one of the tetracyclines are also effective. In view of the possibility of anaphylactic reactions, adrenaline, a steroid and antihistamine should be available at the time of a penicillin injection. Destruction of the bacteria may result in a Herxheimer reaction, with acute but transient exacerbation of the lesions.

Gonorrhoea

This is a venereal disease characterized by infection of mucous membranes by *Neisseria gonorrhoea*, an organism more commonly known as the gonococcus.

It may occur either in the male, the female, or the newborn, and has an incubation period of about 3 to 10 days.

Gonorrhoea in the male is of acute onset but may be followed by chronic manifestations.

In the acute condition the organisms settle in the glands of the mucous membrane of the urethra, producing a purulent discharge (urethritis) accompanied by painful or scalding micturition.

In the female not only the urethra but also the vulva, vagina and cervix may become infected. However, sometimes the initial infection may pass unnoticed.

The **treatment** of acute gonorrhoea consists of administering one of the antibiotic drugs. Some strains of the gonococcus are relatively resistant to penicillin but a single large injected dose of penicillin (up to 5 mega-units) with probenecid 2 g orally will cure the disease in 24 hours in most cases. Streptomycin and kanamycin have the advantage that they will not mask the development of syphilis which might have been contracted at the same time but which owing to the longer incubation period is not apparent at the time the patient seeks treatment. A single dose of 1 or 2 g of streptomycin by intramuscular injection is usually effective but some strains of gonococci are resistant. If single dose oral therapy is used, 2 g of ampicillin with 1 g of probenecid may be employed. Cephalexin is another antibiotic which is useful in gonorrhoea when penicillin is likely to be ineffective or is contra-indicated. A single dose of 3 g for men and 2 g for women is effective if probenecid is given at the same time (1 g for men, 0·5 g for women).

The complications in the male include inflammation of the testicle (orchitis) and stricture of the urethra. In the female inflammation of the Fallopian tubes (salpingitis) and peritonitis may develop and result in infertility. Inflammation of joints (acute or chronic gono-coccal arthritis) may occur in either sex.

The lesion which commonly affects the newborn is inflammation of the eyes (**ophthalmia neonatorum**) resulting from infection during the infant's passage through the birth canal.

It is for this reason that the eyes of babies are carefully cleaned immediately after birth and antiseptic drops may be instilled. Ophthalmia neonatorum is a very serious condition which may result in permanent blindness.

Gonococcal ophthalmia requires the most careful isolation. If only one eye is affected, the other must be covered with a glass shield kept in position with strapping. Pus should not be permitted to collect under the eyelids which should be opened and irrigated very frequently (1–2 hourly). Sulphacetamide (Albucid) or penicillin drops are often employed.

Soft sore (chancroid) is a local venereal ulceration not common in this country due to Ducrey's bacillus. It is treated with sulphona-mides or one of the antibiotics (streptomycin, tetracycline).

Non-specific urethritis is probably caused by a virus. The urethritis may be accompanied by an acute arthritis, skin lesions and conjunctivitis, the condition then being known as *Reiter's syndrome*. The arthritis usually resolves completely but sometimes becomes chronic and causes joint deformities. Antibiotics are ineffective in many cases but tetracycline is commonly prescribed.

Lymphogranuloma inguinale

Another name for this venereal disease is 'Climatic Bubo'. It is mostly confined to the tropics. It is due to infection by a large virus which causes a small local lesion followed by considerable enlargement and eventual abscess formation in the inguinal lymph nodes. These swellings are called buboes. If untreated, pus is discharged from the abscesses which heal slowly and cause much local scarring in the skin and also internally.

The infection in its earlier stages responds well to a sulphonamide drug, streptomycin or tetracycline.

Granuloma venereum

This is a chronic ulcerating disorder of the skin of the genitalia and nearby parts, commonest in tropical areas. It is treated with streptomycin or tetracycline.

Trichomoniasis

The organism **Trichomonas vaginalis** causes an unpleasant greenish vaginal discharge. It may be successfully treated with metronidazole ('Flagyl') 200 mg orally 3 times a day for 7 days. The consort should receive a similar course of treatment at the same time, as his urethra may harbour parasites which could re-infect the vagina.

The control of venereal disease. Of vital importance is the tracing of contacts and the follow-up of cases. Specially trained social workers are necessary for these difficult tasks.

15 Occupational Health (Industrial Disease)

The many occupations involved in modern civilization bring with them dangers to life and health including trauma which may occur in mines and the use of machinery and electricity.

The most obvious other risks are those which involve the use of chemical substances which may enter the body by the paths of:

Inhalation.

Ingestion.

Innoculation and surface contact.

Any of the major systems of the body may be involved, i.e. the skeletal system, lungs, cardio-vascular system, blood, alimentary system, liver, nervous system and the skin. Workers may be involved not only in the factory but also in the open air.

Chemical hazards involve those workers handling any of the following products:

Elements: lead   chromium

arsenic   manganese

phosphorus   beryllium

Compounds: coal-tar derivatives including trinitrotoluene (TNT), tar and asphalt. Also corrosive poisons (strong acids and alkalis), and many others.

Among those substances causing pathological conditions are those due to inhalation of industrial dust, e.g. silicosis and asbestosis (pneumoconiosis) which may seriously affect the lungs of miners and workers using asbestos.

Agricultural workers may be exposed to the effects of modern insecticides and fertilizers (e.g. organo-chlorine and dinitro compounds), apart from infections such as anthrax and tetanus.

Doctors, nurses and scientists, unless adequately protected by immunization, may be at risk in respect of infectious diseases and also from x-rays and radioactive substances unless proper protection is provided.

In so far as environmental conditions such as noise and the vain repetition of monotonous duties are concerned, the special senses and general psychology may be involved. The former may lead to deafness, the latter to industrial and domestic discord.

The subject is so extensive that it is not possible here to give a full account. It is, however, particularly important in taking the history of any malady that enquiries should always be made into the possibility of an industrial cause.

Many of the problems which may arise are covered by the Factory Acts and, obviously all aspects of prevention are of utmost importance.

Treatment of any of the conditions when they arise will vary according to circumstances.

The Nurse and the Law

Occasional references have been made to a few matters which have a Medico-legal significance. These concern both the doctor and to some extent the nurse, both student and qualified.

It is not intended here to go into any details but only to *remind* the nurse of the possibilities of the situation.

First of all, for example, in the day-to-day duties of complying with the requirements of the Misuse of Drugs Regulations (p. 503) and the Factory Act (see above), the nurse has some responsibilities and should be aware of the main rules.

The nurse may be in the position of an ordinary citizen in a Court of Law. In which case, the nurse will be expected to give evidence on oath on matters of fact only. On the other hand, in addition to this, a qualified nurse may be asked to give an opinion on a professional matter and be regarded as an expert witness.

16 Causes of Sudden Death

Sudden or unexpected death apart from suicide, murder and violent injury may occur as the result of failure in function of the circulatory, respiratory or nervous systems, and the modes of death are sometimes referred to as syncope, asphyxia or coma.

1. Circulatory system

(*a*) Disease of the coronary arteries resulting in the sudden onset of coronary artery thrombosis (p. 150) is a fairly common cause of rapid death.

(*b*) The only valvular disease of the heart likely to cause sudden death is that of aortic stenosis.

(*c*) Rupture of an aneurysm of the aorta results in rapid death and in such instances bleeding may occur into the pericardium, the trachea or oesophagus.

(*d*) Pulmonary embolism. Any large blood clot dislodged from a vein will be carried to the right side of the heart and on into the pulmonary artery. If such a clot is sufficiently large it will block the pulmonary artery completely and cause cessation of the pulmonary circulation, a condition which is incompatible with life. Sudden death may, therefore, occur from this cause. Clotting in veins is called phlebothrombosis (p. 157) and is not uncommon after abdominal operations, especially those on the pelvis. Unexpected sudden death several days after an operation is often due to this cause. In a few cases the use of contraceptive pills appears to contribute to the occurrence of thrombosis and subsequent embolism.

(*e*) Vagal arrest. Sudden death, as from fright, is sometimes due to complete vagal inhibition (overactivity of the vagus nerve) of the heart. Fright may also cause death by stimulating a gross over-secretion of adrenaline, which causes ventricular fibrillation.

2. Respiratory system

Asphyxia resulting in rapid death may occur from blockage of the larynx or trachea by any foreign body. This includes aspiration of vomited material, which is especially liable to take place in an unconscious patient, e.g. during or after anaesthesia. Pressure on the air passages by a tumour which has suddenly increased in size or altered its position may have similar results. Severe haemoptysis, e.g. from a ruptured aneurysm or advanced tuberculosis, may prove fatal.

Sudden death may occur in bronchial asthma; sometimes intemperate use of an aerosol inhaler (containing adrenaline or isoprenaline) is responsible.

3. Nervous system

The commonest affection of the nervous system resulting in sudden death is cerebral haemorrhage. Embolism or thrombosis and subarachnoid haemorrhage may also prove fatal. Occasionally, a cerebral tumour causes the rapid onset of death in coma.

4. Other causes

Sudden death may occur as a result of any severe injury to the body or brain, from haemorrhage, electric shock or poisoning. Interference with the pelvic organs for the purposes of producing criminal abortion sometimes causes death from shock or air-embolism. Anaphylactic reactions and over-sensitivity to some drugs e.g. penicillin may have fatal results.

The signs of death

1. Cessation of respiration and the circulation. The pulse cannot be felt and no heart sounds are heard with the stethoscope or when the ear is placed on the precordium.

2. An ashy white pallor or cadaveric appearance of the body.

3. Eye changes. The eyeball appears dull, feels soft and sinks back. The pupil does not react to light and the corneal reflex is lost.

4. The muscular reaction to mechanical or electrical stimulation rapidly disappears.

5. Coldness. The body loses heat at a rate largely dependent on external conditions. As a general rule the temperature falls about 1 °C per hour and the body is quite cold in about 12 hours.

6. Rigor Mortis or general stiffening of all the muscles of the body usually commences in about 4 hours and last about 24 hours.

7. Hypostasis or post-mortem staining is due to the collection of blood in the most dependent parts of the body during the process of cooling but does not as a rule come on until about 8 hours after death.

8. Putrefaction may appear from 1 to 3 days after death.

9. Characteristic changes occur in the electrocardiogram and electroencephalogram.

17 Notes on Some Important Drugs

The subject of drugs is of considerable importance to the nurse since their administration is one of her routine duties, which carries with it great responsibility on account of the powerful nature of many preparations. Absolute accuracy of measurement is essential in every case, and in the event of any doubt entering the nurse's mind about the correctness of a dose or drug which she is about to give, there must be no hesitation in referring the matter to a senior officer.

The sale and supply of certain dangerous substances, especially those which may lead to the formation of drug habits (addiction), are controlled by law (The Misuse of Drugs Regulations). In hospital, these drugs must be kept under lock and key, and it is the duty of the nurse to see that any register, for which she is responsible, is accurately completed. The following are some of the substances to which the act applies. Opium, morphine and their preparations; diamorphine (heroin); cocaine; pethidine and methadone ('Physeptone'); A number of other analgesics are also included, e.g. 'Dromoran', 'Dilaudid', 'Proladone'.

The care and distribution of some other drugs are controlled by The Poisons Act. This group includes most of the alkaloids and barbiturates.

Care must be taken that all bottles and containers are clearly and correctly labelled. The nurse will be wise to reject any unlabelled bottle even though she imagines herself to be familiar with its contents. Drugs for internal administration should be kept in a cupboard separate from those used for external application and the latter should be dispensed in coloured and different-shaped bottles.

The main points to remember in administering medicines are:

1. Punctuality, having special regard to the instructions before or after meals and the method of administration, e.g. with or without water, etc.

2. To shake the bottle carefully after reading the label and before measuring the dose.

3. To observe and report any signs of overdose or intolerance (see digitalis, p. 129).

4. To have hypodermic injections and dangerous drugs checked by a second person.

5. To make certain that the patient actually takes pills or tablets, especially in psychiatric cases.

The British Pharmacopoeia (BP) is a list of 'official' drugs and their doses. Another book containing a number of useful preparations is known as the British Pharmaceutical Codex (BPC). The British National Formulary (BNF) is used in connection with the Health Act and contains many of the preparations commonly employed and useful explanations of their actions. There are, however, a large number of therapeutic agents having special trade names and prepared by various firms of manufacturing chemists which are not included in these lists but information on these can be obtained from publications such as MIMS. Generally speaking proprietary preparations are more expensive than similar substances in the BNF.

The fact that the same drug may be known by several different names is a difficulty which doctors, nurses and pharmacists all have to face, but 'official' names should be used when possible.

Another problem is that, in the prescription of doses, both the Apothecaries' measures and the Metric system are used in such a way that no guidance can be given which will aid memory. On a broad basis it may be stated that traditional preparations such as a mixture (15 ml, ½ fl oz) and linctus (8 to 2 ml, 120 to 30 minims) have standard doses: whereas newer and very powerful drugs, the dosage of which is very small, are often prescribed in milligrams and administered in tablet form.

In Britain all doses should now be in metric units. 'Official' preparations (i.e. those in the BP, the BPC and the BNF) are all formulated so that the unit dose is 5 ml for linctuses, elixirs and paediatric mixtures, and 10 ml for adult mixtures.

Injections given from ampoules are often measured in cubic centimetres (cc) or millilitres (ml), which for practical purposes are the same amount.

Methods of administration

Therapeutic substances are administered or applied in a number of different ways.

By mouth (*per os*) or under the tongue (sublingual).

By the rectum (*per rectum*).

By injection:

   (*a*)   hypodermic,   (*b*)   intramuscular,   (*c*)   intravenous, (*d*) intrathecal.

By inhalation and insufflation.

By the skin (*a*) application, (*b*) ionization.

Their comparative rapidity of action is, in most cases, in the following order: intravenous injection, inhalation, intramuscular and hypodermic injection, sublingual and by the mouth.

The use of drugs in pregnancy

It must be emphasized that many of the drugs in common use may have an adverse effect on the fetus whether taken in the early months or later. Basically, the pregnant woman should not take any drug unless it is absolutely necessary for her own condition, e.g. epilepsy, and that whatever dose is selected should be carefully controlled by a medical practitioner.

Drugs acting on the stomach

Antacids. These are used in the treatment of peptic ulcer and are also given in other types of dyspepsia when it is necessary to neutralize the hydrochloric acid in the stomach, e.g.

Aluminium hydroxide, 'Aludrox', 0·6 g (10 grains).

Magnesium trisilicate (0·5 to 2 g).

Magnesia (magnesium oxide).

The average dose of these substances is 2 to 4 g (30 to 60 grains). Mixtures containing them are made up to 10 ml.

Special antacid tablets which are allowed to dissolve slowly in the mouth are in common use, e.g. 'Nulacin', 'Gelusil'.

Drugs such as atropine, belladonna and propantheline ('Probanthine') also diminish gastric secretion and movement.

Drugs derived from liquorice have a healing effect on peptic ulcers. Examples are carbenoxolone ('Biogastrone' and, in a special capsule, 'Duogastrone') and 'Caved-(S)'.

Carminatives. These drugs aid the expulsion of gas from the stomach by increasing the tone of its muscle and by stimulating its movements. The bitters also have this action.

   e.g.   (i)   Oil of peppermint 0·2 ml ($\frac{1}{2}$ to 3 minims).

   (ii) Aromatic spirit of ammonia (spiritus ammoniae aromaticus or sal volatile, 4 ml, 15 to 60 minims).

Emetics. It has been seen (p. 210) that vomiting is a reflex mechanism controlled by the vomiting centre in the medulla. Drugs which produce vomiting may do so either as a result of their action on the stomach or by direct stimulation of the vomiting centre.

Emetics are used to remove the contents of the stomach and may be valuable when the organ is distended. They may be employed in cases of poisoning due to substances other than caustics. Their use is dangerous in the latter condition because the violent contractions of the organ may cause rupture of its walls if they have been severely damaged by a corrosive substance.

Emetic drugs are rarely used except in emergency and in most cases it is preferable to wash out the stomach with normal saline after passing a stomach tube.

The emetics acting directly on the stomach include: ipecacuanha, zinc sulphate (1 g, 15 grains in warm water), salt and water, mustard and water (8 g in 150 ml of warm water).

An emetic acting on the medulla and given by injection is apomorphine 6 mg ($\frac{1}{10}$-grain).

Anti-emetics. These are drugs which help to control nausea and vomiting and may also be used in Menière's disease. They include travel-sickness remedies, e.g.

(*a*) Drugs of the anti-histamine type, viz.:
    Promethazine ('Avomine')
    Cyclizine ('Marzine') } 25–50 mg.
    Dimenhydrinate ('Dramamine')

(*b*) Drugs of the phenothiazine type, viz.:
    Promazine ('Sparine') } 25–50 mg.
    Chlorpromazine ('Largactil')
    Perphenazine ('Fentazin'), 2–8 mg.

(*c*) Metoclopramide ('Maxolon'), 10 mg.

'Dramamine' and all the drugs listed under (*b*) and (*c*) may be given intramuscularly, which is advantageous in patients who cannot retain anything in their stomachs.

Cyclizine and similar drugs are reported to have caused fetal abnormalities in animals and, therefore, should be used with great caution if at all in early pregnancy.

Drugs acting on the intestine

(a) **Aperients.** These are drugs used to increase intestinal movement and promote evacuation of the bowels. Aperients may be divided into 3 classes according to the power of their action, but it must be remembered that any drug may pass into another class if given in unusually small or large doses.

1. Laxatives are substances which slightly increase the action of the bowels by increasing peristalsis, e.g. (i) Wholemeal bread, fruits, especially figs and prunes, which leave adequate roughage. (ii) Magnesia 8 g (30 to 120 grains). (iii) Liquid paraffin 30 ml ($\frac{1}{4}$ to 1 fl oz), which acts mainly as a lubricant. (iv) Syrup of figs, 8 ml (30 to 120 minims).

2. Simple purgatives. These cause mild irritation of the intestinal mucous membrane, with an increase in its secretion, and active peristalsis of the intestinal muscles, e.g., rhubarb, senna (e.g. 'Senokot'), cascara sagrada, phenol-phthalein, castor oil, saline aperients such as sodium sulphate (Glauber salts), magnesium sulphate (Epsom salts, 16 g, 30 to 240 grains), bisacodyl ('Dulcolax') tablets.

3. Drastic purgatives which cause greatly increased intestinal secretion and irritation of the mucous membrane followed by severe diarrhoea and colic, e.g. calomel, jalap, colocynth, are no longer used.

Pituitary extract and carbachol are drugs which given by hypodermic injection stimulate intestinal peristalsis and aid evacuation.

4. Suppositories. Glycerine or bisacodyl ('Dulcolax') suppositories are useful in many cases.

(b) Drugs used to decrease intestinal movement and spasm. A mixture containing kaolin and morphine or opium is often given to check diarrhoea (Mist. Kaolini et Morphiniae). Diphenoxylate ('Lomotil') is also useful.

Atropine, belladonna and propantheline are of value in reducing both gastric and intestinal spasm.

(c) Drugs used to destroy intestinal parasites. These have been mentioned in the treatment of intestinal worms (p. 245).

Thread-worms—Piperazine ('Antepar' and 'Pripsen'), viprynium ('Vanquin').

Round-worms—Piperazine, 4 grams; tetrachlorethylene (up to 3 ml).

Tape-worms—Niclosamide ('Yomesan'), dichlorophen ('Anthiphen'). Extract of male fern (extractum filicis, 6 ml, 45 to 90 minims); mepacrine (1 g).

Hook-worms—Bephenium ('Alcopar'), 5 g; tetrachlorethylene.

(d) Intestinal antiseptics. Attempts are sometimes made to check bacterial growth in the intestine. Sulphaguanidine, sulphasuxidine and other sulphonamides, tetracyclines, neomycin, 'Colomycin' and streptomycin all act as intestinal antiseptics when given by mouth. Chloramphenicol is used in typhoid fever. Substances such as charcoal and kaolin are used to absorb intestinal toxins and gases.

Drugs acting on the circulatory system

1. Digitalis. The following are the preparations of digitalis which are commonly employed, especially in the treatment of atrial fibrillation (pp. 104, 129).

Digitalis leaves (folia). Dose: 30 to 100 mg. ($\frac{1}{2}$ to $1\frac{1}{2}$ grains).
Digoxin ('Lanoxin'). Dose: 0·25 to 1 mg.
Digitoxin ('Nativelle's digitalin'). Dose: 0·1 to 1 mg.
Lanatoside C ('Cedilanid'). Dose: 0·25–1 mg.

2. Drugs which raise the blood pressure. These may act either by increasing the force of the cardiac contraction or by constricting the blood vessels and are circulatory stimulants, given by injection, e.g. adrenaline (1 in 1000, 0·5 ml, 2 to 8 minims), noradrenaline, pituitary extract (0·5 to 1 ml). Mephentermine ('Mephine') and metaraminol ('Aramine') are more commonly employed.

3. Drugs which lower the blood pressure. (Hypotensive drugs.) E.g. reserpine ('Serpasil'), pentolinium ('Ansolysen'), guanethidine ('Ismelin'), methyldopa ('Aldomet'), clonidine ('Catapres'), debrisoquine ('Declinax'), bethanidine ('Esbatal').

It is important to remember that diuretics such as chlorothiazide, increase considerably the effect of hypotensive drugs, the dose of which may have to be halved when they are given together.

4. Drugs which dilate the coronary arteries. These act by dilating the blood vessels and are used especially in angina pectoris, e.g. tablets of glyceryl trinitrate (trinitrin) 0·5 mg. They must be chewed slowly and allowed to dissolve in the mouth. Amyl nitrite 2 ml (2 to 5 minims) by inhalation.

'Mycardol' is a similar drug having a more prolonged action.

5. Drugs which dilate peripheral arteries. E.g. Tolazoline ('Priscol'), 'Ronicol', 'Hexopal'.

Drugs acting on the blood

Anti-anaemic Drugs (haematinics)

Iron deficiency anaemia:
    (*a*) By mouth.
        Ferrous sulphate: 200 mg, (3 grains), thrice daily.

Ferrous gluconate: 300 mg, (5 grains), thrice daily.

Iron and ammonium citrate: 2 g, (30 grains), three times daily.

(b) Intravenously.

The total dose infusion (TDI) of 'Imferon' provides all the required iron in one or two infusions. The drug is diluted with normal saline or 5% dextrose solution. A history of asthma contradicts 'Imferon TDI'.

(c) By intramuscular injection, e.g. 'Imferon', 'Jectofer'.

Pernicious anaemia:

Cyanocobalamin (Vitamin B_{12}). Average dose: 250 to 1000 micrograms. Usually given by intramuscular injection. Oral therapy is unreliable.

Preparations include 'Cytamen', 'Distivit'.

Megalocytic anaemia e.g. in sprue, coeliae disease and in pregnancy; folic acid 5–20 mg daily.

Drugs acting on the respiratory system

1. Those stimulating the respiratory centre. When the respiratory centre is stimulated the depth and frequency of the respirations are increased. This is often necessary in cases of poisoning, during anaesthesia and in cardiac failure. The following drugs have this effect: nikethamide, 'Vandid', amiphenazole ('Daptazole'), carbon dioxide gas. Nalorphine is used when the depression is due to morphine.

2. Those depressing the respiratory centre. These drugs diminish the depth and slow the rate of respiration. They also reduce the excitability of the centre and are therefore effective in diminishing cough. Opium, morphine and diamorphine (heroin), codeine may be used for this purpose. Anaesthetics (ether, chloroform, etc.) and alcohol in large doses have a similar effect.

3. Drugs which loosen bronchial secretion. These are known as **expectorants.** After absorption from the alimentary tract that are partially excreted by the respiratory mucous membrane and either loosen or increase the secretion of mucus from its surface. They are of value in bronchitis and aid expectoration, e.g. Ammonium salts, squills, ipecacuanha, potassium iodide.

'Bisolvon', 8 mg tds by mouth, reduces the viscidity and volume of mucus in chronic bronchitis.

4. Drugs which decrease bronchial secretion. These include belladonna, atropine and stramonium.

5. Drugs which relax spasm of the bronchial muscles (bronchodilators). These are used especially in asthma and bronchitis. They include adrenaline, isoprenaline, ephedrine, atropine, stramonium and lobelia.

Aminophylline and choline theophyllinate ('Choledyl') are also useful.

Adrenaline. Active principle of the medulla of suprarenal gland, also prepared synthetically (see p. 461).

ACTION AND USES.

1. Asthma: relaxes spasm of bronchial muscles.
2. Allergy: e.g. urticaria and anaphylactic shock.
3. Shock: raises blood pressure by constricting blood vessels.
4. Some cases of cardiac arrest.
5. Local haemorrhage: e.g. epistaxis, bleeding tooth-socket. Applied locally on a gauze plug it acts as a haemostatic by constricting blood vessels.

ADMINISTRATION

1. Subcutaneous injection: 0.13 to 0.5 ml (2 to 8 minims). Strength: 1 in 1,000 solution.
2. Inhalation or spray from an atomizer.
3. Special preparations with an adrenaline-like action can be given sub-lingually. They should be allowed to dissolve slowly under the tongue. Dose: 10 to 20 mg ($\frac{1}{6}$ to $\frac{1}{3}$ grain) or $\frac{1}{2}$ to 1 tablet of isoprenaline sulphate.

Drugs acting on the urinary system

1. Those rendering the urine alkaline, e.g. the alkaline carbonates and bicarbonates and potassium citrate.

2. Those rendering the urine acid, e.g. acid sodium phosphate, ammonium chloride.

3. Diuretics. These are drugs which increase the excretion of urine and their main use is in cases of generalized oedema, especially that due to chronic heart failure. The **mercurial** diuretics, e.g. Neptal, are now obsolete.

Non-mercurial diuretics which can be given orally include chlorothiazide ('Saluric'), 0.5 to 2 g daily and chlorthalidone ('Hygroton') 100–200 mg on alternate days. Also frusemide ('Lasix'), triamterine ('Dytac') and ethacrynic acid ('Edecrin'). Some of these drugs also tend to lower blood pressure.

In view of the possibility of potassium depletion it is advisable to give potassium chloride at the same time.

Spironolactone ('Aldactone A'), 25 mg, is a synthetic steroid which has a diuretic action and which may be given at the same time as chlorothiazide or frusemide to enhance their action.

4. Urinary antiseptics. Certain drugs are excreted in the urine and exert an antiseptic action on the renal tract, e.g. sulphonamides, 'Furadantin' and various antibiotics, also occasionally sodium mandelate (p. 344). Trimethoprim is complementary to sulphonamides in its action, attacking bacterial metabolism at a different stage. Co-trimoxazole ('Septrin', 'Bactrim') is a sulphonamide-trimethoprim combination.

Drugs acting on the central nervous system

1. Those which stimulate the nervous system. These are drugs which stimulate the higher nervous centres and tend to keep the patient awake. They are used sometimes to counteract the side-effect of other drugs which tend to make the patient drowsy, e.g. phenobarbitone. They also help to reduce the appetite and may be given in the treatment of obesity. However, they tend to be habit-forming and their use should generally be avoided.

When inhaled they reduce nasal congestion and have been used in the treatment of nasal catarrh.

Amphetamine sulphate ('Benzedrine'), 2·5 to 10 mg.

Dexamphetamine sulphate ('Dexedrine'), 2·5 to 10 mg.

Methyl amphetamine ('Methedrine'), 2·5 to 10 mg.

2. Drugs which depress the nervous system. (a) ANTI-CONVULSANT DRUGS. These are used in the treatment of epilepsy and fits (p. 363).

(b) ANALGESIC DRUGS. These are drugs which are given to relieve pain. The drug selected usually depends on the severity of the pain and whether or not a hypnotic action is also desired. The milder analgesics may be combined with hypnotic drugs, e.g. one of the barbiturates, if necessary. For very severe pain, morphine or one of the allied drugs is used.

Acetyl-salicylic acid, Aspirin; Calcium acetylsalicylate, 'Disprin': 1 g, (5 to 15 grains), 'Paynocil'.

Codeine, codeine phosphate: 60 mg ($\frac{1}{6}$ to 1 grain).

This may be used alone, but is often combined in a table with aspirin and paracetamol (Tab. Codeinae Composita, 'Veganin'). Dose: 1 to 2 tablets.

Dihydrocodeine ('DF 118'), 10–60 mg.

Paracetamol ('Panadol').

Dextropropoxyphene ('Doloxene'): 65 mg.

Dextromoramide ('Palfium'): 5 mg.

Pentazocine ('Fortral'): 30 mg IM.

Methadone ('Physeptone', etc., CD). Dose: 5 to 10 mg ($\frac{1}{12}$ to $\frac{1}{6}$ grain). By mouth or intramuscular injection. This is a powerful analgesic, which is likely to produce nausea, vomiting and faintness if given to ambulant patients. It should, therefore, only be used on patients who are confined to bed or at night. It has little hypnotic effect.

Pethidine (CD). Dose: 25 to 100 mg. It may be given by mouth or hypodermic injection and is a powerful analgesic with little hypnotic effect.

Morphine (CD). Dose: 8 to 20 mg ($\frac{1}{8}$ to $\frac{1}{3}$ grain). This is a well-known derivative of opium which is a drug of addiction. It is usually given by hypodermic injection but may also be injected intravenously or a tablet may be allowed to dissolve under the tongue. Small doses are also contained in some mixtures, e.g. Mist. Kaolini et Morphinae used in the treatment of diarrhoea and in Linctus Scillae Opiatus (Gee's linctus).

The main action is to depress the central nervous system whereby pain is abolished and sleep induced. In addition, secretions from glands, intestinal movements, and the respiratory centre are also depressed so that the mouth becomes dry, constipation may follow its administration, and breathing becomes slow and shallow.

N.B.—Nalorphine ('Lethidrone'), 10 mg, by intravenous injection is given in morphine poisoning.

Preparations containing opium

Tincture of opium. Dose: 2 ml (5 to 30 minims).

Ipecacuanha and opium powder (Pulv. Ipecac. et Opii—Dover's Powder). Dose: 0·6 g (5 to 10 grains).

Nepenthe. Dose: 2·5 ml (20 to 40 minims). This is usually given by mouth, but sterile solutions are available for injection.

Preparations of morphine

Morphine sulphate: 8 to 20 mg ($\frac{1}{8}$ to $\frac{1}{3}$ grain).

Solution of morphine hydrochloride (Liq. Morph. Hydrochlor.). Dose: 2 ml (5 to 30 minims).

Morphine suppository contains 15 mg ($\frac{1}{4}$ grain).

Papaveretum. This contains some of the alkaloids of opium including 50% morphine. It is the basis of various proprietary preparations such as 'Omnopon'.

'Omnopon' 20 mg ($\frac{1}{3}$ grain) is equivalent to morphine 10 mg ($\frac{1}{6}$ grain).

Either morphine or 'Omnopon' may be combined with scopolomine (hyoscine). 0·6 mg, $\frac{1}{100}$ grain, as a pre-operation sedative.

Diamorphine (Heroin). Dose 10 mg ($\frac{1}{12}$ to $\frac{1}{6}$ grain). This drug has an addiction similar to morphine but is even more likely to produce addiction. It is usually given by injection.

Linctus diamorphinae: 8 ml (30 to 120 minims), is sometimes used for a troublesome cough. 5 ml contain 3 mg ($\frac{1}{20}$ grain of diamorphine.

(*c*) HYPNOTICS AND TRANQUILLIZERS. Hypnotics are given with a view to producing sleep. Some hypnotic drugs also have analgesic properties.

(*a*) Potassium bromide is now obsolete.

(*b*) Chloral hydrate 2 grams (5 to 30 grains). Dichloralphenazone, ('Welldorm').

(*c*) Paraldehyde. Dose: by mouth—8 ml (30 to 120 minims).
per rectum—30 ml ($\frac{1}{2}$ to 1 fl oz).
intramuscularly—5 to 10 ml.

(*d*) The barbiturates. This is a very large group of drugs which have a powerful action in producing sleep by depressing the nervous system. Many preparations have been made which differ somewhat in their chemical composition. These include phenobarbitone (Luminal), Nembutal (pentobarbitone), Soneryl (butobarbitone) and Amytal (amylobarbitone).

(*e*) Tranquillizers are intended to relax a person without making him drowsy, e.g. chlordiazepoxide ('Librium') and diazepam ('Valium').

Chlorpromazine ('Largactil') and promazine ('Sparine') act as tranquillizers and anti-emetic drugs. They may be given either by mouth or injection.

Drugs acting on the eye

1. Drugs contracting the pupil (myotics), e.g. eserine (physostigmine).

2. Drugs dilating the pupil (mydriatics), e.g. atropine, homatropine, cocaine. The latter also acts as a local anaesthetic.

3. Antiseptic and antibiotic eye drops.

4. Steroid drops, e.g. hydrocortisone.

N.B.—It is important to remember that some drugs given for other conditions may adversely affect vision or even cause serious damage to the retina or optic nerve.

Anti-histamine drugs

These are mainly used for the relief of allergic symptoms such as hay fever, urticaria and other skin conditions. Their action in asthma is unreliable.

Phenindamine ('Thephorin') (25 to 50 mg).
Promethazine ('Phenergan') (25 to 75 mg).
Diphenhydramine ('Benadryl') (50 mg).
Chlorcyclizine ('Histantin') (50 to 100 mg).
Antazoline ('Antistin') (100 mg).
Mepyramine ('Anthisan') (100 mg).
Chlorpheniramine ('Piriton') (4 mg).

Some of them have a slightly depressing action and tend to make the patient drowsy especially if taken with alcohol.

They may also be applied locally as creams or ointments but may cause dermatitis in sensitive persons.

Anti-coagulants (see p. 159).

Heparin: 10,000 units intravenously every 4 to 6 hours. Phenindione ('Dindevan'). Dose: 25 to 100 mg twice daily. Nicoumalone ('Sinthrome') is also used: initial dose 8–16 mg. Warfarin ('Marevan'): initial dose 30 to 40 mg.

Heparin dosage is controlled by estimations of the clotting time. The dosage of the other drugs, which are all given orally, is controlled by prothrombin estimations.

Over-dosage with heparin is treated by injecting protamine sulphate 50 to 100 mg intravenously. For over-dosage of the other anticoagulants, blood transfusion and injections of vitamin K_1 are given.

Anti-malarial drugs. These include:

Proguanil ('Paludrine'): 100 to 200 mg ($1\frac{1}{2}$ to 13 grains) daily.
Pyrimethamine ('Daraprim'): 25 mg once weekly for prophylaxis.
Chloroquine ('Nivaquine'): 300 mg of base once weekly for prophylaxis. For treatment: 600 mg stat, 300 mg 6 hours later and then 300 mg daily for 2 days.
Quinine sulphate: 600 mg (1 to 10 grains).
Primaquine: 15 mg of base daily for 14 days.

Atropine. Dose: 0·25–1 mg ($\frac{1}{240}$ to $\frac{1}{60}$ grain) by hypodermic injection. Atropine is the alkaloid derived from the plant **Belladonna** or Deadly Nightshade. Their main actions are:

1. To diminish the secretions of the sweat glands, salivary glands and those of the bronchial mucous membrane.
2. To diminish spasm of the muscles of the stomach, intestines and bladder.
3. To dilate the pupil of the eye.
4. To paralyse the vagus nerve so that the rate of the heart is increased.

USES. *External.* Glycerine of belladonna and belladonna plaster may be applied for the relief of pain of all sorts, including pleurisy, neuralgia, phlebitis and arthritis.

Internal. Atropine or belladonna may be given to lessen abdominal pain due to spasm of the stomach or intestinal muscles and to check peristalsis. It may be used during the treatment of peptic ulcer. It is given intravenously in the treatment of bradycardia following a myocardial infarction.

Atropine is also given before general anaesthesia to check the excessive secretion of mucus which is especially liable to follow the inhalation of ether.

PREPARATIONS

Guttae Atropinae (eye drops), 1%.

Oculentum Atropinae (eye ointment), 1%.

Hyaluronidase ('Hyalase'). This is an enzyme which can be prepared from various animal tissues. Its main action is to alter the permeability of connective tissues such as are found in the subcutaneous areas. This increases the spread and absorption of substances given by subcutaneous injection.

It is, therefore, used particularly to enable infusions of saline and other substances to be given subcutaneously, especially when the intravenous route is difficult or impossible.

The sulphonamides

The sulphonamides were discovered several years before the antibiotics and in some cases (e.g. infections of the renal tract) they are still useful. Their main action is bacteriostatic, that is they prevent the multiplication of bacteria so that the natural defences of the body can overcome the infection. Many different types have been developed so that they may be classified according to their main uses.

Those used for general infections may also be employed for the other purposes mentioned.

(a) Sulphonamides used for general infections. The most important are: sulphadimidine ('Sulphamezathine') and sulphadiazine.

Others include: Sulphathiazole and sulphafurazole ('Gantrisin'). Trisulphonamide ('Sulphatriad') is a mixture of sulphadiazine, sulphathiazole and sulphamerazine.

'Midicel', 'Lederkyn' (sulphamethoxypridazine) and sulphaphenazole ('Orisulf') are long-acting proprietary preparations, a single dose of which is sufficient to cover 24 hours.

Among the general infections which may be sensitive to the sulphonamides are those caused by streptococci, pneumococci, meningococci and gonococci. Sulphadiazine is particularly valuable in meningococcal meningitis.

(b) Sulphonamides used for urinary infections. In addition to the sulphonamides mentioned above, the following are particularly active against the *Escherichia coli*, the commonest organism infecting the urinary tract:

Sulphamethizole ('Urolucosil'), (100–200 mg), sulphacetamide ('Albucid') and sulphafurazole ('Gantrisin').

A combination of a sulphonamide with trimethoprim as in cotrimoxazole ('Septrin', 'Bactrim') is very effective in urinary tract infections. It is also useful in bronchitis and in septicaemias.

(c) Sulphonamides used for intestinal infections. The sulphonamides previously mentioned are soluble and, therefore, absorbed into the bloodstream from the alimentary canal. There are a number of insoluble sulphonamides which are not absorbed in any quantity and continue to act on sensitive bacteria throughout the whole length of the bowel. This is of advantage in the treatment of bacillary dysentery and other intestinal infections in which a general effect is not required. There is less risk of urinary crystallization with these sulphonamides in these conditions in which much fluid may be lost by diarrhoea. They include: sulphaguanidine, phthalylsulphathiazole ('Sulfathalidine'), succinylsulphathiazole ('Sulfasuxidine'), and phthalylsulphacetamide ('Enterocid').

Salicylazosulphapyridine ('Salazopyrin') is a special sulphonamide used in the treatment of ulcerative colitis.

(d) Sulphonamides for local use. Sulphonamides are sometimes applied to the skin in the form of ointments but they may cause sensitization and dermatitis. Eye drops and eye ointments are used in conjunctivitis.

Toxic effects. These include headache, nausea and vomiting.

Occasionally skin rashes and agranulocytosis occur. Unless sufficient fluid is given at the same time some sulphonamides tend to crystallize in the urine causing haematuria and even suppression of urine. This is particularly likely to occur if dehydration is present as a result of diarrhoea or excessive sweating.

Antibiotics

Each of the many available antibiotics has its own sphere of activity against the common bacteria. Unfortunately they all have certain disadvantages.

1. Bacterial resistance. Many bacteria soon develop resistance to one particular antibiotic. This is particularly true of staphylococci.

2. Toxic effects. Gastro-intestinal disturbances and skin rashes are not uncommon.

3. Super-infection. This applies specially to broad-spectrum antibiotics given by mouth which by killing off the normal bacteria of the alimentary canal permit the growth of other insensitive organisms, e.g. staphylococci and candida (monilia).

4. Skin sensitivity may develop in nurses and doctors handling these drugs, especially penicillin and streptomycin and also if they are applied in ointments.

Penicillin

This substance, which was the first of the antibiotics to be employed, is the active principle of a mould (*Penicillinum notatum*). Although it has a wide range of action not all bacteria are affected by it and even some of those which are can eventually develop some degree of resistance to it, e.g. staphylococci.

The organisms most sensitive to pencillin are:

staphylococcus	gonococcus
streptococcus	treponeme of syphilis
pneumococcus	anthrax bacillus
meningococcus	gas gangrene organisms

Among those which are unaffected are:

colon bacillus	tubercle bacillus
whooping-cough bacillus	viruses

Penicillin acts partly by preventing the growth of bacteria in the body and thereby permitting the natural defences of the individual to overcome the infection (bacteriostatic action), and partly by actually killing the organisms (bactericidal action).

Many types of penicillin are available:

A. Natural penicillins

1. Benzyl penicillin (soluble or crystalline penicillin G.) which is used for all types of injection and local application.

2. Procaine penicillin which is more slowly absorbed and is given in doses of 300,000 units daily by intramuscular injection. In order to get a more rapid effect this may be combined with a similar dose of soluble penicillin.

3. Benzathine penicillin ('Penidural') and benethamine penicillin which are only slowly absorbed, so that a single intramuscular injection may give an effective blood level lasting several days.

4. Phenoxymethyl penicillin (penicillin V), which is suitable for oral administration.

B. Synthetic penicillins

These include phenethicillin ('Broxil'), methicillin ('Celbenin'), cloxacillin ('Orbenin'), ampicillin ('Penbritin'), amoxycillin ('Amoxil') and carbenicillin ('Pyopen'). These may be used when the organism is found to be insensitive to other forms of penicillin and other antibiotics.

Penicillin may be administered in the following ways:

1. Intramuscular injection of 250,000 to 1 million units of soluble penicillin may be given 6 to 8 hourly.

Procaine penicillin, 300,000 units in 1 ml once or twice daily.

2. Intravenous injection. Soluble penicillin may be injected intravenously in doses similar to or greater than those given by intramuscular injection. (1,000,000 units is called one Mega unit.)

3. Intrathecal injection may be used in certain cases of meningitis (p. 386).

4. Intrapleural injection may be used in the treatment of empyema (p. 294).

5. Local application. Penicillin may be used either in the form of a solution, a cream or a powder. In the latter instance it is often mixed with a sulphonamide and may be blown with an insufflator on to raw surfaces or into wounds twice daily. Solutions may be used for the irrigation of wounds or sinuses and as eye drops. The use of local applications is, however, discouraged because of the risk of sensitivity reactions.

Examples of diseases in which penicillin may be used are:

pneumonia	actinomycosis	anthrax
gonorrhoea	gas gangrene	meningitis
carbuncles	bacterial endocarditis	syphilis

Toxic effects. Penicillin is usually non-toxic even in high dosage. Some patients, however, develop hypersensitivity (allergic) reactions including fever and skin rashes, which may be treated with antihistamine drugs and the application of calamine lotion. Very rarely, severe or even fatal anaphylactic shock may occur. This is treated by the immediate intravenous injection of hydrocortisone hemisuccinate 100 mg, and antihistamine e.g. chlorpheniramine ('Piriton') 10 mg i.v. and subcutaneous injection of adrenaline (1 : 1000, 0·5 ml).

Before giving penicillin by any route it is, therefore, essential to enquire about previous sensitivity and also if the patient is subject to asthma or other allergic conditions. Desensitization may be difficult and is only indicated in exceptional circumstances.

The tetracycline group of antibiotics

These include: (*a*) tetracycline ('Achromycin').

                (*b*) chlortetracycline ('Aureomycin').

                (*c*) oxytetracycline ('Terramycin').

These are very valuable antibiotics which can be given by mouth and by intravenous injection. Tetracycline may also be given intramuscularly. They are effective in most of the conditions which can be treated by penicillin and, in addition, may be used for bronchitis, mycoplasma pneumonia, *Escherichia coli* infections, influenza, whooping-cough and amoebic dysentery. They are sometimes called broad-spectrum antibiotics. These antibiotics, however, can cause staining of milk teeth if given during infancy, or administered to the mother during pregnancy. Some patients develop diarrhoea.

Erythromycin

Erythromycin has a similar action but bacterial resistance develops rapidly to this drug. Its main uses are in staphylococcal infections which are resistant to other antibiotics and in patients allergic to penicillin.

Oleandomycin ('Romicil') and *Spiramycin* ('Rovamycin') are in the same group and have similar antibacterial activity.

Novobiocin ('Albamycin') is also active against staphylococci and is sometimes used in combination with erythromycin.

'Fucidin' is used almost exclusively to treat staphylococcal infections. It is rapidly absorbed from the gastro-intestinal tract. Injections are available.

Colomycin is an antibiotic active against *Esch. coli*, Salmonella, *Haemophilus* and other organisms and is used particularly in gastro-intestinal and urinary infections.

Nystatin has no action on ordinary bacteria but is effective against candida (monilia) and similar yeast infections.

Griseofulvin is used in the treatment of fungus infections of the skin (ringworm).

Chloramphenicol ('Chloromycetin')

This has a special value in the treatment of typhoid fever and influenzal meningitis. It has a bitter taste and is supplied in the form of capsules containing 250 mg and rectal suppositories. Cases of aplastic anaemia have followed its use and the total adult dose should not exceed 25 g over a period of 10 days. Although chloramphenicol is effective in whooping-cough, gonorrhoea, some cases of pneumonia and urinary infection, its use in these conditions is rarely justified in view of the risk of producing aplastic anaemia.

The average dose of chloramphenicol and the tetracyclines is 500 mg followed by 250 mg every 6 hours, but this may be increased in severe infections. Minor toxic effects such as nausea or vomiting are sometimes observed. The usual course of treatment lasts for 4 or 5 days. If prolonged beyond this, vitamin B should be given as these drugs may interfere with its formation in the intestines.

Streptomycin

Streptomycin is an antibiotic administered in a similar manner to penicillin, namely, by intramuscular or intrathecal injection. Its main use is in pulmonary tuberculosis and other forms of tuberculous infection such as tuberculous meningitis, miliary tuberculosis and tuberculous laryngitis. The average dose for an adult by intramuscular injection is 1·0 g daily in a single dose and treatment may be continued for many weeks. Tubercle bacilli develop resistance to streptomycin but this is delayed or prevented if para-aminosalicylic acid (PAS) or isoniazid (INH) are given at the same time. Toxic symptoms such as vertigo which may be permanent, are not infrequently observed about the third week of treatment and are more common in elderly patients. In handling the drug care should be taken to avoid it coming in contact with the skin as dermatitis may be produced in some cases. It is of value in the rare influenzal meningitis and is of use in some cases of gonorrhoea, urinary infection and gastro-enteritis for which short courses are given.

Viomycin, cycloserine, ethionamide and *thiacetazone* are drugs which may be used in tuberculosis when the organism has become resistant to streptomycin. They are, however, more toxic. Other drugs include ethambutol and capreomycin.

Bacitracin is an antibiotic derived from *bacillus subtilis*, which has a limited use against streptococci, staphylococci and some other organisms. It has a toxic effect on the kidneys and is only given by injection in selected cases when other antibiotics have failed. (Dose: 100,000 units daily.) It may be applied locally to infected wounds with safety.

The following table indicates the effectiveness of sulphonamides and antibiotics against the common organisms.

Organism	Penicillin	The Tetra-cyclines	Chlor-amphenicol	Strepto-mycin	Sulph-onamides
Streptococcus	+ + +	+ + +	—	—	+ +
Staphylococcus	+ +	+ +	—	—	+
Pneumococcus	+ + +	+ + +	—	+	+ +
Meningococcus	+ + +	+ +	—	—	+ + +
Gonococcus	+ + +	+ +	+	+	+ +
S. typhi	—	—	+ +	—	—
B. anthracis	+ + +	+ + +	—	—	+
E. coli	—	+ +	+ +	+	+
H. influenzae	—	+ +	+	—	—
H. pertussis	—	+	+ +	—	—

Cortisone and allied steroids

Cortisone and hydrocortisone are among the hormones produced by the adrenal glands. Since their discovery a number of synthetic compounds of similar chemical composition having similar physiological and therapeutic effects have been manufactured. The synthetic steroids are more potent than the naturally occurring hormones and consequently are given in smaller dosage. In addition, by slight variations in the chemical structure certain undesirable side effects have been reduced. Among the most important are:

Natural hormones: Cortisone (50–200 mg)
Hydrocortisone.

Synthetic steroids: Prednisone and prednisolone (5–20 mg daily)
Triamcinolone (2–16 mg daily)
Betamethasone (0·5 to 5 mg daily)
Fludrocortisone (0·1 to 0·3 mg daily)

Many proprietary preparations are available.

(*a*) Cortisone, prednisone and prednisolone are used mainly for internal administration.

Among the conditions in which they may be used, especially if other forms of therapy have not been effective are:

1. *Rheumatic and connective tissue (collagen) diseases:*
   rheumatoid arthritis   polyarteritis nodosa
   rheumatic fever   lupus erythematosus

2. *Allergic disorders:*
   severe asthma   drug sensitivity
   status asthmaticus   serum sickness

3. *Skin diseases:*
   pemphigus vulgaris   dermatitis
   erythema multiforme

4. *Endocrine disorders:*
   Addison's disease   pituitary disorders
   post-adrenalectomy

5. *Blood diseases:*
   haemolytic anaemia   purpura

6. *Other disorders:*
   ulcerative colitis   temporal arteritis
   shock   sarcoidosis
   nephrotic syndrome   delirium tremens

(*b*) Hydrocortisone, although it can be given internally and, in grave emergency such as anaphylactic shock, by intravenous injection, is used mainly for local application and local injection into and around joints. For this purpose doses of 0·25–1 ml (25 mg per ml) may be used. The acetate is used for local injections and is not suitable for intravenous use. Hydrocortisone sodium succinate (hemisuccinate) and hydrocortisone sodium phosphate are the preparations for intravenous injection.

Among the conditions in which local injection is used are:

rheumatoid arthritis	bursitis
osteo-arthritis	'tennis elbow'
traumatic arthritis	keloid scars

Retention enemas may be used in ulcerative colitis (50–100 mg in 5 oz of 1% methyl cellulose or normal saline).

Hydrocortisone lotion and skin ointments may be used for such conditions as:

allergic skin disorders	pruritus
eczema of various types	contact dermatitis

Hydrocortisone eye drops (1%) and eye ointment (2·5%) (to both of which an antibiotic may be added) for

blepharitis	interstitial keratitis
conjunctivitis	iritis

Their use is contra-indicated in acute corneal ulcer.

Contra-indications and toxic effects

Among the effects of these hormones and steroids are:

1. An alteration in carbohydrate metabolism leading to an increase in the blood sugar, so that they must be used with caution in diabetics who will probably require an increased dose of insulin during their administration.

2. They reduce the ability of connective tissue cells to multiply and so tend to suppress the natural reaction to inflammation and to delay healing. Their use may therefore be particularly dangerous in tuberculosis unless covered by antituberculous drugs.

3. They increase the secretion of hydrochloric acid in the stomach thus, together with the previous effect, tend to cause peptic ulcers or to delay their healing.

4. In large doses they produce iatrogenic Cushing's syndrome, viz. a swollen round 'moon face', excess of hair and a tendency to acne.

5. They cause disturbances of electrolyte and water metabolism. In particular, there may be water and sodium retention leading to oedema and excessive potassium excretion. These effects are less marked with the synthetic steroids than with cortisone.

6. In some cases the blood pressure is raised, and sometimes mental disturbances are caused.

7. Their administration tends to suppress the natural secretion of the adrenals while they are being given, so that the drugs should be withdrawn gradually over a period of several weeks or months in order that the glands may recover their natural functions.

When prolonged courses or large doses are given the following precautions may be desirable:

1. Daily weight, urinary output and blood pressure records.
2. Observation for oedema, 'moon face' and thrombosis of leg veins.
3. Diet: high protein, restricted fat and carbohydrate.
4. Drugs: potassium chloride to prevent potassium depletion,
   aluminium hydroxide to prevent peptic ulcer,
   antibiotics in the presence of infection,
   sedatives to minimize mental disturbances,
   anabolic steroids to counteract the catabolic (breaking-down) effect of cortisone and its analogues,
   calcium tablets to replace the calcium lost from bone made osteoporotic by steroids.

Corticotrophin (ACTH) is a hormone obtained from the anterior lobe of the pituitary gland which stimulates the cortex of the suprarenal to secrete cortisone. It may be given by intramuscular injection:

(*a*) Water-soluble form, 25 to 50 mg every 4 hours.

(*b*) Gel-compound form, 25 to 50 mg every 12 to 24 hours.

Tetracosactrin ('Synacthen') is a synthetic agent which has the same action as corticotrophin; it is used particularly in the investigation of suspected Addison's disease.

Alcohol

Alcohol is a substance of wide social usage but it must also be regarded as a potential poison and a drug of addiction. Its use as a therapeutic measure has been steadily decreasing in medical practice although it probably has a limited sphere of usefulness.

Its main pharmacological actions may be summarized thus:

1. It is a central nervous system depressant. The apparent stimulating effect in the first instance is due to abolition of the normal mental control of the higher centres of the brain thereby removing inhibitions and anxiety. Progressively its toxic effects precipitate disturbance of behaviour, inco-ordination of muscular movements and speech and, finally, coma which may prove fatal.

2. It acts as a peripheral vaso-dilator which gives rise to a general feeling of warmth. In the stomach this may temporarily improve the appetite.

3. It is readily metabolized into carbon dioxide and water, providing a number of Calories. It is, therefore, to some extent of food value especially as it is quickly absorbed from the stomach.

4. Excessive intake has a diuretic action, hence the headache and dry mouth due to dehydration in a 'hang-over'.

5. Continued intake is liable to cause defective absorption of vitamins, in particular those of the B complex.

The clinical effects of alcohol

Although many people consume moderate quantities of alcoholic liquor without any obvious harmful effect the clinical manifestations of excess may be considered as:

(*a*) acute and (*b*) chronic alcoholism.

Acute alcoholism. The symptoms of progressive drunkenness are too obvious and well known to require further description. Several special points should, however, be remembered.

(*a*) It may precipitate an epileptic fit or migraine in persons subject to these conditions.

(*b*) Alcohol greatly increases the effect of barbiturates, narcotics and some other drugs.

(*c*) It may obscure cerebral or other injury sustained in the inebriated state, sometimes with fatal results.

(*d*) In any case it is unwise to administer it as 'first aid' treatment as the odour of the breath may cause the false impression that the individual is drunk rather than suffering from some organic lesion.

Treatment. In the early stages, before unconsciousness, the simplest measure is to induce vomiting by tickling the back of the throat followed by drinking at least a pint of water which may be repeated at intervals. In comatose patients gastric lavage after ensuring that there is no respiratory obstruction and using an endotracheal tube to avoid the inhalation of vomitus. Intravenous glucose, injections of nikethamide and vitamin B may be helpful.

The post-alcoholic syndrome ('hang-over') may be helped by further intake of water or fruit juice sweetened with sugar or glucose and moderate doses of paracetamol or aspirin. The associated anorexia is usually self-limiting. Whether further small doses of alcohol ('the hair of the dog') are helpful is a matter of individual experience.

Chronic alcoholism. While it must be admitted that some individuals consume considerable quantities of alcohol over many years without ever being obviously intoxicated and without it having any obvious adverse effects, in others many serious conditions may develop. These include:

(*a*) Effects on the nervous system, e.g. neuritis, muscular incoordination ('the shakes'), progressive mental deterioration (alcoholic dementia), insomnia, hallucinations and delirium tremens.

(b) Cirrhosis of the liver and its associated symptoms.

(c) Chronic gastritis associated with dyspeptic symptoms, vomiting, anorexia and malnutrition.

(d) Vitamin deficiency, particularly B_{12}, which may be associated with optic neuritis and visual defects.

(e) Degeneration of the heart (alcoholic cardiomyopathy).

Treatment. The management of alcohol dependence is essentially a matter for experts and often requires institutional treatment. Gradual reduction of intake covered by sedative drugs help to minimize withdrawal symptoms. Special drugs such as 'Antabuse' or aversion therapy with apomorphine, given to produce vomiting every time an alcoholic drink is taken, are sometimes employed.

'Alcoholics Anonymous' is a worldwide organization which is of value to the reformed, but once an individual has been weaned from the habit a single drink may restart the addiction.

Medical uses and abuses. It is not always wise to cut off the supply of alcohol from a patient suffering from an acute disease who is accustomed to its use. In some cases of bronchopneumonia and gastro-enteritis in young babies small doses of brandy often induce sleep and act as an easily absorbed foodstuff. A small drink at night sometimes helps the insomnia of the elderly but appropriate sedatives, if necessary, are less expensive!

Its use should be forbidden in cases of infective hepatitis, jaundice and peptic ulcer and when it might potentiate the action of any other drugs which are being taken. On the other hand if it produces a feeling of well-being in the terminal stages of cancer or similar fatal conditions its use is certainly justified.

DRUG ADDICTION

Drug addiction in some form has been widespread throughout the world for centuries. This is exemplified by the universal use of alcohol in some form, opium smoking and the chewing of coca leaves (cocaine) in some native areas.

In the Western World, apart from alcohol, the addictive use of other drugs has, until recently, been relatively restricted but the possibilities were foreseen some years ago when the Dangerous Drugs Act and various Poisons Acts were introduced whereby certain drugs could only be legally obtained on medical prescription.

In some instances addiction has had an 'iatrogenic' cause. That is that for perfectly legitimate reasons a patient has been put on a drug, e.g. morphine, for the relief of symptoms by a doctor but after a time has been unable to give it up, even though the original reason for its use has ceased.

However, in recent years the problem has magnified very seriously, especially as there are now so many new drugs available which produce addiction.

Addiction or drug dependence may be defined as the compulsive need to continue taking a drug in order to maintain a physical or psychological feeling of well-being and outlook to which the victim has been accustomed by its use. Sudden withdrawal leads to intolerable symptoms, while prolonged use may cause permanent serious mental and physical deterioration.

The general implications of illicit drug taking and methods of distribution are well known and need no further reference.

The substances most commonly involved are:

1. Cannabis (marijuana or hashish).
2. Amphetamines (dexedrine, drinamyl, methedrine).
3. Barbiturates.
4. Hypnotics and opiates (morphine, heroin, pethidine and cocaine).
5. Hallucinogens (LSD, mescaline, some synthetic glues etc.).

Some of these drugs may be taken by mouth, others are given by self-injection, either subcutaneously or intravenously, or may be inhaled.

Cannabis. This is obtained from a plant which is easily grown. The strength of the product can, however, vary considerably in its potency and even if its use is started on the milder forms it so often leads to the use of other even more dangerous drugs such as heroin. It is usually smoked in the form of 'reefer' cigarettes. In itself, in strict moderation, it probably produces no serious physical effects similar to chronic bronchitis and lung cancer caused by tobacco. Nevertheless, the feeling of well-being and excitement resembling drunkenness are in themselves undesirable and excessive and long-term use leads to brain damage and psychological changes.

Amphetamines. These cause wakefulness, loss of appetite and alternating periods of elation and depression leading to dependence on increasing doses.

Barbiturates. These do have a temporary calming effect but also give rise to an unpleasant 'hang-over' which prompts the taking of further doses of these and other drugs to avoid lassitude and depression.

Hypnotics and opiates. Morphine and heroin, which is prepared from it, are highly addictive and are sometimes described as 'hard drugs'. Both have very valuable temporary medical uses but soon produce dependence requiring ever increasing doses. Their illicit use leads to self-neglect in all forms, physical and mental deterioration and often early death. Pethedine is similar in action. Cocaine being expensive and difficult to obtain does not now appear to be a major problem.

Hallucinogens. They produce the most dangerous 'trips'. Although not strictly addictive and do not produce dependence, their effect is to produce nightmare-like states during which the victim may perform acts not only dangerous to himself, e.g. jump off high buildings believing that he can fly, but could involve murder. The habitual user will suffer personality changes and general deterioration in work and character.

Treatment. This is always difficult especially as addicts tend to be of unstable personality. Assuming an addict appreciates the position and is seriously willing to undertake a cure, special centres for treatment are available.

In most instances abrupt withdrawal of the drug is not possible. Therefore, it must be legitimately supplied in reducing doses and, where necessary an alternative drug given such as methadone which is less addictive and can itself be reduced in dose until both can be eliminated. There is always a danger that an addict may obtain supplies from more than one doctor outside special centres and 'trade-in' any excess for profit.

Psychotherapy and rehabilitation are of great importance. At the present time the problem of this social evil is great and the results of treatment limited in success in spite of legal and medical efforts.

Symptoms produced by over-dosage of certain drugs

Arsenic. Faintness, nausea, incessant vomiting which may be bloodstained, epigastric pain, diarrhoea and tenesmus. Thirst and burning in the throat, restlessness, cramps in the legs followed by severe collapse with cold, clammy skin and weak pulse.

Atropine and belladonna. Dryness of the mouth and throat with dysphagia because food is not properly lubricated. Dryness of the skin, followed sometimes by an erythematous rash. Rapid pulse. Dilatation of the pupils with some defect in vision because of paralysis of accommodation. Delirium and, later, coma. Occasionally, purging and frequency of micturition.

Cocaine. Pallor, faintness, giddiness. Dilatation of the pupils, weak pulse, nausea and vomiting, collapse and, sometimes, convulsions.

Digitalis. See p. 129.

Morphine and Opium. Giddiness, drowsiness increasing to coma. Slow breathing due to depression of the respiratory centre in the medulla, slow pulse. Pupils contracted to pin-point size. Absent tendon and other reflexes. Skin cold, countenance livid, temperature subnormal.

Quinine. (Generally due to idiosyncrasy.) Ringing in the ears, slight to severe deafness, headache, giddiness, disturbances of vision. In very severe cases, collapse and death from cardiac and respiratory failure.

Salicylates. (Aspirin, etc.) Symptoms are similar to those produced by quinine. In addition, nausea, vomiting, delirium, flushed face, weak and irregular pulse, rapid, sighing respiration and, occasionally, erythematous rash.

Strychnine and Nux Vomica. Sense of suffocation, twitching of muscles followed by tetanic convulsions and opisthotonos which may last a minute or two. Pulse rapid, temperature may rise. Muscles of face contracted to resemble a grin (risus sardonicus), eyes staring. Increasing exhaustion between convulsions. Consciousness and mental faculties unaffected. Death from asphyxia or exhaustion.

Anticoagulants. Haemorrhage: haematuria, haematemesis, retroperitoneal haematoma (extremely painful), cerebral haemorrhage, etc.

Purgatives. Chronic diarrhoea with loss of water (dehydration) and potassium (hypokalaemia), perhaps causing a very grave illness.

Antihypertensive drugs. Postural hypotension.

Oxygen. Retrolental fibroplasia, causing blindness in neonates; carbon dioxide narcosis in chronic bronchitics in respiratory failure.

Phenacetin. Renal damage.

Barbiturates. Confusional states in the elderly; coma and death (often suicidal).

Phenothiazines (e.g. chlorpromazine). Parkinsonian-like syndromes.

Streptomycin. Permanent vertigo.

Dihydrostreptomycin. Deafness.

Chlorpropamide, and other antidiabetic drugs. Hypoglycaemic coma.

Vitamin D. Hypercalcaemia and renal damage.

Cytotoxic drugs. Serious bone-marrow depression, causing thrombocytopoenia, agranulocytosis and aplastic anaemia.

18 Poisoning

A poison may be administered accidentally or intentionally (murder or suicide), but in every suspected case it is the duty of the nurse to preserve all bottles, etc., from which the poison may have been obtained, together with vomitus, urine and stools. All these may be of importance in determining the nature and amount of poison taken.

Toxic substances may enter the body by the inhalation of poisonous gases, by the mouth, by injection and some by absorption through the skin (e.g. agricultural chemicals), and the onset of symptoms may be very rapid or delayed. Most of the drugs and therapeutic substances used in medical practice can act as poisons if not employed in the proper doses. There are also many toxic substances used in industry and agriculture which can be dangerous.

In a case of poisoning it is clearly desirable to know the actual substance involved but in practice this information may not be immediately available. It must be remembered that more than one toxic substance may have been taken. In any case there are comparatively few actual specific chemical antidotes which can be used and, therefore, prompt symptomatic first aid treatment is of great importance.

Special 'Poison Information Centres' exist which can advise on the identification of the toxic substance and the treatment necessary.

The aims of treatment:
1. To remove the poison from the body and increase the rate of elimination.
2. To treat dangerous symptoms, e.g. respiratory depression.
3. To neutralize the poison by giving a chemical antidote which renders it inert if this is possible.

Inhaled poisons. The most common type is that due to carbon monoxide which is present in domestic coal gas and the exhaust fumes of motor cars. If the patient is in a gas-laden atmosphere obviously the first thing to do is to remove him into fresh air. The main object then is to remove the residual gas from the lungs and to maintain respiration.

1. See that the natural airways are clear and that the tongue is pulled forward.

2. Perform artificial respiration.

3. Administer oxygen with 5% carbon dioxide which is also a powerful stimulant of the respiratory centre. Hyperbaric oxygen is valuable if this is available.

Ingested poisons. Except in cases of corrosive poisoning and poisoning with paraffin and petroleum products, when special care is necessary, it is generally desirable to empty the stomach as soon as possible either by inducing vomiting or by gastric lavage especially in cases of salicylate poisoning. Vomiting may be provoked by tickling the fauces or by giving a simple emetic such as a desertspoonful of salt or mustard in a tumbler of warm water, assuming that the patient can swallow.

When gastric lavage is carried out the patient is placed in the prone position with the head lower than the trunk and overhanging the end of a couch or table. After passing a stomach tube the gastric contents should first be aspirated with a syringe and retained for examination. This should be followed by lavage with tap water or some other solution if specially indicated. One litre is usually sufficient. Massive lavage with large quantities may do more harm than good.

It must always be remembered that in a deeply unconscious patient there is a risk of inhaling the gastric contents. It may be necessary to introduce a cuffed intratracheal tube in order to prevent this.

1. Poisons having a local action

(a) Corrosives. These include the mineral acids (hydrochloric, sulphuric and nitric, also battery fluid and acetic acid), and caustic alkalis (potash, soda and ammonia). They are characterized by their destructive action on the parts with which they come in contact.

Symptoms. Staining and corrosion of the mouth and lips. Vomiting, often of blood, mucus and shreds of destroyed tissue. Dysphagia, thirst, dyspnoea. Severe shock, weak rapid pulse and abdominal pain. If death does not ensue, there may be subsequent narrowing of the oesophagus or pylorus as a result of scarring. A stomach tube is not passed in these cases because of the risk of perforating the damaged organ.

CORROSIVE ACIDS. Give in 1 pint of water, magnesia, chalk, soap suds, white wash, ceiling plaster, washing soda or whiting. Tracheostomy may be necessary.

CAUSTIC ALKALIS. Give citric or tartaric acid, vinegar (30 to 100 ml in water) or the juice of 6 lemons.

When corrosive or irritant poisons have been taken, demulcents such as the whites of 3 eggs in 1 pint of water, olive oil, milk, or thick gruel are given after the administration of the appropriate antidote, in order to soothe the inflamed mucous membrane. Further symptomatic treatment is given as required.

(b) Irritants. These cause intense inflammation of the parts affected and the symptoms and results are similar to but less severe than those produced by the corrosives. Gastric lavage may, therefore, be employed. Many disinfectants, such as strong lysol, and iodine, also metallic poisons and phosphorus, are included in this group.

Injected poisons. These can usually only be treated symptomatically. In some instances a specific antidote is available.

Symptomatic treatment

In most cases of poisoning the important effects requiring treatment are:

1. Respiratory failure and asphyxia.
2. Circulatory failure.
3. Renal failure and electrolyte disturbance.
4. Cerebral depression and coma.
5. The prevention of subsequent pneumonia.

Respiratory failure and asphyxia. Barbiturates in particular depress the respiratory centre and in addition render it insensitive to the stimulus of carbon dioxide resulting in anoxia, hypotension and hypothermia. It is important, therefore: (a) To maintain a clear airway by clearing the fauces of vomit or mucus and by keeping the tongue forward. For this purpose a rubber airway may be helpful. Sometimes tracheal intubation is desirable. Occasionally bronchial toilet by bronchoscopy and possibly tracheostomy are necessary.

(b) To supply sufficient oxygen to increase its concentration in the alveoli and to maintain adequate ventilation of the lungs. Oxygen or oxygen with 5% carbon dioxide is administered. Artificial respiration may be essential. In the first instance mouth to mouth breathing may be employed. When available a positive pressure apparatus may be needed.

(c) Stimulation of the respiratory centre may be considered necessary if a respirator is not available. For this purpose nikethamide or 'Vandid' may be employed. Analeptic drugs such as bemegride are now regarded as contraindicated.

(*d*) Peritoneal dialysis or haemodialysis may be necessary.

Circulatory failure. Blood pressure may be raised by the intravenous injection of 'Aramine' or 'Mephine'. Severe cases may need noradrenaline.

Conscious patients suffering pain and shock after corrosive poisoning may require morphine or pethidine.

Renal failure and electrolyte disturbances. Care must always be taken not to overload the circulation with fluid and to risk the production of pulmonary oedema, but intravenous fluids may be necessary if the patient is dehydrated or remains unconscious for a long period. It may be possible to estimate the concentration of the poison in the blood and at the same time to estimate the electrolytes which can then be corrected if abnormal.

In the case of some poisons it is possible to reduce the concentration in the blood by the use of 'forced diuresis' or an 'artificial kidney' (dialysis). Intravenous mannitol, given slowly, is sometimes employed.

Cerebral depression and coma. The treatment of this state is essentially one of good nursing (see p. 360).

Some poisons, e.g. atropine, cause delirium and convulsions. In such cases an intramuscular injection of sodium amytal or paraldehyde may be necessary.

Sometimes penicillin or a similar antibiotic is given to unconscious patients with a view to preventing the development of pneumonia.

N.B.—All cases of suicidal poisoning should receive psychiatric treatment after recovery.

Antidotes

Following gastric lavage and symptomatic treatment the following specific antidotes may be needed:

Arsenic and heavy metals	Dimercaprol (BAL)
Cyanides	Amyl nitrite inhalations
	Intravenous sodium nitrite (10 ml of 3%)
	IV sodium thiosulphate (50 ml of 50%)
Iodine	Thin starch paste. Sodium bicarbonate. Magnesia

Iron Salts	Gastric lavage with 1% sodium bicarbonate, followed by oral 'Desferal' (5 G in 100 ml water) of which intravenous or intramuscular injections may follow.
Morphine	IV nalorphine, 5 to 10 mg
'Mushroom' poisoning	Atropine, nikethamide Antiphallinic serum
Salicylates (Aspirin)	Gastric lavage with weak bicarbonate solution. Forced alkaline diuresis. Dialysis with artificial kidney.
Household detergents	Milk.

19 Intensive Care and Resuscitation

There are many patients for whom a period of special medical and nursing care may make the difference between life and death. Although to some extent this may be effected in side wards and cubicles or even in a general ward, such arrangements have many disadvantages which are overcome in a special intensive care unit.

The concept of *intensive care* implies the specialized nursing of certain gravely ill patients in one area where resuscitation facilities are concentrated and which has its own specially trained staff.

An intensive care unit (ICU) may be general or special. Special units may be designed for patients with myocardial infarction (Coronary Care Units) or respiratory failure. Other special units may be designed for major postoperative care or for accident victims. The two sexes are commonly nursed in the same ward; this permits the concentration of the greatest nursing skill in one area. The nursing staff of the unit are trained in special observations and techniques. They should be able to recognize (but not necessarily to identify) abnormal cardiac rhythms displayed on an oscilloscope and know how to obtain a permanent recording on paper. They need to be familiar with the care of tracheostomies and with mechanical ventilators.

The unit should preferably be supplied with piped oxygen because large volumes of this gas are likely to be used and personnel will have plenty to do other than to change oxygen cylinders.

Apparatus in the unit includes mechanical ventilators (positive or positive-negative pressure types), power-operated suckers, laryngoscopes and endotracheal tubes, electrical cardioverters (defibrillators) and cardiac pacemakers. Equipment for peritoneal dialysis is necessary. Cut-down packs and often a thoracotomy set are usually among the items stocked in the unit.

In a coronary care unit it is vital that dysrhythmias are immediately recognized and the patient's electrocardiogram is therefore continuously displayed on an oscilloscope. Frequent ventricular extra-systoles may indicate the imminence of ventricular fibrillation and therefore demand suppression, usually with lignocaine (1–2 mg per minute by intravenous infusion). Patients with ventricular fibrillation should be electrically defibrillated as soon as possible; if defibrillation cannot be performed immediately, the circulation must be sustained by external cardiac massage, with artificial ventilation if necessary.

One method of signalling dysrhythmias is for an alarm bell to ring if the patient's heart rate changes beyond pre-set limits. The electronic monitors which do this, however, have so far been un-satisfactory because they give too many false alarms. The attentive nurse remains the best monitor. The nurse is relied upon also to observe the patient's colour (especially cyanosis), peripheral circula-tion and personal comfort. Patient distress cannot be monitored by a machine and makes a good nurse essential. Distress may be due to pain, anxiety, an obstructed airway or a full bladder, among other causes.

Arterial blood pressure may be recorded either with an external cuff or via an intra-arterial cannula. Central venous pressure may be monitored through a polyethylene catheter introduced via a neck vein so that its tip lies in the superior vena cava or in the right atrium.

The normal range of central venous pressure is + 4 to + 10 cm of water above the right atrium (measuring from the mid point of the antero-posterior diameter of the thorax at the level of the 4th costal cartilage as reference or 'zero' level). Abnormally low values are found after haemor-rhage and elevated values occur after over-transfusion, in heart failure, and with cardiac tamponade (compression of the heart by fluid in the peri-cardial sac).

Many coronary patients have been saved from death by recogni-tion of dangerous dysrhythmias, immediate recognition of cardiac arrest, and prompt use of resuscitative techniques including electrical cardioversion.

ARTIFICIAL RESPIRATION

The cessation of breathing does not necessarily mean that death will ensue, especially if the heart continues to beat.

Normal respiration is under the control of the respiratory centre situated in the medulla oblongata whence impulses pass via the phrenic nerve to the diaphragm and by various other spinal nerves to the other muscles of respiration.

Breathing may cease if the respiratory centre is damaged by drug over-dosages, injury or disease, and also if the nerves to the respiratory muscles are affected so that no impulse can pass along them.

It must be emphasized that the function of respiration is to obtain interchange of gases in the alveoli of the lungs. In order that this may be effective it is essential that the lungs are properly ventilated. In other words, the depth of respiration is a much more important factor than the rate. In shallow rapid breathing the column of air obviously only moves in and out of the trachea and bronchi, little exchange only occurring in the alveoli.

Artificial respiration may, therefore, be required in the following conditions:

(a) Affections of the respiratory centre.

1. Over-dosage with anaesthetics and poisoning with hypnotic drugs, e.g. morphine, alcohol, barbiturates.
2. Carbon monoxide poisoning.
3. Electric shock.

(b) Affections of the nerves of respiration.

1. Paralysis due to the action of diphtheria toxin.
2. Paralysis due to poliomyelitis, the virus of which may damage the anterior horn cells of the motor nerves in the spinal cord or nuclei of cranial nerves in the brain-stem (bulbar type).
3. Certain other diseases of the nervous system.

(c) 1. Asphyxia.
2. Apparent drowning.

In many cases of the first and last groups (a and c) breathing can be re-established by the use of artificial respiration for a few minutes or hours, and the ordinary first-aid methods, including 'mouth to mouth' breathing, may be employed with success. In cases of the second group (b), however, artificial respiration may be necessary for several days, weeks, or even many months, and this can only be maintained by mechanical means.

(a) The tank or cabinet type of respirator which consists of a metal tank equipped with a mattress. The patient's head projects through a soft rubber diaphragm which forms an airtight collar around the neck. There are also port holes through which a bed pan can be passed or an enema administered.

By means of bellows driven by an electric motor the air pressure within the chamber is made to alternate between normal atmospheric pressure and a slight negative pressure. When the pressure within the chamber is negative the chest of the patient expands and air is taken into the lungs: with the return to normal pressure the thorax contracts and air is expired.

The depth of respiration is controlled by a pressure gauge, 12 to 18 cm of water being the usual negative pressure employed. The rate of artificial respiration can be adjusted by the speed of the pump at about 20 per minute. Great care must be taken not to produce over-ventilation of the lungs.

A patient may live and be nursed in this apparatus indefinitely.

(b) The cuirass type respirator which consists of a rubber bag enclosed in canvas which is fixed round the patient's chest and alternately inflated and deflated by means of an electric pump, so that the thorax is alternately compressed and relaxed. The speed and force of compression can also be controlled.

(c) The rocking bed apparatus;

(d) The positive pressure or positive-negative machine, which is used to inflate the lungs through either an endotracheal or a tracheostomy tube.

Cardiac resuscitation (cardiac arrest)

Death will occur if the heart has ceased to pump adequate amounts of oxygenated blood to the brain. However, prompt resuscitative measures may maintain life until the heart resumes its function either spontaneously or with the help of drugs or an electric shock from a 'defribillator'. Since the brain suffers irreversible damage after about 3 minutes without an adequate blood supply, it follows that resuscitation, if it is to be successful, must be started at once by the person on the spot. In hospital this is likely to be the nurse rather than a doctor. The doctor should, of course, be sent for immediately.

The initial steps in resuscitation are the performance of artificial respiration, preferably by the mouth to mouth method, in order to oxygenate the blood, together with external cardiac massage. The patient is placed on his back on a hard surface. It may be possible to lay the patient on the floor or else to insert a board under the lower part of the chest. The neck is fully extended preferably over a rolled object, such as a dressing gown, in order to obtain a clear airway and to prevent the tongue from falling back. The nurse then stands or kneels by the side of the patient, closes the nostrils with the left hand at the same time supporting the jaw. The mouth is kept open with the right hand while the nurse blows her own expired air into the mouth of the patient at the rate of approximately fifteen breaths per minute, removing her own mouth between breaths.

Preferably another nurse will place one hand over the lower end of the sternum with the other on top of the first and will compress the sternum at the rate of sixty pressures per minute.

Pressure must be adequate but care must be taken not to use too much force which might fracture the ribs. Unless the operator is very heavy or powerful the weight of the individual leaning forward over the patient is adequate. In the case of children or very small adults one hand on the sternum is sufficient. For small babies the thorax should be grasped by one hand, with the fingers behind and gently squeezed by pressure applied by the thumb placed in the middle of the sternum. The lower end should be avoided in order to minimize possible damage to the underlying liver.

If the cardiac massage is successful the pulse will return and the pupils which initially are likely to be dilated should contract.

If the operator is single-handed, having placed the patient in a suitable position and assured a clear airway, cardiac massage should be commenced and after each fourth compression of the chest air should be blown into the patient's lungs, thus combining cardiac massage with mouth to mouth breathing.

In the meantime, unless the patient can be moved to an intensive care unit, a resuscitation trolley containing a laryngoscope, endo-tracheal tubes and defibrillator together with an electrocardiograph should be obtained, also such drugs as the medical staff may require, such as adrenaline, calcium chloride and sodium bicarbonate for intravenous injection.

These measures should be adopted in the case of any patient who unexpectedly shows signs of cardiac collapse, unless he is known to be suffering from an incurable disease, but in any case of doubt they must be commenced at once if they are to be effective.

20 Some Test Questions

These questions do not include those involving anatomy and physiology and nursing details but are intended to indicate the main medical problems considered in this book.

CHAPTER 1. INTRODUCTION

1. What diseases do you know which may be caused by virus infection? Give an account of any one of the diseases you mention.
2. Describe a rigor. In what conditions may rigors occur? Describe the treatment of this symptom.
3. State briefly what you know about: allergy, hay fever.
4. What infectious diseases may be controlled by immunization? What measures are taken to achieve a high level of immunity in the population?
5. A young woman is admitted to hospital with persistent pyrexia. (*a*) What are the possible causes of this condition? (*b*) What preventive measures may be taken and why? (*c*) What investigations may be made?
6. Give an account of the regulation of body temperature. What is meant by fever? Give an account of the effects of fever on the body. Describe the nursing management of a patient with a temperature of 40 °C (104 °F).

CHAPTER 2. INFECTIOUS DISEASES

1. Describe the symptoms and course of the disease in a patient suffering from typhoid fever.
2. Describe the symptoms, complications and treatment of:
   Scarlet fever
   Measles   } (any one of these may be asked)
   Whooping-cough

3. State what you know about each of the following diseases:
   (*a*) rubella; (*b*) mumps; (*c*) chicken-pox.
4. State briefly what you know about:
   (*a*) the rash in small-pox
   (*b*) Koplik's spots
   (*c*) vaccination.

CHAPTER 3. DISEASES OF THE CIRCULATORY SYSTEM

1. Describe the observations you would make when taking the radial pulse. What are the common abnormalities which may occur and what conditions may cause them?
2. Describe how blood pressure is measured. Give an account of the symptoms and treatment of high blood pressure and mention any complications which may result from this condition.
3. What do you understand by atrial (auricular) fibrillation? Give an account of the causes of this condition and describe the symptoms and treatment.
4. What are the common causes of chronic (congestive) heart failure? Describe the signs and symptoms and state briefly the treatment which may be given to relieve the patient.
5. What are the common causes of heart disease? Discuss the management and treatment of congestive heart failure.
6. What is meant by ascites? Enumerate the causes of this condition and describe the treatment of ascites due to chronic heart failure.
7. Describe an attack of angina pectoris. What may cause this condition? State what you know about the treatment of an attack and the advice which may be given to a patient in order to prevent recurrences.
8. What do you understand by acute myocardial infarction (coronary artery thrombosis)? Give an account of the symptoms, treatment and nursing care of a patient suffering from this condition.
9. Give an account of the treatment of hypertension. With what conditions may a rise in blood pressure be associated and what are its complications?
10. Define the terms 'thrombosis' and 'embolism'. Give examples of each and describe any steps which may be taken to prevent their occurrence.
11. Describe the symptoms, treatment and nursing care of a patient

suffering from pulmonary embolism. In what circumstances may this condition arise?

12. Describe a case of acute rheumatic fever in a young adult. What complications may occur? Give an account of the medical treatment and nursing care of this condition.

13. Describe a case of chorea and give an account of the medical and nursing treatment of a patient suffering from this condition.

14. State briefly what you know about:

mitral stenosis;	atrial (auricular) fibrillation;
aneurysm;	angina pectoris;
venesection:	sedimentation rate (ESR).

CHAPTER 4. DISEASES OF THE BLOOD

1. Classify the common types of anaemia which may occur and mention their causes and treatment.

2. Describe the signs, symptoms and treatment of pernicious anaemia. What do you know about the cause of this disease? State briefly what you know about:

leukaemia;	polycythaemia;
agranulocytosis;	glandular fever.
purpura;	

3. A child is suffering from acute leukaemia. (a) What symptoms and signs may be present? (b) What medical and nursing care may be required? (c) What advice and help may be given to anxious relatives?

4. For what reasons may a transfusion of blood be given? What precautions are taken to prevent complications? What observations should be made by a nurse before, during and after the transfusion?

CHAPTER 5. DISEASES OF THE ALIMENTARY SYSTEM, ETC.

1. What may cause difficulty in swallowing? State how a case of dysphagia may be examined and investigated.

2. Describe the symptoms of a gastric ulcer. What complications may occur? Give a brief account of the medical treatment of this condition.

3. What may cause vomiting of blood? Describe the medical and nursing care of a patient who has had a severe haematemesis.

4. What is meant by 'pyloric stenosis'? In what circumstances can this condition occur? Give an account of the symptoms and treatment of an infant suffering from pyloric stenosis.

5. Describe the symptoms, treatment and nursing care of an infant of one year suffering from gastro-enteritis. What precautions should be taken to prevent the spread of this infection in a hospital ward?

6. Describe the causes and symptoms of acute gastro-enteritis. Give an account of the treatment and nursing care of a young adult suffering from this condition.

7. What is meant by melaena? Give a brief account of the causes of this condition and state how a severe case would be treated and nursed.

8. Mention the abnormalities which might be seen on naked eye examination of the faeces. Indicate how your observations might assist in diagnosis.

9. What information may be obtained from inspection of: (a) vomit, (b) faeces, (c) sputum?

10. Describe the abnormalities which may be found in the faeces and discuss their significance.

11. What is meant by the term 'constipation'? State what may give rise to this condition and discuss its treatment.

12. Discuss the management of chronic constipation.

13. Describe the symptoms of ulcerative colitis and give an account of the nursing and treatment of this condition.

14. What is meant by 'jaundice'? State the common causes of this symptom and describe how you would test for bile in the urine.

15. State briefly what you know about:

thrush;	pentagastrin test;
parotitis;	sigmoidoscopy;
thread-worms;	barium enema;
cirrhosis of the liver;	cholecystogram.

CHAPTER 6. DISEASES OF THE RESPIRATORY SYSTEM

1. Give an account of the causes, symptoms, complications and treatment of acute tonsillitis.

2. What conditions may cause haemoptysis? Describe the treatment and nursing care of a severe case. Mention any investigations which may be carried out to ascertain the cause of this symptom.

3. What are the causes of acute bronchitis? Describe the symptoms and the medical and nursing care of this condition.

4. An elderly patient suffering from chronic bronchitis has been admitted to hospital. (a) What are the common complaints of

such a patient? (b) What factors may be important in producing chronic bronchitis? (c) Describe the nursing management of such a patient.

5. Describe an attack of bronchial asthma. State what you know about the causes and treatment of this condition.

6. Give an account of the causes, symptoms, complications and treatment of pneumonia.

7. What are the symptoms of pulmonary tuberculosis? Describe the main methods which are employed in (a) the diagnosis, (b) prevention, (c) the treatment of this disease.

8. State what you know about cancer of the lung, including the symptoms and the methods which may be employed in investigating a suspected case.

9. State briefly what you know about:

tonsillitis;
quinsy;
laryngitis;
Cheyne-Stokes breathing;

bronchiectasis;
bronchoscopy;
Mantoux test.

CHAPTER 7. DISEASES OF THE URINARY SYSTEM

1. What observations and tests may a nurse carry out on the urine? Indicate how these may be of value to the physician in his diagnosis and treatment.

2. Discuss the significance of the following abnormal constituents which may be found in the urine: (a) albumin; (b) blood; (c) sugar; (d) acetone.

3. What may cause the appearance of blood in the urine? How may this be recognized and what investigations might be carried out to ascertain the cause of the bleeding?

4. Give an account of the causes, symptoms and treatment of acute pyelitis.

5. Give an account of the symptoms, complications, treatment and nursing care of a patient suffering from acute nephritis.

6. What are the signs and symptoms of uraemia? Mention the causes of this condition and discuss its treatment.

7. State briefly what you know about:

albuminuria;
hydronephrosis;
renal colic;

blood urea;
intravenous pyelogram.

CHAPTER 8. DISEASES OF THE NERVOUS SYSTEM

1. What observations would you make on a patient who has been found unconscious? Indicate how these might be of assistance in arriving at a diagnosis.
2. What are the common causes of prolonged unconsciousness? Describe the management and discuss the treatment of any one of these conditions.
3. Describe an epileptic fit. State how you would deal with a patient during such a fit. Give an account of the medical treatment and the advice given to the patient between attacks.
4. State what you know about poliomyelitis.
5. Describe the signs and symptoms of meningitis. Mention the types of this disease which may occur and indicate the treatment and nursing care required.
6. Given an account of the symptoms and treatment of meningococcal meningitis. What other types of meningitis may occur? Mention any special treatment these types may require.
7. Describe a case of tuberculous meningitis. How may such a patient be treated and nursed?
8. What is meant by the term 'apoplexy'? Mention the causes and symptoms of this condition and describe its medical and nursing treatment.
9. What is meant by 'hemiplegia'? Give a brief account of the causes of this condition and state how you would nurse a case during the early stages.
10. A woman of 40 is in hospital with advanced disseminated (multiple) sclerosis. (a) Describe the nursing management. (b) If the patient wishes to return home what social services are available to her? (c) What advice might then be given to the relatives?
11. What are the common causes of insomnia? Describe what may be done to alleviate this condition.
12. State briefly what you know about:

migraine;	delirium;
paralysis agitans;	hysteria;
multiple sclerosis;	prolapsed ('slipped') disc.

CHAPTER 9. AUTO-IMMUNE DISEASE

1. What do you understand by the term 'Auto-immune disease'? Give examples and add a note on treatment.

CHAPTER 10. DISEASES OF JOINTS, ETC.

1. Give an account (or describe a case) of rheumatoid arthritis. Describe the medical and nursing care of a patient during the acute stages of the disease.

CHAPTER 11. DISORDERS OF METABOLISM AND DEFICIENCY DISEASES

1. Enumerate the conditions which may result from deficiency of the various vitamins. Give an account of the symptoms and treatment of (a) rickets, (b) scurvy.
2. What is meant by dehydration? Describe how this condition may be recognized, prevented and relieved.
3. Describe the symptoms, complications and treatment of diabetes mellitus.
4. Give an account of the symptoms and complications of diabetes mellitus. State how a case of diabetic coma would be treated.
5. Compare and contrast the symptoms which might be observed in (a) diabetic coma; (b) from insulin overdosage. How may these conditions be distinguished. Describe the treatment of one of them.
6. State briefly what you know about:
   ketosis;   dehydration.
   gout;

CHAPTER 12. DISEASES OF THE DUCTLESS GLANDS

1. Describe a case of thyrotoxicosis. State what you know about the treatment of this disease.
2. State what you know about myxoedema.
3. Write an account of diseases of the adrenal gland.
4. Write short notes on (a) diabetes insipidus, (b) Simmond's disease.

CHAPTER 13. DISORDERS OF THE SKIN

1. What would lead you to suspect the presence of: (a) scabies; (b) pediculosis. Outline the treatment of these conditions.
2. State briefly what you know about:
   acne;   psoriasis;
   scabies;   urticaria;
   impetigo;   erythema nodosum;
   pediculosis;   herpes zoster.

CHAPTER 14. VENEREAL DISEASE

1. Name three diseases which may be transmitted by sexual intercourse. What factors may contribute to an increase in these diseases and what might be done to prevent them?
2. Write brief notes on the three stages of syphilis. How may the disease be treated?
3. Give an account of the symptoms and treatment of gonorrhoea.

CHAPTER 15. CAUSES OF SUDDEN DEATH

1. Mention some of the conditions which may cause the sudden death of a patient in a hospital ward. Indicate any steps which might be taken to minimize these dangers.

CHAPTER 16. DRUGS

1. State briefly what you know about the following drugs:

antacids;	diuretics;
anticoagulants;	propranolol
analgesics;	paraldehyde;
aspirin;	iron;
digitalis;	phenobarbitone;
atropine;	streptomycin;
adrenaline;	vitamin B_{12}.

2. What symptoms may arise as a result of over-dosage with the following drugs:

insulin;	atropine;
digitalis;	phenobarbitone;
sodium salicylate;	morphine.

MISCELLANEOUS

Write a short essay on any one of the following:
The measures which may be adopted to alleviate pain; rehabilitation; occupational therapy; the care of the elderly; the role of the social worker; pain in the chest; cough; fits; headache; vomiting; ascites; jaundice; oedema; constipation; oxygen therapy; venereal disease; anaemia; uraemia.

Tables

APOTHECARIES WEIGHT
(Formerly used in dispensing)

20 grains	= 1 scruple (℈)	
3 scruples	= 1 drachm (ʒi)	= 60 grains
8 drachms	= 1 ounce (℥i)	= 480 grains
12 ounces	= 1 pound	= 5760 grains

Care must be taken to distinguish these from the domestic avoirdupois weights and from fluid measures.

AVOIRDUPOIS WEIGHT

16 drachms = 1 ounce (oz) =	437 grains	= 28·35 G
16 ounces = 1 pound	= 7000 grains	= 0·45 Kg
14 pounds = 1 stone	= 6·5 kilograms	

APOTHECARIES FLUID MEASURE

60 minims	= 1 fluid drachm =	4 ml (approx.)
8 fluid drachms	= 1 fluid ounce	= 30 ml (approx.)
20 fluid ounces	= 1 pint	= 0·57 litre
2 pints	= 1 quart	= 1·13 litre
4 quarts	= 1 gallon	= 4·54 litres

THE METRIC SYSTEM

The unit of weight is one gram, which is the weight of one millilitre of water.

1 microgram	= 1 millionth part of 1 gram
1000 micrograms	= 1 milligram = $\frac{1}{60}$ grain
10 milligrams	= 1 centigram = $\frac{1}{6}$ grain
10 centigrams	= 1 decigram = 1·5 grain
10 decigrams	= 1 gram = 100 centigrams = 15 grains
1000 grams	= 1 kilogram = 2·2 (2$\frac{1}{4}$) pounds

1 millilitre (ml) = 1 cubic centimetre (cc) or 15 minims approx.
1000 millilitres = 1 litre = 1·75 (1$\frac{3}{4}$) pints = 35 fluid ounces

MEASURES OF LENGTH, AREA AND VOLUME

1 inch	= 2·54 cm
12 inches = 1 foot	= 0·3 metre
36 inches = 1 yard	= 0·91 metre
16·5 feet	= 5·0 metres
3·38 feet	= 1 metre
1 sq inch	= 6·45 sq cm
1 sq foot	= 0·09 sq metre
1 cu inch	= 1·64 cu cm
1 cu foot	= 0·03 cu metre

Approximate equivalents

The following are the approximate equivalents used in dispensing.

Grains	Milligrams	Grains	Milligrams
15	1000 (1 g)	$\frac{1}{10}$	6
12	800	$\frac{1}{12}$	6
10	600	$\frac{1}{25}$	2·5
5	300	$\frac{1}{60}$	1
3	200	$\frac{1}{120}$	0·5
1	60	$\frac{1}{150}$	0·4
$\frac{1}{2}$	30	$\frac{1}{200}$	0·3
$\frac{1}{3}$	20	$\frac{1}{300}$	0·2
$\frac{1}{4}$	15	$\frac{1}{600}$	0·1
$\frac{1}{6}$	10		

Minims	Millilitres	Fluid ounces	Millilitres
5	0·3	$\frac{1}{2}$	15
15	1	1	30
20	4	20 (1 pint)	600

DOMESTIC MEASURES

1 teaspoonful is just over 60 minims or 5 ml.

1 desertspoonful is about 120 minims or 8 ml.

1 tablespoonful is about half a fluid ounce.

1 tumblerful is just over half a pint.

These measures are very inaccurate and should not normally be used.

N.B.—A standard 5 ml spoon is now issued to patients and the unit dose of linctuses and paediatric mixtures has been adjusted to this. Adult mixture doses are 10 ml.

Thermometric equivalents

°C	°F	°C	°F
0·0	32·0	38·8	101·84
15·5	60·0	39·0	102·20
18·5	65·0	39·2	102·56
35·0	95·0	39·4	102·92
36·0	96·80	39·6	103·28
36·2	97·16	39·8	103·64
36·4	97·52	40·0	104·0
36·6	97·88	40·2	104·36
36·8	98·24	40·4	104·72
37·0	98·60	40·6	105·08
37·2	98·96	40·8	105·44
37·4	99·32	41·0	105·80
37·6	99·68	42·0	107·60
37·8	100·04	43·0	109·40
38·0	100·40	44·0	111·20
38·2	100·76	49·0	120·0
38·4	101·12	100·0	212·0
38·6	101·48		

To convert °C to °F multiply by $\frac{9}{5}$ and add 32.
E.g. 37 °C $\times \frac{9}{5} = 66 \cdot 6 + 32 = 98 \cdot 6$ °F.
To convert °F to °C subtract 32 and multiply by $\frac{5}{9}$.
E.g. 100 °F $- 32 = 68 \times \frac{5}{9} = 37 \cdot 7$ °C.
N.B.—Water boils at 100 °C (212 °F).

Normal blood values

Haemoglobin	14·8 grams/100 ml $= 100\%$
Men	14–18 grams/100 ml.
Women	12–16 grams/100 ml.
Red blood cells	
Men	5·0–6·4 millions/cu mm.
Women	4·2–5·6 millions/cu mm.
White blood cells	
Adults	
Total	4,000–11,000/cu mm.
neutrophils	60–70%
lymphocytes	25–30%
monocytes	5–10%
eosinophils	1–4%
basophils	0–1%

Platelets	150,000–500,000/cu mm.
ESR (Westergren)	
Men	up to 15 mm in one hour
Women	up to 25 mm in one hour
Serum sodium	135–150 mEq/1.
Serum potassium	3·6–5·6 mEq/1.
Serum chloride	96–108 mEq/1.
Serum bicarbonate (alkali reserve)	22–30 mEq/1.
Serum calcium	9·0–11·0 mEq/1.
Serum inorganic phosphorus	2·5–4·5 mEq/1.
Blood urea	15–40 mg/100 ml.
Serum uric acid	up to 6·5 mg/100 ml.
Capillary blood sugar (fasting)	Folin-Wu method 70–120 mg/100 ml.
	True blood sugar 60–105 mg/100 ml.
Serum cholesterol	125–250 mg/100 ml.
Serum triglyceride	up to 150 mg/100 ml.
Serum PBI	4–8 micrograms/100 ml.
Serum bilirubin	0·1–0·8 mg/100 ml.
Thymol turbidity	0–4 units
SGOT	up to 40 R-F units/ml.
SGPT	up to 35 R-F units/ml.
Serum LDH	100–450 units/ml.
Alkaline phosphatase	3–13 KA units/100 ml.
Acid phosphatase	1–5 KA units/100 ml.
Serum proteins	
Total	5·5–8·0 g/100 ml.
Albumin	3·3–5·6 g/100 ml.
Globulin	1·6–3·1 g/100 ml.
Fibrinogen	0·2–0·4 g/100 ml.

LATIN PHRASES AND ABBREVIATIONS SOMETIMES USED IN
PRESCRIBING

Ana	āā.	of each
Ante cibum (cibos)	a.c.	before food (meals)
Ad libitum	ad lib.	to the amount desired
Aequales	aeq.	equal
Alternis diebus	alt. die.	alternate days (every other day)
Alternis noctibus	alt. noct.	alternate nights
Aqua	aq.	water
Bis die	b.d.	twice a day
Bis in die	b.i.d.	
Cras mane	c.m.	tomorrow morning
Cras nocte	c.n.	tomorrow night
Cum	c̄.	with
Ex aqua	ex. aq.	in water
Hac nocte	h.n.	this night
Mitte	m.	send
Nocte et mane	n. et m. (nmque)	night and morning
Nomen proprium	n.p.	proper name of a drug on a prescription
Omni mane	o.m.	every morning
Omni nocte	o.n.	every night
Parti affectae	p.a.	to the affected part
Post cibum (cibos)	p.c.	after food (meals)
Pro oculis	p.oc.	for the eyes
Pro re nata	p.r.n.	as the occasion arises (to be repeated when required)
Quater in die	q.i.d.	4 times a day
Quantum sufficit	q.s.	a sufficient quantity
Repetatur	rep.	let it be repeated
Semissis	ss. or fs.	half
Si opus sit	s.o.s.	if necessary (a single dose)
Statim	stat.	at once
Ter die sumendum	t.d.s.	to be taken 3 times a day
Ter in die	t.i.d.	3 times a day

Derivation of words

Aerophagy	(Greek) *aer* = air, *phagein* = to eat or swallow
Aetiology	(Greek) *aieta* = cause, *logos* = discourse
Allergy	(Greek) *allos* = another, *ergon* = energy
Anaemia	(Greek) *an* = negative, *haima* = blood
Anasarca	(Greek) *ana* = throughout, *sarx* = flesh
Ante-	(Latin) = before
Anti-	(Latin) = against
Bacillus	(Latin) = a rod
Bruit	(French) = a noise
Chole-	(Greek) = bile
Coccus	(Greek) = a berry
Diphtheria	(Greek) *diphthera* = membrane
Dyspepsia	(Greek) *dys* = bad, *peptein* = to digest
Endo-	(Greek) *endon* = within
Erythema	(Greek) = a redness
Fusiform	(Latin) *fusus* = a spindle, *forma* = shape or form
Hyper-	(Greek) = over
Hypo-	(Greek) = under or less
Macro-	(Greek) = large
Micro-	(Greek) = small
Metron	(Greek) = measure (-meter)
Mye-	(Greek) *myelos* = marrow
Myo-	(Greek) = muscle
-oscopy	(Greek) *scopein* = to inspect
-ostomy	(Greek) *stoma* = opening
-otomy	(Greek) *temnein* = to cut
Otorrhoea	(Greek) *ous* = ear, *rein* = to flow
Pathognomonic	(Greek) *pathos* = disease, *gnomonicos* = showing
Pathology	(Greek) *pathos* = disease, *logos* = discourse
Peri-	(Greek) = around
Phobia	(Greek) *phobos* = fear
Poly-	(Greek) = many
Pre-	(Latin) = before
Pro-	(Greek) = before
Pye-	(Greek) *pyelos* = pelvis (e.g. pyelitis)
Pyo-	(Greek) *pyon* = pus
Retro-	(Latin) = stepping back, behind
Spirochaete	(Greek) *speira* = coil, *chaite* = hair
Supra-	(Latin) = above
Trans-	(Latin) = across

Calorie value of various foodstuffs

	Grams per Ounce, (30 g) Foodstuff			Calories per Ounce (30 g)
	Carbohydrate	Protein	Fat	
Miscellaneous				
Alcohol	—	—	—	7
Bacon	0	4	18·5	181
Beef	0	8	6	86
Bread	14	2·5	0·5	70
Butter	0	0	25	225
Cheese (Cheddar)	1	8	10	134
Chicken	0	5·5	4·5	65
Cream (40%)	1	1	12	120
Cream (20%)	1	1	6	65
Egg (1 = 2 oz)	0	6	6	78
Fish	0	6	0	24
Ham	0	4	9·5	104
Macaroni	21	4	0	97
Milk	1·5	1	1	20
Mutton	0	7	6·4	90
Oil or Lard	0	0	28	252
Sugar	28	0	0	112
Cereals				
Beans (Haricot)	16	7	0·5	95
Cornflour	20	1·8	1·2	104
Oatmeal	20	4·5	2	116
Peas (dried)	17·4	7	0	100
Rice	21	2·3	0	100
Sago	24	0	0	96
Tapioca	24	0	0	96

Calorie value of various foodstuffs

	Grams per Ounce, (30 g) Foodstuff			Calories per Ounce (30 g)
	Carbohydrate	Protein	Fat	
Vegetables				
Asparagus	1	0·5	0	7
Beetroot	3	0·5	0	14
Cabbage	1·3	0·4	0·1	9
Carrots	3	0·3	0	13
Celery	1	0·3	0	5
Lettuce	0·8	0·3	0·1	6
Onions	3	0·4	0	14
Parsnips	4	0·4	0	18
Potatoes	6	1	0	30
Rhubarb	1	0·2	0	6
Tomatoes	1	0·2	0	6
Fruits				
Apples	4	0·1	0·2	18
Bananas	6	0·4	0·2	29
Cherries	4·5	0·3	0·2	23
Dates	22·3	0·6	0·8	101
Grapes	5·4	0·3	0·4	28
Grapefruit (half)	10	0	0	40
Oranges (1 = 2 oz)	10	0	0	40
Pears	4	0·2	0	18
Plums	6	0·3	0	25
Prunes	21	0·6	0	86
Strawberries	2	0·3	0	10

Some Common Abbreviations

		Page
IVP	Intravenous pyelogram	325
IZS	Insulin-zinc suspension (c.f. PZI)	445
MAOI	Monoamine oxidase inhibitor	407
MDR	Misuse of Drugs Regulations	503
MOH	Medical Officer of Health (obsolete), see DCP	—
MSU	Mid-stream urine	317
NHS	National Health Service	—
P_{CO_2}	Partial pressure of carbon dioxide	274
P_{O_2}	Partial pressure of oxygen	274
PAS	Para-amino salicylic acid (sodium amino-salicylate)	305
PBI	Protein-bound iodine	457
PCV	Packed cell volume	187
PPM	Parts per million	—
PUO	Pyrexia of unknown origin	18
PZI	Protamine zinc insulin	445
RV	Residual volume (of air)	275
SLE	Systemic lupus erythematosus	412
TAB	Typhoid, Paratyphoid A and B (vaccine)	47
TLC	Total lung capacity	275
VC	Vital capacity	275
WR	Wassermann reaction	495

Index